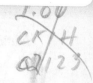

Living Vegetarian

2nd Edition

by Suzanne Babich, DrPH, MS, RDN

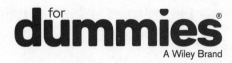

A Wiley Brand

Living Vegetarian For Dummies®

Published by: **John Wiley & Sons, Inc.,** 111 River Street, Hoboken, NJ 07030-5774, www.wiley.com

Copyright © 2023 by John Wiley & Sons, Inc., Hoboken, New Jersey

Published simultaneously in Canada

For general information on our other products and services, please contact our Customer Care Department within the U.S. at 877-762-2974, outside the U.S. at 317-572-3993, or fax 317-572-4002. For technical support, please visit www.wiley.com/techsupport.

Wiley publishes in a variety of print and electronic formats and by print-on-demand. Some material included with standard print versions of this book may not be included in e-books or in print-on-demand. If this book refers to media such as a CD or DVD that is not included in the version you purchased, you may download this material at http://booksupport.wiley.com. For more information about Wiley products, visit www.wiley.com.

Library of Congress Control Number: 2022946107

ISBN 978-1-119-90311-6 (pbk); ISBN 978-1-119-90312-3 (ebk); ISBN 978-1-119-90313-0 (ebk)

SKY10036382_100422

Contents at a Glance

Recipes at a Glance

Entreés

Salads

Side Dishes

Soups

Table of Contents

Introduction

Vegetarianism has come a long, long way.

As a child, I wore a button that said, "Real People Wear Fake Furs." I'd picked it up at the Ann Arbor Street Art Fair when my older sister was in college at the University of Michigan. It was the late '60s, and it wasn't much longer before my mother announced to our family that from then on, she would be a vegetarian. She never said why — and we never asked! — but for the next several years, the former Wisconsinite ate cheese omelets or cheddar-cheese-and-pickle sandwiches on whole-wheat toast for dinner while the rest of us ate the meat she prepared for us. That is, of course, until my siblings and I followed her lead and, one by one, without fanfare, we followed Mom's model and became vegetarians ourselves.

My dad worried we'd miss vital nutrients. He chided my mother for planting the idea. Mom, a registered nurse, was considered a bit odd by her hospital colleagues. By now, it was the early '70s, and vegetarians lived on communes or wore Birkenstocks and long hair on college campuses. They weren't kids and working, middle-aged moms.

A competitive swimmer in high school, I hoped that a vegetarian diet would boost my endurance and athletic performance, as Olympic gold medalist Murray Rose claimed it had for him. It didn't help enough, but it did pique my interest in nutrition and set me on the path to a career in dietetics. It would be many years, however, before the scientific community came around to the idea that a diet of grains, fruits, vegetables, legumes, seeds, and nuts can be adequate — never mind superior — to a diet centered on animal products.

In college, I learned about vegetarianism in a lesson on fad diets. At that time, in the early 1980s, a blood cholesterol level of 300 mg/dl was considered normal, and patients in the coronary care unit in the hospital got bacon and eggs and white toast for breakfast.

My grandmother worried that I wouldn't get enough iron if I didn't eat red meat. She thought that my slender body wasn't "healthy" enough in size as compared to her old-world, European standards. For baby boomers like me, this was the environment for vegetarians in North America 40 to 50 years ago.

Everything is different now.

Slowly, over the last 30 years, the Academy of Nutrition and Dietetics (AND) — long the conservative holdout on such matters — went from cautious at first, to later tentative at best, to now clearly stating in its position papers that vegetarian diets confer health advantages. U.S. government dietary recommendations now explicitly acknowledge the vegetarian alternative and advise all Americans to make fruits, vegetables, grains, and legumes the foundation of a healthy diet. It's as close as the government can come to a stamp of approval for a plant-based diet as it balances science with the economic interests of the powerful meat and dairy industries.

As a practicing nutritionist and vegetarian, I've observed these changes taking place over decades. The progress has been steady, and at this point, I think we can say that vegetarianism has become mainstream in much of the world.

The scientific rationale for eating a plant-based diet is thoroughly documented. The advantages for everyone and everything on our planet are compelling. The next task is helping people everywhere make the transition to an eating style that, while culturally mainstream today, is still outside the personal experience of the majority of people. Accomplishing this requires education as well as the political will to initiate and enforce public policies that make it easier for you and me to sustain lifestyles that support health.

To sum it up: Living vegetarian is an excellent way to meet today's dietary recommendations for good health. It's also critical to protecting and supporting the environment. Of course, it's also the ethical "right thing to do." There's every reason in the world to start living vegetarian. This book is for everyone who wants a head start on making the switch.

About This Book

This book is for vegetarians and prospective vegetarians, too — for anyone curious about what a vegan is, for those who still have questions about where vegetarians get their protein, for parents who are wringing their hands because Junior has "gone vegetarian," and for Junior to give to Mom and Dad so that they won't worry.

This book is for vegetarians and nonvegetarians alike. Whether you want to control or prevent diseases such as diabetes and coronary artery disease, manage your weight, save money, or help keep the planet healthy and the animals happy, this book has what you need. That's because the secret to living well is eating well, and to eat well, you need to make plant foods the foundation of your diet.

It's the simple truth.

Don't feel you need to read the chapters in this book in order or read the book from cover to cover. It's designed to make sense and be helpful whether you surf it or read it in its entirety. Throughout the text, you'll find cross-references to guide you to other parts of the book where you can find related information.

Foolish Assumptions

If you're holding this book, you or someone who loves you bought or borrowed this book to gain a better understanding of how to live a vegetarian lifestyle. I'm assuming that this book is appropriate for a variety of purposes, including:

» Dipping your toe into the topic. If you just want a little more information to help you decide whether living vegetarian may be something you'd like to consider doing, this book is appropriate for you.

» Digging in deeper. You may already have a general sense of what's involved in living vegetarian, but you want more in-depth advice and understanding of how to go about it. This book is for you.

» Sharing the knowledge. If you know someone with an interest in going vegetarian — or someone who may simply be curious and interested in finding out more — this book is a reliable resource.

» Refreshing your own knowledge. Longtime vegetarians may benefit from the up-to-date information in this book.

» Having a reference on hand. Health professionals often encounter vegetarians in their work and have to give them medical or dietary advice. If you're a health professional and you have no personal experience with a vegetarian lifestyle, this book may be helpful as an accurate and quick reference.

You can make some assumptions about me, too:

» I know what I'm talking about. I'm a registered dietitian/nutritionist with a master's degree in human nutrition and a doctorate in public health. I'm an expert on vegetarian nutrition and have lived a vegetarian lifestyle myself for nearly 50 years.

>> My advice is practical. It's informed by my own experience of living vegetarian for most of my life, as well as many years of experience counseling individuals on special diets, including both vegetarians and nonvegetarians.

>> I'm not giving individualized advice. As much as I wish it were possible, books aren't an appropriate means of dispensing medical or dietary advice tailored to individual needs. I can give you general information that provides you with a good foundation of knowledge about the topic. However, if you have specific issues you need help with — particularly medical conditions that require you to follow a special diet — you should get additional, individualized guidance from a registered dietitian. I include information in Chapter 1 about how to locate a dietitian with expertise in vegetarian diets.

Icons Used in This Book

Another fun feature of *For Dummies* books is the clever icons that flag helpful nuggets of information. Each icon denotes a particular type of information. Here's what each icon means:

TIP

Tips are insights or other helpful clues that may make it more convenient or hassle-free for you to follow a vegetarian diet.

REMEMBER

When you see this icon, the information that follows is a rule-of-thumb or another truism you should keep in mind.

WARNING

If you see this icon, the information is meant to help you avoid a common pitfall or to keep you from getting into trouble.

TECHNICAL
STUFF

This is information that, while interesting, isn't vital to your understanding of the topic. In other words, some of you may skip it, but it's there if you care to find out more.

Where to Go from Here

The science of nutrition is complicated, but being well-nourished is a relatively simple matter. It's even easier to do if you eat a wholesome, plant-based diet. That's where this book comes in.

If you want a clearer understanding of what vegetarianism is, start with the foundational information in Chapter 1. If you have a child or teenager who's interested in becoming vegetarian, check out Chapter 21. If you're ready to whip up some tasty vegetarian meals, head straight to Part 3 — you can start with the breakfast recipes in Chapter 9 or skip straight to the dessert recipes in Chapter 14 (I won't tell!).

Whether you go vegetarian all the way or part of the way, moving to a more plant-based diet is one of the smartest moves you can make. I hope this book helps. Best wishes to you as you take the first step!

1

Being Vegetarian: What It's All About

Review the basic information you need to help you get started, including the various types of vegetarian diets and the reasons many people make the switch.

Understand nutrition issues pertaining to meatless diets, including how to ensure you get what you need from whole foods.

Examine the pros and cons of taking vitamin and mineral supplements.

Consider some good-sense advice about living the vegetarian lifestyle, including how to plan for meatless meals, and practical ways to master the behavioral changes that are a part of the transition to a new eating style.

Chapter **1**

Vegetarianism 101: Starting with the Basics

Mention a vegetarian diet, and many people visualize a big hole in the center of your dinner plate. They think that to be a vegetarian, you have to like lettuce and carrot sticks — *a lot.* Just contemplating it leaves them gnawing on their knuckles.

Nothing could be further from the truth, however.

Vegetarian diets are diverse, with an abundance of fresh, colorful, and flavorful foods. For anyone who loves good food, vegetarian meals are a feast. That may be difficult for nonvegetarians to imagine. Vegetarian diets are common in some parts of the world, but they're outside the culture and personal experience of many other people.

That's why I start with the basics in this chapter. I tell you about the many forms a vegetarian diet can take and the reasons people choose to go meat–free. I give you a quick overview of what's involved in planning and making vegetarian meals, and I introduce some important considerations for making the transition to a meat–free diet a little easier.

Vegetarian Label Lingo: Who's Who and What They Will and Won't Eat

Most of us are pretty good at describing a person in just a few words:

> "a social media influencer"
>
> "a Gen-Xer"

It's like the saying goes: "A picture (or label) paints (or says) a thousand words."

People use labels to describe vegetarians, with different terms corresponding to different sets of eating habits. A lacto ovo vegetarian eats differently than a vegan eats. In some cases, the term used to describe a type of vegetarian refers to a whole range of lifestyle preferences, rather than to just the diet alone. In general, though, the specific term used to describe a vegetarian has to do with the extent to which that person avoids foods of animal origin. Read on for a primer on vegetarian label lingo, an explanation of what I call the vegetarian continuum, and an introduction to vegetarian foods.

From vegan to flexitarian: Sorting out the types of vegetarianism

In 1992, *Vegetarian Times* magazine sponsored a survey of vegetarianism in the United States. The results showed that almost 7 percent of Americans considered themselves vegetarians.

However, a closer look at the eating habits of those "vegetarians" found that most of them were eating chicken and fish occasionally, and many were eating red meat at least a few times each month. Most vegetarian organizations don't consider occasional flesh-eaters to be vegetarians.

As a result, the nonprofit Vegetarian Resource Group (VRG) in 1994 began sponsoring national polls on the prevalence of vegetarianism, wording the interview questions in such a way as to determine the number of people who *never* eat meat, fish, poultry, or byproducts of these foods. (The organization continues to conduct periodic polls, and you can find the results online at www.vrg.org/nutshell/faq.htm#poll.)

Over the years, the number of people who fit the VRG definition of vegetarian has increased from between 2 and 3 percent of the adult population in the U.S. in the

1990s to 6 percent of U.S. adults in 2020. That means the percentage of people in the U.S. who are consistently vegetarian has tripled over the past 30 years.

Of course, the U.S. population has also increased substantially in the past 30 years. So, while the percentage of vegetarians has tripled, the absolute number of vegetarians has increased even more. Consider that the U.S. adult population in 1994 was 194,484,890. Two percent of that number is 3,889, 698. The U.S. adult population in 2020 was 256,662,010. Six percent of that number is 15, 399,721. That means the actual number of vegetarians in the U.S. has quadrupled since the mid-1990s!

Many others are cutting back on meat consumption. A 2020 VRG poll found that 54 percent of American adults say that they sometimes or always eat vegetarian meals when they eat out. Does that make them "part-time" vegetarians?

The fact is, people interpret the term *vegetarian* in many different ways.

Many people use the term loosely to mean that they're consciously reducing their intake of meat. The word *vegetarian* has positive connotations in general, especially among those who know that vegetarian diets confer health benefits. In fact, the same 2020 VRG poll found that when making food choices, a majority of Americans consider the most important factors to be taste, cost, and health, in that order. Vegetarians say their primary considerations are health, animal welfare, the taste of the food, cost, ethics, and the environment.

So what about these true vegetarians? Who are they and what do they eat (or not eat)?

REMEMBER

The definition of a vegetarian most widely accepted by vegetarian organizations is this: A vegetarian is a person who eats no meat, fish, or poultry.

Not "I eat turkey for Thanksgiving" or "I eat fish once in a while." A vegetarian consistently avoids all flesh foods, as well as byproducts of meat, fish, and poultry. A vegetarian avoids refried beans made with lard, soups made with meat stock, and foods made with gelatin, such as some kinds of candy and most marshmallows.

The big two: Lacto ovo vegetarian and vegan

Vegetarian diets vary in the extent to which they exclude animal products. The two most common types of vegetarianism are:

>> Lacto ovo vegetarian: A lacto ovo vegetarian diet excludes meat, fish, and poultry but includes dairy products and eggs. According to a 2020 VRG poll,

half of U.S. adult vegetarians — 3 percent of American adults — fall into this category. Lacto ovo vegetarians eat such foods as cheese, ice cream, yogurt, milk, and eggs, as well as foods made with these ingredients.

>> Vegan: Technically, the term vegan (pronounced vee-gun) refers to more than just the diet alone. A vegan is a vegetarian who avoids eating or using all animal products, including meat, fish, poultry, eggs, dairy products, and any foods containing byproducts of these ingredients. A 2020 VRG poll found that of the 6 percent of U.S. adults who are consistently vegetarian, half of them are vegan. Vegans also use no wool, silk, leather, and any nonfood items made with animal byproducts. Some vegans avoid honey, and some don't use refined white sugar, or wine that has been processed using bone char or other animal ingredients. Needless to say, vegans also don't eat their dinner on bone china. (For more details on veganism, see the nearby sidebar.)

TECHNICAL STUFF

In academic nutrition circles, *strict vegetarian* is the correct term to use to describe people who avoid all animal products but who don't necessarily carry animal product avoidance into other areas of their lives. In practice, however, the term vegan is usually used by both strict vegetarians and vegans, even among those in the know. In other words, technically, the term strict vegetarian refers to diet only. The term vegan encompasses both food and other products, including clothing, toiletries, and other supplies.

MORE THAN A DIET: VEGANISM

Maintaining a vegan lifestyle in our culture can be difficult. Most vegans are strongly motivated by ethics, however, and rise to the challenge. A large part of maintaining a vegan lifestyle has to do with being aware of where animal products are used and knowing about alternatives. Vegetarian and animal rights organizations offer information and materials to help.

Sometimes vegans unwittingly use a product or eat a food that contains an animal byproduct. Knowing whether a product is free of all animal ingredients can be difficult at times. However, the intention is to strive for the vegan ideal.

So a vegan, for instance, wouldn't use hand lotion that contains lanolin, a byproduct of wool. A vegan wouldn't use margarine that contains casein, a milk protein. And a vegan wouldn't carry luggage trimmed in leather. Vegans (as well as many other vegetarians) also avoid products that have been tested on animals, such as many cosmetics and personal care products.

The list goes on: Semi-vegetarian, flexitarian, and others

Lacto ovo vegetarian and vegan are the two primary types of vegetarian diets, but there are more labels for near vegetarians, including the following:

>> A *semi-vegetarian* is someone who's cutting back meat intake, in general.

>> A *flexitarian* is basically the same as a semi-vegetarian. It refers to someone who's generally cutting back on meat but may eat meat from time to time, when it's more convenient or on a special occasion.

>> A *pescatarian* is someone who avoids red meat and poultry but eats fish or seafood.

>> A *pesco pollo vegetarian* avoids red meat but eats chicken and fish.

>> A *pollo vegetarian* avoids red meat and fish but eats chicken.

These terms stretch the true definition of a vegetarian. None of these actually qualify as vegetarian diets, but they indicate the person is moving towards a more *plant-based* diet.

In fact, *plant-based* is a term that is used commonly now, as in "they eat a plant-based diet" or "the menu is plant based." Someone who eats a plant-based diet may or may not be consistently vegan or even vegetarian. However, they are probably striving to make the majority of their diet come from foods of plant origin.

Ultimately, if you really want to be sure you understand what someone eats, you need to ask them for details. Labels may give you a clue, but they may be interpreted differently by different people.

Don't leave out: Lacto vegetarian, raw foods, fruitarian, and macrobiotic diets

The list actually goes even further. A *lacto vegetarian* excludes meat, fish, and poultry, as well as eggs and any foods containing eggs. So a lacto vegetarian, for instance, wouldn't eat the pancakes at most restaurants because they contain eggs. A lacto vegetarian does eat dairy products such as milk, yogurt, and cheese.

Another adaptation of a vegetarian diet is a *raw foods diet*, which consists primarily of uncooked foods — fruits, vegetables, sprouted grains and beans, and plant sources of fat, including avocados, nuts, seeds, and oils. Though raw foodists never cook foods in an oven or on a stovetop, some of them eat ingredients that have been dehydrated in the sun.

In practice, most raw foodists in North America actually eat a *raw vegan* diet. The proportion of the diet that comes from raw foods is typically anywhere from 50 to 80 percent. Most raw foodists aim for a diet that's 100 percent raw, but what they can realistically adhere to still includes some amount of cooked food.

Still another adaptation, the *fruitarian diet,* consists only of fruits, vegetables that are botanically classified as fruits (such as tomatoes, eggplant, zucchini, and avocados), and seeds and nuts. Planning a nutritionally adequate fruitarian diet is difficult, and I don't recommend the diet for children.

Macrobiotic diets are often lumped into the general category of vegetarian diets, even though they may include seafood. This diet excludes all other animal products, however, as well as refined sugars, tropical fruits, and "nightshade vegetables" (for example, potatoes, eggplant, and peppers). The diet is related to principles of Buddhism and is based on the Chinese principles of yin and yang. Therefore, macrobiotic diets include foods common to Asian culture, such as sea vegetables (including kelp, nori, and arame), root vegetables (such as daikon), and miso. Many people follow a macrobiotic diet as part of a life philosophy. Others follow the diet because they believe it to be effective in curing cancer and other illnesses, an idea that has little scientific support.

The vegetarian continuum: Going vegetarian a little or a lot

Pop quiz: What would you call a person who avoids all flesh foods and only occasionally eats eggs and dairy products, usually as a minor ingredient in a baked good or dish, such as a muffin, cookie, or veggie burger?

Technically, the person is a lacto ovo vegetarian, right? But this diet seems as though it's leaning toward the vegan end of the spectrum.

As a nutritionist, I see this kind of variation — even within the same category of vegetarian diet — all the time. One lacto ovo vegetarian may eat heaping helpings of cheese and eggs and have a high intake of saturated fat and cholesterol as a result. In fact, this type of vegetarian may have a nutrient intake similar to the standard American diet— not so good. Another lacto ovo vegetarian may use eggs and dairy products, but only in a very limited fashion — as condiments or minor ingredients in foods. This person's nutrient intake more closely resembles that of a vegan.

What am I getting at? That labels are only a starting point, and they have limitations. Even if you know generally what type of vegetarian a person is, you may see a lot of variation in the degree to which the person uses or avoids animal products.

Many new vegetarians find that their diets evolve over time. At the start, for example, many rely heavily on cheese and eggs to replace meat. Over time, they learn to cook with grains, beans, and vegetables, and they experiment with cuisines of other cultures. They decrease their reliance on foods of animal origin, and gradually, they consume fewer eggs and dairy products. Some eventually move to a mostly vegan (or strict vegetarian) diet.

You might say that vegetarian diets are on a continuum, stretching from the standard American, meat-centered diet on one end to veganism on the other (see Figure 1-1). Most vegetarians fall somewhere in between. Some may be content staying wherever they begin on the continuum, while others may progress along the spectrum as they hone their skills and develop new traditions, moving from semi-vegetarian, or lacto ovo vegetarian, closer to the vegan end of the spectrum.

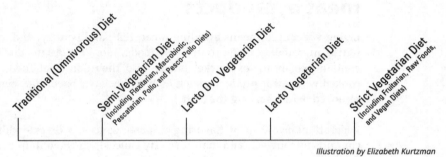

FIGURE 1-1:
The vegetarian continuum.

Illustration by Elizabeth Kurtzman

Common foods that happen to be vegetarian: Beyond mac and cheese

Your eating style is a mind-set. For proof, ask someone what she's having for dinner tonight. Chances are good that the answer is, "We're grilling steaks tonight," or, "I'm having fish." Ever notice how no one mentions the rice, potato, salad, vegetables, bread — or anything other than the meat?

Many vegetarians eat these common foods — side dishes to nonvegetarians — in larger quantities and call them a meal. Others combine them in new and delicious ways to create main courses that replace a burger or filet. Your skills at assembling appealing vegetarian meals will improve over time.

Until they do, going vegetarian doesn't have to mean a whole new menu. Many vegetarian foods are actually very familiar to nonvegetarians as well. Some examples include:

>> Falafel (common in Middle Eastern restaurants)

>> Pasta primavera

>> Salad

>> Tofu (especially at Chinese restaurants)

>> Vegetable lasagna

>> Vegetarian chili

>> Vegetarian pizza

>> Veggie burger

When meat-free isn't vegetarian: Bypassing meat byproducts

Living vegetarian means avoiding meat, fish, and poultry, and it includes eliminating ingredients made from those foods, too. Vegetarians don't eat soups that contain beef broth or chicken stock, and they don't eat foods that have been cooked with meat products, such as ham hocks or bacon fat, even if the meat is removed before serving the dish.

Vegetarians avoid meat flavoring in pasta sauces, Worcestershire sauce (which contains anchovies), and many stir-fry sauces, which contain oyster sauce. They don't eat marshmallows and some candies, which contain gelatin made from the cartilage and skins of animals. In Chapter 5, I cover all this in more detail, listing foods that may contain hidden animal products.

Going Vegetarian Benefits Everyone

Some people go vegetarian for the simple reason that they don't like meat. They chew and chew, and they still have a glob of aesthetically unpleasant flesh in their mouth. Some people just like vegetables better.

Others go vegetarian because they recognize the link between diet and health, the health of ecosystems on our planet, the welfare of animals, or the ability of nations to feed hungry people. Whichever issue first grabs your attention, the other advantages may reinforce your resolve.

Eating for health

Many people view their health (or lack thereof) as something that just sort of happens to them. Their bad habits catch up with them, or they have bad genes. Their doctor just gave them a clean bill of health, and then they had a heart attack out of the blue. (Well, we all have to die of *something.*) Who could have foreseen it? They lived reasonably — everything in moderation, right? What more could they have done?

A lot, most likely. You may be surprised to discover how much power you wield with your knife and fork. The fact is that vegetarians generally enjoy better health and longer lives than nonvegetarians.

In comparison with nonvegetarians, vegetarians are at lower risk for many chronic, degenerative diseases and conditions. That's because a diet composed primarily of plant matter has protective qualities. I cover the diet and health connection in more detail in Chapter 2.

Protecting our planet

A disproportionate amount of the earth's natural resources is used to produce meat and other animal products. For example:

>> It takes about 25 gallons of water to grow 1 pound of wheat, but it takes about 390 gallons of water to produce 1 pound of beef.

>> A steer has to eat 7 pounds of grain or soybeans to produce 1 pound of beef.

Animal agriculture — the production of meat, eggs, and dairy products — places heavy demands on our land, water, and fuel supplies, and in some cases, it contributes substantially to problems with pollution. You should understand how your food choices affect the well-being of our planet. I discuss the issues further in Chapter 2.

Compassionate food choices

Many people consider a vegetarian diet the right thing to do. Their sense of ethics drives them to make very conscious decisions based on the effects of their food choices on others. You may feel the same way.

In Chapter 2, I describe more fully the rationale for considering the feelings and welfare of animals used for their flesh, eggs, or milk. I also discuss the implications of food choices for world hunger. A strong argument can be made for living vegetarian as the humane choice — not just in terms of the effect on animals, but also because of what it means for people, too.

Meatless Meals Made Easy

Making vegetarian meals doesn't have to be time-consuming or difficult. Despite all the gourmet cooking magazines and high-end kitchen supply stores around, you and most other people probably don't anticipate spending much of your free time making meals.

Not to worry. You can make the best vegetarian meals quickly, using basic ingredients with simple techniques and recipes.

Mastering meal planning and prep

After decades of counseling individuals on many types of diets, I've found one thing to be universally true: Nobody follows a structured meal plan for very long. Though it may be helpful for some to see a sample meal plan, following rigid diet plans doesn't work well for most people. That's because you, like me, probably juggle a busy schedule that requires a fair amount of flexibility in meal planning.

You find a good deal of advice in this book that pertains to planning and preparing meatless meals in the most efficient way possible. In general, though, your meals should follow the guidelines I present in Chapter 7.

REMEMBER

The best way to prepare meals with a minimum of fuss is to remember the key word — simple.

You need very little equipment and only basic cooking skills — boiling, baking, chopping, and peeling — to prepare most vegetarian foods. The best recipes include familiar, easy-to-find ingredients and have short ingredient lists.

The recipes I include in this book in Part 3 are a great place to start in addition to the menus in Chapters 25 and 26. You may also find, as you dig a little further into living vegetarian, that you don't have to rely on recipes at all to prepare great meals. My hope for you is that you gain confidence in your ability to put ingredients together in simple and pleasing ways so that you can quickly and easily assemble delicious, nutritious vegetarian meals.

Shopping strategies

Grocery shopping doesn't take exceptional skills, but smart shopping habits can help ensure that you have the ingredients you need on hand when you need them. Because you probably don't have lots of free time to spend roaming the supermarket, you want to shop efficiently, too.

A few tips to keep in mind:

>> **Keep a list.** Post on your refrigerator — or another convenient spot — a running list of ingredients you need to pick up the next time you're at the store. You'll be less likely to forget a key item, and you'll be less likely to spend impulsively, too.

>> **Shop for locally grown, seasonal foods.** Stop at your local farmer's market or roadside vegetable stand. Fruits and vegetables grown near your home taste better and retain more nutrients than foods that spend days on a truck being shipped across the country after being picked.

>> **Mix it up.** Visit different grocery stores from time to time to take advantage of new food items and varied selections across stores. Ethnic markets and specialty shops can give you good ideas and offer some interesting new products to try.

In Chapters 6 and 7, I describe various commonly used vegetarian ingredients, and I give advice about shopping and stocking your vegetarian kitchen.

Mixing in some kitchen wisdom

If the idea of creating meatless meals is new to you, harboring some concerns about your ability to plan and prepare good-tasting meals is understandable. Until you've had some experience, you may mistakenly believe that living vegetarian means buying lots of specialty products or spending hours chopping vegetables.

Not true. Going vegetarian — done well — will simplify your life in many ways. You'll have fewer greasy pans to wash, and your stovetop and oven should stay cleaner longer. Foods that contain fewer animal ingredients are likely to be less of a food safety concern than those that contain meat, eggs, and dairy products.

And living vegetarian costs less.

Of course, you can spend as much time and money as you want to on your meals. Living vegetarian, though, is all about basic foods prepared simply. The staples — fruits, vegetables, grains, and beans — are generally less expensive than animal-based ingredients and easy to use.

Cooking creatively

Vegetarian meals invite creativity.

After you're free of the idea that a meal has to be built around a slab of meat, the variety really begins. After all, you can put together plant ingredients to make a meal in an almost endless number of ways. Plant ingredients come in varied colors, textures, and flavors. The sampling of recipes I include in this book (see Part 3 for these recipes) are an introduction to what's possible. Don't hesitate to experiment with these — add a favorite herb or substitute Swiss chard for kale.

You'll soon be spoiled by the variety and quality of vegetarian meals. After you've practiced living vegetarian for a while, you'll find that you don't have space on your plate for meat anymore, even if you still eat it! The vegetarian foods are so much more interesting and appealing.

Assembling meals: The no- or low-cook option

News flash: You don't have to be a great cook to go vegetarian. In fact, you don't have to cook at all, if you don't want to.

The extent to which you opt to peel and chop fruits and vegetables and simmer soups on the stove is largely a matter of what you like to do. Like all of us, the effort you devote to cooking may also depend on how much time you have, how many people live with you, and how much money you have to spend on food.

There are many economical, delicious, nutritious, and convenient ready-to-eat foods and pre-prepared ingredients available today. They require little more than heating in the microwave or arranging on a plate. They can free you to spend more time on other activities you enjoy and less on meal preparation. I explain further in Chapters 6 and 7. Suffice it to say, when it comes to meal planning, you have options.

Embracing a Meat-Free Lifestyle

At this point, you may be distracted by such thoughts as, "I need a degree in nutrition to get this right," or, "I wonder whether I'll be vegetarian enough." Your mind may be leaping ahead to such concerns as, "Will my family go along with this?" In this section, I help you put issues like these into perspective.

Taking charge of your plate

You have no reason to be afraid to stop eating meat. I haven't touched a hamburger in more than 45 years, and I'm alive and well.

In the opening of his book *Baby and Child Care* (Gallery Books), Dr. Benjamin Spock, a legendary figure to baby boomers like me, wrote these famous words: "Trust yourself. You know more than you think you do." You may not have studied the Krebs cycle or be able to calculate your caloric needs, but if you're reading this book, you probably have enough gumption to get your diet mostly right.

Mostly right is usually good enough.

REMEMBER

The science of nutrition is complicated, but being well nourished is a fairly simple matter. It may sound strange coming from a nutritionist, but you really have no need to worry about nutrition on a vegetarian diet. Vegetarian diets aren't lacking in necessary nutrients.

Poor nutrition is a function of lifestyle — vegetarian or not. The greatest threats? Junk foods and a lack of attention to the foods you need most to support health — particularly fruits, vegetables, whole grains, and legumes.

Your public persona: Affirming your choice

Vegetarianism has become mainstream in recent years. If you live in an urban setting or near a college town, chances are good that a number of your friends or coworkers are vegetarians of one sort or another.

Other people aren't so lucky. If you find yourself feeling isolated because you're the only vegetarian you know, keep a few points in mind:

» **You're unique.** Only about 6 percent of the adult population is truly vegetarian at this time. If you feel a little different, it's because you are. You'd fit right in if you lived in India or any other culture in which vegetarianism has been a tradition for thousands of years.

» **You alone decide what to eat.** You may be different from most people, but you should feel confident in your decision to live a vegetarian lifestyle. It's better for your health and the environment, and it's a nonviolent choice. A vegetarian diet is the thinking person's diet.

» **You owe no one an explanation.** Stand tall and take comfort in knowing that you're on the cutting edge of the nutritional curve.

Cohabitating harmoniously

REMEMBER

The most important things to do if you want your partner, children, parents — or anybody else you live with — to be happy in a vegetarian household are:

>> **Take a low-key approach.** Arguing, chastising, and cajoling are seldom effective in gaining buy-in from other people. In fact, being pushy is likely to get you the opposite result. Explain your rationale to adults and older children, and then let them decide for themselves what they will or won't eat.

>> **Model the preferred behavior.** The choices you make and the way in which you live send the most compelling — and noticeable — message.

Vegetarian diets are a great idea for kids. Establishing health-supporting eating habits early in life can help your children maintain good eating habits into adulthood. I include detailed information about managing the nutritional aspects of vegetarian diets for kids of all ages in Part 5.

Setting realistic expectations

Making any lifestyle change requires you to master new skills and change long-standing habits, and that takes time. Don't be too hard on yourself if you experience a few occasional setbacks.

REMEMBER

Experiment with new recipes, try vegetarian foods in restaurants, and invite friends to your house for meals. Read all you can about meal planning and vegetarian nutrition. With practice and time, you'll gain confidence and get comfortable with your new lifestyle. Think of this as a long-term goal — it took me several years before I felt like an expert at it.

Educating yourself with reliable information

This book gives you a solid introduction to all things vegetarian, but don't stop here. It's helpful to hear (or read, or view) the same subject matter presented differently by various sources. It takes most people several rounds before they absorb and understand a new subject well.

I mention good resources throughout this book, but I also list several of the best all-around resources for vegetarians of any skill level in the upcoming sections.

The Vegetarian Resource Group

The Vegetarian Resource Group (VRG) is a U.S. nonprofit organization that educates the public about the interrelated issues of health, nutrition, ecology, ethics, and world hunger. The group publishes the bimonthly *Vegan Journal* (previously *Vegetarian Journal*) and provides numerous other printed materials for consumers and health professionals. The organization provides the materials free of charge or at a modest cost in bulk, and many are available in Spanish. VRG's health and nutrition materials are peer-reviewed by registered dietitian nutritionists and physicians. VRG also advocates for progressive changes in U.S. food and nutrition policy. (Full disclosure: I served as a nutrition adviser to VRG for about 25 years.)

You can reach VRG at P.O. Box 1463, Baltimore, MD 21203; phone 410-366-8343; email: vrg@vrg.org, website: www.vrg.org. From VRG's website you can download and order materials, including books, handouts, reprints of articles, recipes, and more. The site also includes links to hundreds of other resources and organizations dedicated to plant-based diets.

The North American Vegetarian Society

The North American Vegetarian Society (NAVS) is best known for its annual vegetarian conference, Vegan Summerfest, which is usually held on the campus of the University of Pittsburgh at Johnstown, in Pennsylvania, in July. This casual, family-oriented conference draws a friendly, international crowd of several hundred people of all ages and with diverse interests. Nonvegetarians are welcome. Vegan Summerfest is an excellent opportunity to sample fabulous vegetarian foods, meet other vegetarians, attend lectures, and pick up materials from a variety of vegetarian organizations.

You can contact NAVS at P.O. Box 72, Dolgeville, NY 13329; phone 518-568-7970; email: navs@telenet.net, website: https://navs-online.org.

The Physicians Committee for Responsible Medicine

The Physicians Committee for Responsible Medicine, also called PCRM, is a nonprofit organization of physicians and others who advocate for compassionate and effective medical practices, research, and health promotion, including vegetarian diets.

Visit PCRM online at www.pcrm.org. You can also contact the organization at 5100 Wisconsin Avenue, NW, Suite 400, Washington, D.C. 20016-4131; phone 282-686-2210 or send a message via email directly through the organization's website.

Vegetarian Nutrition, a Dietetic Practice Group of the Academy of Nutrition and Dietetics

The Vegetarian Nutrition Dietetic Practice Group (VNDPG) is a subgroup within the Academy of Nutrition and Dietetics (AND) for dietitians with a special interest in vegetarian diets. The group publishes a quarterly newsletter, and other consumer nutrition educational materials are available online at www.vndgp.org. (Full disclosure: I was VNDPG's founding chair in 1992 and was a member for more than 20 years.)

TIP

The AND also offers a referral service for people who need individual nutrition counseling. To find the name and contact information of a registered dietitian nutritionist in your area with expertise in vegetarian diets, go online to www.eatright.org/find-a-nutrition-expert.

Other great resources

TIP

If you're looking for even more information on the vegetarian lifestyle, consider the following:

>> **The Vegan Society** in the United Kingdom at www.vegansociety.com. Find information here about vegan lifestyles from our friends in the U.K.

>> **The Vegan RD** at www.theveganrd.com. This site includes information provided by registered dietitian nutritionists who are experts in vegan and vegetarian diets.

All of the websites listed here will lead you to other great resources to help you learn more about vegetarian lifestyles. Pull up a comfy chair and start reading!

IN THIS CHAPTER

» Discovering reasons to adopt a vegetarian lifestyle

» Putting vegetarianism into the broader public health perspective

» Choosing a vegetarian diet for your good health

» Rejecting meat to help save the planet

» Becoming a vegetarian for ethical reasons

Chapter **2**

Vegetarians Are Sprouting Up All Over: Why Meatless Makes Sense

Sometimes, what you don't know won't hurt you. Other times, what you do know can help you and others . . . a lot.

Vegetarian diets are like that. You can find many compelling reasons why living vegetarian is a good thing to do. One of those reasons may pique your interest, and after you discover more, other reasons may reinforce your resolve. When you think about it from all angles, a vegetarian diet makes a lot of sense.

What you eat is a highly personal decision. Many factors, including a variety of psychological and social issues, affect your capacity to make changes in your lifestyle. That's why many people who adopt a vegetarian lifestyle see their diet evolve over time. Consider the rationale for adopting a vegetarian diet, and do what you can to move in that direction at a pace that's right for you.

In this chapter, I share some details about the prevalence of vegetarianism. I describe how eating a vegetarian diet promotes your overall health and the health of the planet. I also explain why ethics and compassion for animals compel many people to make the switch. In Chapter 5, I share some additional advice on how to help you along in the transition to being meat-free.

You're in Good Company

Contemplating a move to a more plant-based diet? You're not alone. In fact, you may be among an elite group of deep thinkers with the determination it takes to live a lifestyle outside cultural norms. That takes courage and tenacity, but it's a decision more people are making.

The percentage of people in the U.S. who are consistently vegetarian has steadily increased over the past few decades. That figure stands at about 6 percent of the adult population, according to a 2020 Harris Poll conducted for the nonprofit Vegetarian Resource Group (VRG).

The number of people eating a vegan diet also continues to rise. The VRG estimates that half of the vegetarians in the U.S. eat a vegan diet free of all animal products, including meat, fish, poultry, eggs, dairy products, and byproducts of these foods. Women are more likely than men to be vegetarian, and they are also more likely than men to be vegan.

Among nonvegetarians, the number of people actively cutting back on their meat intake is also increasing, fueling the explosion of meatless food products in supermarkets and the regular sight of vegetarian options on mainstream restaurant menus. More than half of all American adults, for example, report that they always or sometimes order vegetarian meals when they eat out. Half of that group are ordering vegan meals.

The numbers are nearly equal for men and women, and even by political parties — Democrats, Republicans, and Independents. You can read the full 2020 Harris Poll results, conducted for the VRG, online at `www.vrg.org/journal/vj2020issue4/2020_issue4_poll_results.php`.

FAMOUS VEGETARIANS YESTERDAY AND TODAY

If you're thinking about going vegetarian, you may be interested to know that you're joining an illustrious group of like-minded individuals.

Considering the small number of people who are consistently vegetarian, it's remarkable how many well-known personalities throughout history have chosen the lifestyle. The list includes philosophers, artists, intellectuals, entertainers, political leaders, sports figures, and many more. (I cover vegetarian diets for athletes in Chapter 22.)

The following list includes some of the better-known people throughout the centuries who have advocated or live a vegetarian lifestyle:

- Hank Aaron: Professional baseball player
- Louisa May Alcott: Author
- Susan B. Anthony: Suffragist
- Fiona Apple: Singer-songwriter
- Travis Barker: Musician
- Mayim Bialik: Actor and game show host
- David Bowie: Singer-songwriter and actor
- Berke Breathed: Cartoonist
- James Cromwell: Actor and activist
- Leonardo da Vinci: Artist, scientist, inventor
- Jenna Dewan: Actor and dancer
- Peter Dinklage: Actor
- Thomas Edison: Inventor
- Billie Eilish: Singer-songwriter
- Albert Einstein: Physicist
- Benjamin Franklin: Founding Father, scientist, inventor, philosopher, printer, and economist
- Mahatma Gandhi: Spiritual leader
- Philip Glass: Composer

(continued)

(continued)

- Dustin Hoffman: Actor

- Desmond Howard: Professional football player

- John Harvey Kellogg: Physician and inventor of dry breakfast cereal

- Carl Lewis: Olympic runner

- Tobey Maguire: Actor

- Sir Paul McCartney: Musician

- Martina Navratilova: Professional tennis player

- Sir Isaac Newton: Physicist

- Bill Pearl: Bodybuilder and four-time Mr. Universe

- Plato: Philosopher

- Natalie Portman: Actor

- Pythagoras: Philosopher

- Fred Rogers: Television's "Mister Rogers"

- Albert Schweitzer: Physician and Nobel Peace Prize winner

- Alicia Silverstone: Actress

- Socrates: Philosopher

- Benjamin Spock: Pediatrician and author

- Biz Stone: Twitter co-founder

- Carrie Underwood: Singer

The Population Perspective

Living vegetarian makes good sense when you consider the big picture. What you eat matters individually, but the collective impact of individual food choices also has an effect on the health and well-being of everyone. Think of it as your superpower!

I explain in more detail in this chapter, but vegetarians enjoy health benefits as a result of their food choices. If more people go vegetarian, more of us will enjoy healthier lives. Only 6 percent of Americans are vegetarians today, but what if that number increased to 20 percent . . . or 30 percent?! Think of the money that our health systems and communities could save if people needed fewer medications, fewer medical interventions from preventable, diet-related diseases and conditions, and missed fewer days of work due to illness.

And — wait — there's more!

Our food choices also have the power to clean up and protect Planet Earth. More vegetarian diets would mean fewer cows, chickens, and pigs; less pollution from animal agriculture; and fewer precious resources such as clean, fresh water being wasted to support meat and dairy production. It would mean less methane gas in the atmosphere, thereby reducing the greenhouse effect.

In public health terms, vegetarian diets are a no-brainer — a knife and fork approach to fighting climate change!

Supporting Your Health with a Plant-Based Diet

Scientific consensus today — supported by a large body of research — shows that vegetarian diets generally support health and confer health benefits. That doesn't mean vegetarian diets are foolproof or the Fountain of Youth; if your vegetarian diet largely consists of soda and French fries, you likely won't see any health benefits. But if you follow my basic guidelines for a healthful, meat-free diet, you'll decrease your risk for disease and promote your overall health.

REMEMBER

People often worried in the past about whether vegetarians could get the nutrients they need from a diet without meat, but the tables are turned today. The riskier diet is the one that *isn't* vegetarian.

Protecting yourself from disease

In recent years, the U.S. government, in its "Dietary Guidelines for Americans," as well as Health Canada and leading health organizations, have issued statements acknowledging that well-planned vegetarian diets meet nutritional needs and support health. In fact, vegetarian diets are associated with lower risk for many chronic diseases and conditions, including coronary artery disease, diabetes, high blood pressure, some forms of cancer, obesity, and others.

It's not hard to understand why.

Vegetarian diets tend to be lower in *saturated fat* than nonvegetarian diets. Although you can find saturated fat in some plants, saturated fats come primarily from animal products, particularly high-fat dairy foods and meats. In fact, most of the fat in dairy products is saturated fat.

For example, 58 percent of the fat in whole milk is saturated, and 56 percent of the fat in cheddar cheese is saturated. In ice cream, 61 percent of the fat is saturated, according to data from the U.S. Department of Agriculture.

REMEMBER

Saturated fats are usually firm at room temperature, like a stick of butter. That fact can help you identify foods that may be high in the artery-clogging fats. Foods that are high in saturated fat include red meats, the skin on poultry, butter, sour cream, ice cream, cheese, yogurt made with whole milk, 2 percent milk, and 3.3 percent whole milk. Be aware, though, that coconut oil, palm oil, and palm kernel oil are also high in saturated fat, even though they come from plant sources.

Saturated fats stimulate the body to produce more cholesterol. *Cholesterol* is a waxy substance found in plaque in diseased arteries. Everyone needs some cholesterol, but the human body manufactures a sufficient amount. You don't need more from outside sources, and for people with a predisposition for coronary artery disease, high blood cholesterol levels may contribute to hardening of those tubes that deliver blood and oxygen to your heart.

TECHNICAL STUFF

Cholesterol is produced in the liver, so it's found only in animal products. Foods of plant origin contain no cholesterol. (Have you ever seen a lima bean with a liver?)

WARNING

Lacto ovo vegetarian diets have the potential to be high in saturated fat and cholesterol if you don't limit the eggs and high-fat dairy products you eat. If you switch to a lacto ovo vegetarian diet, try not to rely too heavily on these foods to replace the meat you once ate. (Chapter 1 has definitions of lacto ovo and other kinds of vegetarianism.)

Getting more of what you need — and less of what you don't

Though vegetarians come in all shapes and sizes, vegetarian diets can help people control their weight. In general, vegetarians eat more filling, low-calorie foods, such as fruits and vegetables, than nonvegetarians do. Dietary fiber makes vegetarian foods bulky. *Dietary fiber* is the part of a plant that's only partially digested by your body, or not digested at all. When you eat fiber-rich foods, you tend to get full before you take in too many calories. In that way, foods that are rich in fiber help to control your weight. Read on for more details about the benefits of dietary fiber as well as protein and phytochemicals! All these nutrients play important roles in supporting your health.

Fiber

Dietary fiber does more than help control your weight. It brings several other health benefits, too. For example, fiber can bind with environmental contaminants and help them pass out of the body. Fiber also decreases the amount of time it takes for waste material to pass out of the body, so potentially harmful substances have less time to be in contact with the lining of your intestines.

If you get plenty of fiber in your diet, you're less likely to have constipation, hemorrhoids, and varicose veins. Getting plenty of fiber (and water) in your diet also keeps your stools large and soft and easy to pass. You don't have to strain and exert a lot of pressure to have a bowel movement.

TECHNICAL STUFF

Eating a high-fiber vegetarian diet may prevent you from developing *diverticulosis,* a condition marked by herniations or small outpocketings in the large intestine. These pouches can fill with debris and become inflamed, a serious and painful disease called *diverticulitis.*

Diets high in fiber are associated with lower rates of colon cancer and coronary artery disease than diets low in fiber. If you have diabetes, you can better control your blood sugar by eating a diet that's high in fiber, too.

REMEMBER

American adults get substantially less fiber in their diets than the amount recommended for good health. Lacto ovo vegetarians generally meet or exceed recommended amounts. Vegans get even more fiber in their diets than other vegetarians.

According to government figures, the average fiber intake of U.S. men and women is 17 to 20 grams per day and 15 to 16 grams per day, respectively. For comparison, the amounts recommended in the government's Dietary Guidelines 2020 to 2025 are 28 to 34 grams per day for males, depending on their age, and 22 to 28 grams per day for women, depending on their age.

Vegetarians tend to do very well in the fiber department. Studies have found that average fiber intakes for lacto ovo vegetarians range from 27 to 38 grams per day, and for vegans, the range is higher: 30 to 47 grams per day.

How do they do it? Easy. One cup of oatmeal contains 8 grams of fiber, a medium pear with skin has about 6 grams of fiber, a cup of vegetarian chili has 12 grams of fiber, a slice of whole wheat bread contains 2 grams of fiber, and one cup of chopped, steamed broccoli has about 5 grams of fiber. It adds up quickly when fiber-rich foods are not displaced by fiberless animal products such as meat, eggs, and dairy products.

REMEMBER

Keep in mind that, even though it's good for you to eat a high-fiber diet, it's also important to drink plenty of fluids, particularly water, when your fiber intake is high.

Protein

Most vegetarians get enough protein, but they don't overdo it, and this moderation has its benefits, including less wear and tear on your kidneys. Vegetarians have fewer kidney stones and less kidney disease than nonvegetarians. High intakes of protein from red and processed meats are also linked with higher blood cholesterol levels and more coronary artery disease, as well as a greater incidence of some types of cancer. A good rule of thumb is to aim for a little less than a half gram of protein for every pound you weigh. A 120-pound person, for example, should get about 44 grams of protein per day.

Phytochemicals

Vegetarian diets are rich in the plant components called *phytochemicals* that promote and protect human health. Conversely, meat is low in beneficial phytochemicals such as antioxidants and high in the oxidants that cause your body to produce detrimental *free radicals*.

The more animal products you include in your diet, the less room you have for plant matter. Whether or not you make the transition to a fully vegetarian diet, you can benefit greatly from dramatically increasing the ratio of plant to animal products in your diet (Figure 2-1 shows a standard American diet and the vegetarian goal).

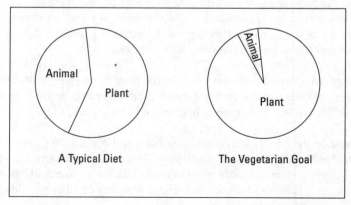

FIGURE 2-1: Plant to animal food source ratios.

Illustration by Elizabeth Kurtzman

In case you're wondering, *free radicals* aren't renegades from the '60s; they're molecules produced as a byproduct of your body's normal metabolism. They're also produced when you're exposed to environmental contaminants such as air pollution and ozone, sunlight and X-rays, and certain dietary components such as fat and the form of iron found in meat. Free radicals speed up the aging process by damaging your cells. They can impair your immune system and cause numerous diseases and illnesses.

Saving the Planet One Forkful at a Time

Choosing to live vegetarian doesn't just benefit your body. When you choose a vegetarian lifestyle, you contribute to the health of the whole planet.

All things considered, vegetarian diets make more efficient use of land, water, and fossil fuel resources than diets that give prominence to meat, eggs, and dairy products.

Calling for climate action

Our world is at a critical juncture in terms of the impact of human activity on the warming of our planet. Globalization and advances in technology, coupled with unchecked growth and consumption, have reached a point of unsustainability. As a result, our planet is permanently warming and growing increasingly polluted, as the amount of farm land and drinkable water decline.

Climate change, if unchecked, threatens to trigger a catastrophic cascade of results that threaten health and well-being, and even the existence of life, on Earth.

You can contribute to fighting climate change and saving the planet. Living vegetarian is a great way to start.

Some scientists consider the world to have entered a new epoch or geological age called the *Anthropocene*. It's a period in the Earth's history in which humans have so utterly taken control of the environment that even the regulating forces of nature cannot correct for the impacts of human activity. One of the unintended negative consequences of human activity on Earth is climate change.

Soil sense

You and I have to take care of the land, or our land won't be able to take care of us. *Animal agriculture* — raising animals for human use — places a heavy burden on the land.

Unfortunately, the amount of land resources needed to raise animals for their meat is far greater than the amount needed to grow enough plant matter to feed the same number of people directly.

Livestock grazing causes *desertification* by eroding the topsoil and drying out the land, preventing it from supporting plant life. Topsoil is being depleted faster than it can be created. Healthy, abundant supplies of topsoil help ensure we have enough farm land to grow the food we need to survive.

The appetite for meat and other animal products also consumes trees and forests, although these trees may not be the ones in your own backyard or your neighbor's. Much of the deforestation happens in Central America and South America, where the number of acres of tropical rain forest cleared to make way for grazing cattle is so big that it's hard to comprehend its enormity.

TECHNICAL STUFF

Think of tropical rainforests as the planet's lungs. One of the many ways that trees help keep the world healthy is by exchanging the carbon dioxide emitted by humans for the fresh oxygen we need to survive. If you didn't have trees, you'd be huffing and puffing as though you had reached the summit of Mount Everest; "breathing through a straw" is how mountain climbers describe the feeling of thinning oxygen. Losing a large percentage of the earth's rainforests has repercussions for every corner of the planet.

REMEMBER

In deforestation, many species of plants and animals are wiped out. These plants and animals hold the keys to scientific discoveries that may benefit humankind. Plants and animals of the rainforests are on the front line, but eventually, the assault on them will reach all of us.

MEAT COSTS EVEN MORE THAN YOU THINK!

If the true cost to society of producing animal products for human consumption were passed on to consumers, fewer people could afford to put these foods on the dinner table as often as they do today. Fortunately, though, for people with a hankering for ham and eggs, government agricultural policies subsidize and protect the production of many of these foods to keep businesses and consumers satisfied with low prices. Of course, the costs don't go away — they're only deferred or shifted. As I point out in this chapter, the production and distribution of animal products makes intensive use of our nonrenewable natural resources and creates byproducts that contaminate our water, air, and soil and harm our health. The cost of meat is sort of like the cost of tobacco to society, which everyone shares in the dollars we spend on health care. As the saying goes, "You can pay me now, or you can pay me later."

Wasting water

When you look at a map of the earth, you see a lot of blue. It's hard to imagine that the earth could be short of water anytime soon. The planet does have a lot of salt-water in the oceans, but one of the greatest threats of animal agriculture is to supplies of *fresh* water.

You can't drink saltwater. The aquifers that lie deep below Earth's surface hold the fresh water needed to irrigate farmland and for drinking. Those giant pools of fresh water are dwindling rapidly because people are sucking up great quantities of the stuff to irrigate huge tracts of land to graze animals that provide a relatively small amount of food. What an inefficient use of a resource as precious as our fresh water!

Furthermore, animal agriculture is polluting both fresh water and saltwater. Pesticides, herbicides, and fertilizers used to grow feed for animals are contaminating water supplies, and nitrogenous fecal waste produced by animals washes into streams, rivers, lakes, and bays. The planet has less clean water than it used to, and the creatures that live in that water are becoming contaminated or are being killed off by the pollution. The problem is accelerating as climate change progresses.

Filching fossil fuels

Animal agriculture is ransacking our planet of fossil fuels. The production of meat, eggs, and dairy products requires intensive use of fossil fuels — including oil, coal, and natural gas — for everything from transporting animal feed and the animals themselves to running farm machinery and operating factory farms where animals are raised. Fossil fuels are also used to make synthetic fertilizers used on factory farms.

Unlike wind, solar, and geothermal sources of energy, fossil fuels aren't readily renewable. After we use our supplies, they're gone. Byproducts such as carbon dioxide and nitrous oxide created by burning fossil fuels for energy also contribute to global warming. Other pollutants, such as methyl mercury from coal-burning power plants, find their way into our water supply, air, and soil and harm the health of humans and other living things.

TECHNICAL STUFF

Emissions from livestock from animal agriculture account for almost one-third of human-caused methane gas emissions, contributing greatly to greenhouse gases responsible for global warming. Moving toward a plant-based diet and plant sources of protein is an important step in reducing greenhouse gas production by reducing the demand for meat and other animal products.

Considering the Ethics

Of course, choosing a vegetarian diet isn't just about improving your own health and well-being. When you adopt a vegetarian diet, you also help to diminish the pain and suffering of those without a voice.

Philosophically speaking

Some of the world's greatest thinkers and philosophers chose or advocated a vegetarian lifestyle, including Pythagoras, Socrates, Leonardo da Vinci, and Benjamin Franklin.

For other people, a vegetarian lifestyle stems from religious or spiritual teachings. Some Christians, for example, interpret the passage Genesis 1:29 from the Old Testament to mean that humans should eat a vegetarian diet: "And God said, behold, I have given you every herb-bearing seed, which is upon the face of all the earth, and every tree, in which is the fruit of a tree yielding seed; to you it shall be for meat."

Members of the Seventh-day Adventist Church are encouraged to follow a vegetarian diet, and about one third of them do. About 8 percent of Adventist vegetarians are also vegan. The Trappist monks, who are Catholic, are also vegetarians, and numerous Eastern religions or philosophies, including Buddhism, Jainism, and Hinduism, advocate vegetarianism. Hindus, for example, consider cows to be sacred.

Vegetarianism is also an ethical choice. Hunger is a good example. For most people in wealthy countries such as the U.S., being hungry is a temporary state of being — the result of skipping a meal because you were in a rush to get out the door in the morning, for example. For less fortunate people in the world, however, hunger is a state of slow starvation with no next meal or snack in sight.

REMEMBER

Despite being a wealthy nation, the U.S. still includes a large number of people who experience hunger, or food insecurity, on a regular basis. Government figures estimate that in the U.S., about 10.5 percent, or 13.8 million Americans, did not have enough to eat in 2020. Some of these people live in *food deserts,* or neighborhoods where access to stores with wholesome, fresh foods, including fruits and vegetables, is limited. For these individuals, choice of diet — vegetarian or not — is a very practical matter. Their first priority is simply getting enough of any food so that they and their families can survive.

Hunger is complicated in terms of ethics, politics, and economics. Many people choose a vegetarian lifestyle as a way of contributing to a more equitable approach to food rationing around the world. In the same sense of knowing that one's lone vote really does count, many people choose to cast their vote in favor of a diet and lifestyle that can sustain the most people.

REMEMBER

In the simplest sense, eating foods directly from the soil — fruits, vegetables, grains, legumes, nuts, and seeds — can nourish many more people than can be fed if the plant matter is fed first to animals and then people eat the animals.

But the appetite of affluent nations for meat and other animal products also creates a market in poor countries for the resources needed to produce those foods. The result is that in low- and middle-income nations, those with power often grow cash crops or livestock feed for export, instead of growing less profitable crops that might feed the local people.

Understanding animal rights and animal welfare

Inhumane treatment of animals compels many people to adopt a vegetarian lifestyle. They consider a meatless diet to be the compassionate choice.

If you share your life with dogs or cats, you know that animals have feelings. You probably also know that cattle, chickens, and pigs don't live in idyllic pastures and barnyards anymore. They live and die in factory farms and slaughterhouses, the likes of which would rival any horror movie.

Male calves born to dairy cows, for instance, are taken from their mothers and raised in confinement for veal. Chickens raised for their eggs live in factory farm conditions in which they are routinely subjected to *debeaking* — the practice of using a machine to cut off the end of a chicken's beak to reduce the pecking damage caused when crowded chickens lash out at one another. All most of us see of the reality are the neat and tidy packages of legs and shoulders on Styrofoam plates wrapped in plastic for sale in the supermarket.

Suffice it to say, some people do allow themselves to think about how animals are treated. They put themselves in the hooves and claws of other creatures, and they take a stand for nonviolence.

In addition to avoiding meat, fish, and poultry, many vegetarians avoid the use of all other animal products. In part, that's because many animal byproducts, such as leather and wool, support the meat industry. The production of other animal products, such as eggs, milk, and other dairy products, is also seen as exploiting those animals, subjecting them to inhumane conditions and treatment, and supporting the meat industry.

TIP

For more information about animal rights, including sources of cruelty-free products, check out the website of People for the Ethical Treatment of Animals (PETA): www.peta.org.

Taking a stand for worker wellness

In addition to considering how animals feel, living vegetarian is also a way to indirectly help people who suffer working in the meat industry. People who work in slaughterhouses and meat processing plants have high rates of physical injury, illness, and mental health problems as a result of the work they do. In fact, during the early weeks of the Covid-19 pandemic, meat packing plants had extremely high rates of Covid cases and deaths because manufacturers wanted to keep up with demand for meat and did not implement adequate safety protocols. If fewer people eat meat, fewer people will be subjected to the toxic work environment of slaughterhouses.

TECHNICAL STUFF

Moral injury is a term that refers to the cognitive or emotional response that some people have when they contribute to, fail to prevent, or witness actions that are at odds with their values or moral code. The term is most often used in the context of those who have participated in military combat and caused the deaths or injuries of other military personnel or civilians. The term is equally valid to describe how people may think or feel about the impact their actions (or inaction) may have on the deaths, injuries, and suffering of animals used for food.

Chapter **3**

Nutrition Know-How for Living Vegetarian

D o you have the old Basic Four Food Groups branded on your frontal lobe? When someone asks you to name foods that provide protein, calcium, and iron, does your mind reflexively retrieve images of rib-eye steaks, cheese wheels, and tall glasses of frothy white cow's milk?

I understand.

You may be savvy enough to know that you can find other food sources of key nutrients, but it's hard to change your mind-set in a culture in which animal products have held center stage for generations.

That's why I devote this chapter to some basic nutrition issues. The information that follows helps to clear up questions and concerns you may have about the nutritional adequacy of a diet that limits or excludes foods of animal origin.

Consuming Enough Protein on a Vegetarian Diet

In all my years of practice as a nutritionist, the number one question people ask about vegetarian diets hasn't changed. They want to know, "Where do you get your protein?"

And you know what? Protein is the nutrient about which vegetarians have the least reason to worry.

Even so, it's not hard to understand why people do worry about protein. We tend to place a lot of emphasis on protein in Western culture. In elementary school, your teacher probably made you cut out pictures of protein-containing foods from magazines and paste them onto poster board. You and your classmates collected pictures of hamburgers, hot dogs, pot roasts, and pizza. Likely absent from that poster were pictures of baked beans and brown rice.

It's certainly important to get enough protein in your diet, but it's not hard to do. There's protein in almost everything you eat, from vegetables, breads and cereals, seeds and nuts, to various kinds of plant milk, and, for those who eat eggs and dairy products, those foods, too.

REMEMBER

In North America and much of the developed world, a cultural bias exists that places the highest value on protein from animal sources. The food industry — in close collaboration with the government — perpetuates policies and practices that maintain the status quo for complex political and economic reasons.

However, getting most or all of your protein from plant sources instead of from animals is easy and better.

In this section, I help you loosen your grip on some misconceptions about the role of protein in human health and tell you all you need to know about protein in meatless diets.

Examining protein facts

To understand how vegetarian diets deliver the protein you need, you first need a solid grasp on what protein is and how your body uses it. That will help illuminate the misunderstandings that persist concerning vegetarian diets and protein.

The word *protein* comes from a Greek word meaning "of first importance." Protein was the first material identified as being a vital part of all living organisms. Proteins make up the basic structure of all living cells, and they're a component of hormones, enzymes, and antibodies.

Most of the protein in your body is in your muscles, but you also have protein in your bones, teeth, blood, and other body fluids. The collagen in connective tissue is a protein, and so is the keratin in hair. The casein in milk, albumin in eggs, blood albumin, and hemoglobin are all examples of proteins.

Protein is a vital part of all living tissues. Proteins are nitrogen-containing compounds that break down into *amino acids* during digestion. Amino acids are the building blocks of proteins and have other functions in the body as well. *Essential amino acids* are amino acids that the body can't manufacture. There are nine of them, and you have to get them from your food.

Most plants contain protein, and some are rich sources. Vegetables, grains, legumes, seeds, and nuts all contain protein. Examples of vegetarian foods that are good sources of protein include

>> Barbecued tempeh

>> Bean burritos

>> Bean soup

>> Cereal and soymilk

>> Falafel (garbanzo bean balls)

>> Lentil soup

>> Oatmeal

>> Pasta primavera

>> Red beans and rice

>> Tofu lasagna

>> Vegetable stir-fry

>> Vegetarian chili

>> Vegetarian pizza

>> Veggie burgers

Plants contain all the essential amino acids in varying amounts. Some plants are high in some essential amino acids and low in others. Getting enough of what you need is easy to do, even if you eat nothing but plant-based foods and your diet contains no meat, eggs, or dairy products at all.

In fact, as long as you get enough calories to meet your energy needs, it's nearly impossible to be deficient in protein. If you ate nothing but potatoes but ate enough potatoes to meet your energy needs, you'd still get all the essential amino acids you need. Now, I don't recommend a potato-only diet. You need other nutrients from food besides protein, and no one food has them all. That's why it's important to include a reasonable variety of foods in your diet.

REMEMBER

However, the practical fact about protein and essential amino acids is that if you eat enough vegetables, grains, legumes, nuts, and seeds (or a reasonable variety of most of those foods), you'll meet or exceed your need for all the essential amino acids.

Debunking old rules about complementary proteins

Despite what you may have heard or read, you don't have to consciously combine foods or *complement proteins* to make sure you get enough protein on a vegetarian diet. The old practice of complementing proteins was based on solid science, but the conclusions that nutritionists drew — and the recommendations they gave — were faulty.

Here's how the idea of complementary proteins works:

Because plant foods are limited in one or more of the essential amino acids, vegetarians have to combine a food that's limited in an amino acid with a food that has an abundance of that same amino acid. The concept is to complement one plant food's amino acid profile with another's, fitting the foods together like puzzle pieces. That way, you have a *complete protein*, with adequate amounts of all the essential amino acids available to the body at the same time.

Nutritionists created complex protein complementary charts that detailed the way foods should be combined, and vegetarians had to be careful to eat their beans with rice or corn and to add milk or cheese to their grains (macaroni and cheese was a big favorite). It was complicated, and the practice made it seem as though vegetarians lived on the brink of nutritional peril if they didn't get the balance right.

Welcome to modern times. We know better now.

Combining the amino acids in foods is no longer recognized as something vegetarians have to do consciously. Your body can do that for you, just like numerous other nutrient interactions that occur without your active intervention. Your job is to do two things:

>> Make sure you get enough calories to meet your energy needs.

>> Eat a reasonable variety of foods over the course of the day.

That's really all there is to it.

Even though it's not necessary to get all essential amino acids in one food, it's interesting to note that soybeans do contain all the essential amino acids. Soy can actually serve as the sole source of protein in a person's diet if that were necessary for some reason.

Getting the protein you need: It's easy to do

Really, you don't have to worry about your protein intake.

Your body can be healthy within a relatively wide range of protein intake, with protein making up anywhere from 10 to 35 percent of the calories in your diet. The human body is more adaptable than you may think.

Okay, if you live on snack cakes and soda, maybe you can end up protein-deficient. But you'd be lacking many vitamins and minerals and other phytochemicals, too. Nevertheless, I know that some of you want to know precisely how much protein you need, so here's a simple way to figure it out:

The rule of thumb for determining recommended protein intake is to aim for 0.8 gram of protein for every kilogram of your body weight. One kilogram is equal to 2.2 pounds. That's body weight (in kilograms) times 0.8 equals grams of protein needed. This formula has a generous margin of error worked into it. In reality, your body actually requires less than this amount. (An exception may be protein requirements for vegans. Although there is no consensus on this point, many vegan nutritionists think vegans should use a factor of 0.9 or even 1.0 to compensate for the lower digestibility of plant proteins.)

So, for example, if you weigh 120 pounds, that equals about 54.5 kilograms (120 pounds divided by 2.2 kilograms). Multiply 54.5 kilograms by 0.8 grams of protein, and you get 43.6 grams of protein, or approximately 44 grams of protein. That's how much protein your body would need each day, and it isn't hard to get.

To see how easy it is to get the protein you need, take a look at the list of foods and their protein contents in Table 3-1. Think about what you eat each day and the portion sizes. Calculate your own protein requirement using this formula and compare it to the amount of protein you eat in a typical day:

Your weight in pounds ____ ÷ 2.2 kilograms = ____ your weight in kilograms ×
0.8 grams protein = ____ your daily protein requirement

TABLE 3-1

Protein Values of Common Foods

Food	Grams of Protein
Animal Products	
1 ounce any type of meat	7
1 ounce cheese	7
1 egg	6
1 cup milk	8
Quarter-pound hamburger (no bun)	25
4-ounce chicken breast	28
10-ounce rib-eye steak	70
3-egg omelet with 2 ounces of cheese	32
Animal Product Alternatives	
1 typical veggie burger	5–25
1 typical veggie hot dog	8
4 ounces tempeh	20
4 ounces tofu (depending on type)	10–12
8 ounces soymilk (plain)	7–10
Legumes (Dried Beans and Peas)	
½ cup most legumes (depending on type)	5–9
½ cup bean burrito filling	6
1 cup black bean soup	6
1 cup vegetarian chili	19
½ cup vegetarian baked beans	6
½ cup garbanzo beans on a salad	7

Food	Grams of Protein
Nuts and Seeds	
1 ounce nuts (depending on type)	4–7
1 ounce seeds (depending on type)	4–11
2 tablespoons tahini (sesame seed butter)	5
2 tablespoons cashew, almond, or peanut butter	4–7
Grains and Grain Products	
1 slice whole-wheat bread (dense style)	2–3
1 medium bran muffin	8
½ cup whole-grain flake cereal	2
½ cup cooked oatmeal	3
1 whole bagel	11
½ cup cooked pasta	4
½ cup cooked rice	2
1 flour tortilla	4
Vegetables and Fruits	
1 cup most cooked vegetables (for example, green beans, tomatoes, cabbage, broccoli)	4
Most fruits	trace amounts

TECHNICAL STUFF

While the recommended protein intake for most adults is 0.8 grams of protein for every kilogram of body weight, it's probably wise for vegans, and any other vegetarians who get most of their protein from whole plant sources, to increase that estimate a smidge to 0.9 grams of protein per kilogram of body weight. That's due to the fact that protein from whole plant sources is less digestible than protein from eggs and dairy products or processed plant foods such as veggie burgers and veggie hotdogs. In everyday life, this small difference in intake isn't likely to translate to a noticeable difference in your diet, though.

The sample one-day menu that follows provides about 1,600 calories and 53 grams of protein. You can see that even if you don't include any animal products at all, it's easy to get all the protein you need.

Breakfast:

1 cup cooked oatmeal, with cinnamon, raisins, and 1 cup plain soymilk

1 slice whole-wheat toast, with margarine and jelly

6 ounces fresh orange juice

Lunch:

Mixed green salad with vinaigrette dressing

1 cup lentil soup

1 chunk cornbread

½ cup fresh fruit salad

Water

Dinner:

4 ounces tofu mixed with Chinese vegetables and brown sauce

1 cup steamed rice

½ cup cooked greens with sesame seeds

Orange wedges

Herbal tea

Snack:

Bagel with plant-based cream cheese

Herbal iced tea mixed with fruit juice

Updating the protein paradigm

Nutrition scientists are deep into discussions today about how best to account for the impact of food production on the environment when making dietary recommendations for the public. Protein is one of the most significant nutrients in discussions about the global warming potential of foods.

So, even though the protein from whole plant foods is not as digestible as the protein from animal sources and processed plant sources, it may be the best over-all when you consider human health and the health of the planet.

Beef, for example, while a rich source of high-quality protein, is a particularly poor choice overall. Beef consumption is associated with increased risk of coronary artery disease and some forms of cancer, and its production places tremendous stress on the environment by the disproportionate use of natural resources and production of greenhouse gases.

Getting your protein from beans and rice or from vegetables instead is not only super for your health, but it's easy on the environment, too.

Taking the bigger picture into account in making dietary recommendations is complex and has political and economic ramifications. Over time, however, it's likely that beans and greens are going to be seen as star performers in the protein games, while animal proteins take the back bench or get booted out of the game altogether.

Moooove Over Milk

Dogs do it. Deer do it. Cows do it. Even chipmunks and raccoons do it. They all produce milk for their babies. So do humans.

But dogs don't drink chipmunk milk. And deer don't drink raccoon milk. That's because milk is species-specific. The milk of each species is tailor-made for its own kind.

So how did people start drinking milk from cows? Even adult cows don't drink cow's milk.

It's an odd state of affairs when you think about it.

Milk is a concentrated source of calcium, and calcium is an essential nutrient for human health. That part is true.

But humans, like all mammals, have no need for milk after infancy. Your body is designed after infancy to get your calcium from other sources in your diet, like plants. Young children gradually stop producing *lactase,* an enzyme present in infancy that permits babies to digest the milk sugar *lactose.*

TECHNICAL STUFF

By adulthood, most people — with the exception of people of Northern European descent — produce much less lactase and have a limited ability to digest milk. This natural condition is called *lactose intolerance.* Most of the world's adults are lactose intolerant to some extent, including the majority of people from Asia, North and South America, Africa, and the Mediterranean.

When people who are lactose intolerant drink milk or eat other dairy products, they often experience symptoms such as gas, bloating, nausea, and diarrhea.

An exception is people of North European ancestry who are thought to have inherited a genetic mutation that allows them to digest milk even as adults.

In the United States — and throughout much of the developed world — powerful dairy industry interests, in collaboration with local, state or provincial, and federal governments, strongly advocate milk consumption for complex political and economic reasons.

They do it despite the fact that most of the world's adults don't digest milk very well. They also push milk despite other health consequences — milk is high in sodium and artery-clogging saturated fat, and it's devoid of beneficial phytochemicals and the dietary fiber largely absent in most people's diets.

In this section, I explain what you need to know about getting calcium the way nature intended — on a vegetarian diet.

Determining who needs milk: The bones of current dietary recommendations

Bone health is a critical consideration for everyone, vegetarian or not. What you eat — or don't — can have a major impact on the strength and resilience of your bones.

Cow's milk is one of the foods that most of us think of when we think "calcium." It's rich in several nutrients, including protein, calcium, potassium, vitamin B12, riboflavin, and others. With the exception of vitamin B12, these nutrients are also plentiful in plant foods.

TECHNICAL STUFF

The Recommended Dietary Allowance (RDA) for calcium is 1,000 milligrams per day for adults ages 19 to 50 years. Although lacto-ovo vegetarians generally have sufficient calcium intakes, it's not difficult for vegans to meet the RDA for calcium, too. Including some fortified plant foods in their diets, such as fortified plant milks, can help.

Understanding the calcium connection

Calcium is vital to a healthy body. Too little calcium in your diet can make you a prime candidate for health problems like *osteoporosis*, the condition that results when the bones begin to waste away and become porous and brittle. Bones in this condition are susceptible to fractures. In the most severe cases, the bones can break with the slightest stress, such as a sneeze or a cough. Osteoporosis is a major health problem that can have life-threatening consequences.

Vegetarians around the world appear to have bone mineral densities that are the same as, or slightly lower than, those of nonvegetarians, though rates of osteoporosis are not higher in vegetarians. Osteoporosis is a very complex disease influenced by many factors, including lifestyle, diet, and genetics. (Your specific risk for osteoporosis needs to be assessed on an individual basis.)

Factors associated with vegetarian diets — high intakes of fruits and vegetables, plenty of vitamins C and K, magnesium, and potassium, for example — may protect against osteoporosis among vegetarians. On the other hand, too-low intakes of protein, vitamin D, or calcium may be risk factors for osteoporosis for some vegetarians.

Making sure you get enough calcium

All vegetarians should err on the side of caution and aim for meeting the levels of calcium intake recommended by the National Academy of Medicine, a unit of the National Academies of Science, Engineering and Medicine (NASEM). Most adults can meet these recommendations by following the meal-planning guidelines I include in Chapter 7.

REMEMBER

Those recommendations call for at least 6 to 8 servings of calcium-rich foods each day. That's not as much food as it may seem. Mountains of broccoli aren't mandatory, but heaping helpings of green leafy vegetables, beans, and other good sources of calcium should be your habit.

Good plant sources of calcium include broccoli, Chinese cabbage, legumes, almonds, dried figs, and dark green, leafy vegetables such as kale, bok choy, collards, and mustard and turnip greens. Other sources are tofu processed with calcium and fortified plant milk or orange juice.

You have lots of delicious ways to work high-calcium foods into your meals. Here are some examples:

>> Bean chili over rice with steamed broccoli and a chunk of cornbread

>> Black bean dip with broccoli and cauliflower florets and carrot sticks

>> Falafel (garbanzo bean balls) in pita pockets and a glass of calcium-fortified orange juice

>> Fig cookies with a glass of fortified soymilk

>> Green beans with slivered almonds

>> Steamed kale with garlic and sesame seeds

>> Stir-fried Chinese vegetables with tofu over rice

Hanging on to the calcium you have

When it comes to your body's calcium stores, what's important is not only getting enough, but also hanging onto what you have.

REMEMBER

Conclusions about how your calcium intake may relate to bone health — and whether or not it increases your risk for hip fracture later in life — is complicated. Your risk may be related to a number of factors, including your genetic background, lifestyle, and various dietary factors. For these reasons, all vegetarians should aim to meet the RDA for calcium.

Help your body hang onto the calcium it already has by paying attention to these points:

TIP

>> **Sodium:** High intakes of sodium may cause your body to lose calcium. Table salt, cheeses, and processed foods contain lots of sodium, as do canned foods such as soups and condiments such as ketchup, mustard, and soy sauce.

   You need some sodium in your diet, but you can get all you need from the sodium that naturally exists in the food supply. You don't have to add sodium to foods. Read the labels on packaged foods and try to limit your sodium intake to no more than about 2,000 milligrams each day (1,500 milligrams is even better) — good advice for vegetarians and nonvegetarians alike.

>> **Tobacco and alcohol:** Avoid tobacco and limit alcohol to not more than two drinks per day. Although the mechanisms are not completely understood, tobacco and excessive alcohol intakes are associated with increased risk of osteoporosis or fracture risk.

>> **Phytates and oxalates:** Substances such as *phytates* and *oxalates*, found in plant foods, inhibit your body's ability to absorb the calcium in the foods that contain them. Whole grains are high in phytates, and raw spinach is high in oxalates, making most of the calcium in these foods unavailable to your body.

   Overall, though, plant foods contain plenty of calcium that your body can absorb. In fact, some research shows that the body better absorbs the calcium in such plant foods as kale, Chinese cabbage, and broccoli than the calcium in cow's milk.

>> **Physical activity:** The more weight-bearing exercise you include in your daily routine, the more calcium you'll keep. People who walk regularly or engage in strength training by using a weight set have denser bones than people who are couch potatoes.

>> **Sunshine:** Your body manufactures vitamin D when you're exposed to sunlight, and vitamin D helps your body absorb calcium.

I should mention one more factor that people often forget. Your body adjusts the absorption of many nutrients, including calcium, according to its needs. In other words, when you need more calcium, your body becomes more efficient at absorbing the calcium that's present in your food. When you need less calcium, your body absorbs less, even if you flood yourself with calcium from dairy products or supplements.

Iron Issues

"Can you list three good food sources of iron?"

When I ask most people that question, they say, "Red meat," and draw a blank after that. Like protein and calcium, most people associate iron with an animal product. But also like protein and calcium, iron is widely available in foods of plant origin.

In this section, I explain what you need to know about getting the iron you need from a vegetarian diet.

Ironing out the basics

Iron is a mineral that forms part of the *hemoglobin* of red blood cells and helps carry oxygen to the body's cells. Iron is also part of the *myoglobin* that provides oxygen to the muscles in your body. When your iron stores are low or depleted, you can't get enough oxygen to your body's cells. A form of *anemia* results, and you may feel very tired.

Before you begin yawning, you might like to know that vegetarians aren't more prone than nonvegetarians to iron deficiency. *Iron-deficiency anemia* happens to be one of the most common nutritional deficiencies around the world, but most of it occurs in developing countries, not in affluent countries, and the cause is usually parasites, not diet. In affluent countries, iron deficiency is most likely to affect children and young people, as well as pregnant and premenopausal women.

Vegetarians need more iron in their diets than nonvegetarians, because the iron from plants isn't absorbed as efficiently as the iron from meat. Most vegetarians get plenty of iron in their diets — in fact, they get more than nonvegetarians — but their bodies' iron stores tend to be lower.

INTRODUCING HEME AND NONHEME IRON

Iron comes in foods in two forms: *heme* and *nonheme* iron. The iron in meat, poultry, and fish is predominantly in the *heme* form. The human body easily absorbs heme iron. In fact, when meat is present in the diet, it increases the amount of iron that you absorb from plant foods as well. This characteristic doesn't necessarily make heme iron a better source of iron, and it may even have drawbacks.

Iron is a potent oxidant that changes cholesterol into a form that's more readily absorbed by the arteries, leading to hardening of the arteries, or *coronary artery disease*. For this reason, men — most of whom are at a higher risk of developing coronary artery disease than most women — are now advised *not* to take daily multivitamin and mineral supplements containing iron.

The form of iron found in plant foods, dairy products and eggs is called *nonheme* iron. Nonheme iron is absorbed less efficiently than heme iron. However, certain other food components — which I discuss in the "Enhancers of iron absorption" section later in this chapter — can radically improve the body's absorption of nonheme iron. These enhancers of iron absorption in plant foods help vegetarians absorb the iron they need.

The RDA for iron varies by age and sex. Generally, the recommendations are higher for premenopausal women than for men and postmenopausal women, because women who menstruate lose more iron than women who don't. The recommendations for adult men and postmenopausal women are only 8 milligrams per day, compared to 18 milligrams per day for premenopausal adult women. The most recent recommendations are also somewhat higher for vegetarians than for nonvegetarians, to compensate for factors in plant foods that may lessen iron absorption.

It's not practical, though, for most people to count the milligrams of iron in their diets. Rather than live life with the calculator open on your cellphone, pay attention to including iron-rich foods in your diet regularly and do what you can to make sure the iron you do eat is well-absorbed. Keep reading as I explain how to do that.

Finding iron in plant foods

Iron is available everywhere you look in the plant world. Rich sources include whole or enriched breads and cereals, legumes, nuts and seeds, some dried fruits, and dark green, leafy vegetables.

REMEMBER

Many of the plant foods that are rich in calcium are also high in iron. The meal ideas that I list in the earlier section "Making sure you get enough calcium" also work if you're trying to ensure that you get enough iron in your diet.

If you're looking for additional iron-rich foods, two good choices are broccoli and Brussels sprouts.

Balancing iron absorption

You may not realize it, but a game of tug of war over iron is going on in your body. That's because certain substances in the foods you eat enhance iron absorption in your body, and other substances inhibit it. Most of the time, the two even out and everything turns out just fine. It pays to understand how the game works, though, so that you can ensure the amount of iron your body is absorbing is just right.

Inhibitors of iron absorption

One of the substances that inhibits your body's ability to absorb iron is the tannic acid in tea. In poor countries where diets are low in vitamin C-rich fruits and vegetables (which enhance iron absorption) and low in iron, a tradition of tea drinking can tip the scales and cause iron deficiency. That doesn't commonly happen in Western countries, where people generally eat a wider variety of foods and have access to plenty of fruits and vegetables.

Other substances that decrease the availability of dietary iron include certain spices, coffee, cocoa; the *phytates* in whole grains, vegetables, and dried beans; and the calcium in dairy products and other high calcium foods and supplements. The reality is, however, that if you eat a reasonable mix of foods, inhibitors and enhancers of iron absorption offset each other and no harm is done.

WARNING

If you're an avid tea drinker, be careful. More than coffee, tea impairs your body's ability to absorb dietary iron. In the American South, it's common for people to drink half a gallon or more of iced tea each day, and quantities of tannins that large may be problematic for some people. Many kinds of herbal tea also contain tannins, though others, including chamomile and citrus fruit teas, do not. If you drink tea, consider drinking it between meals, rather than with meals, to lessen the inhibitory effect of the tannins.

Enhancers of iron absorption

One of the most potent enhancers of iron absorption from a plant source is vitamin C. Healthful vegetarian diets are full of vitamin C. As a vegetarian, if you eat a rich food source of vitamin C with a meal, you can enhance the absorption of the iron in that meal by as much as four times.

You probably eat vitamin C-rich foods with many of your favorite meals and don't even realize it. In each of the following vegetarian meals, a vitamin C-rich food helps the body absorb the iron in that meal:

>> Bowl of black bean soup with sourdough roll; a mixed green salad with tomatoes, green peppers, and onions; and a slice of cantaloupe

>> Bowl of cooked oatmeal with fresh strawberry slices and soymilk

>> Pasta tossed with steamed broccoli, cauliflower, carrots, green peppers, and onions, with marinara (tomato) sauce or garlic and olive oil

>> Peanut butter and jelly sandwich on whole-wheat bread, with orange quarters

>> Tempeh sloppy Joe, with a side of coleslaw

>> Vegetarian chili over brown rice with steamed broccoli or Brussels sprouts

>> Veggie burger with tomato and lettuce and a side of home fries

TIP

Some forms of food preparation may improve the absorption of minerals, including iron, in the diet. For example, iron absorption is better from leavened breads than from unleavened grain products, such as crackers. Fermentation in foods such as sourdough bread and soy products such as miso and tempeh increases the absorption of minerals from those foods. Soaking beans and grains so that they sprout before eating them can also help your body absorb iron and other minerals.

TIP

Other plant components also improve iron absorption, but vitamin C is the most powerful. Using old-fashioned cast-iron skillets, pots, and pans can also increase the amount of iron you absorb, especially when you use them to cook acidic foods, such as tomatoes or tomato sauce. However, most people today prefer to use enamel-coated cast iron cookware, which doesn't confer the same benefit. If you do use the old-fashioned, uncoated type, you should still keep the pots seasoned with cooking oil to help reduce the potential for a metallic taste in foods.

Building B12 Stores

Your body needs vitamin B12 for the proper functioning of enzymes that play a role in the metabolism of amino acids and fatty acids. A vitamin B12 deficiency can cause a form of anemia and a breakdown of the nerves in your hands, legs, feet, spinal cord, and brain.

That's serious stuff for a vitamin that we need in only miniscule amounts. The recommended intake of vitamin B12 for adults is a teeny-weeny 2.4 micrograms per day. Just a fraction of a pinch would be enough to last your entire life.

So what's the big deal about B12?

Getting educated about vitamin B12

For vegetarians, the issue is this: Vitamin B12 is found only in animal products. As far as anyone knows, plants contain little or none. So vegans could risk a vitamin B12 deficiency if their diets didn't contain a source of it.

Vegetarians who eat eggs or dairy products generally don't have as much to worry about, though there is evidence that some lacto ovo vegetarians may have low levels of vitamin B12. Vegetarians who eat eggs and dairy products may get enough vitamin B12 from those foods if they eat them regularly.

WARNING

Vitamin B12 is an issue that vegetarians — particularly vegans — should take seriously, because deficiency can lead to severe and irreversible nerve damage. Despite the need for such a miniscule amount of the vitamin, the stakes are high if you don't get what you need.

TECHNICAL STUFF

It would probably take you a long time to develop a vitamin B12 deficiency. Your body hoards and recycles much of the B12 it gets, which means that your body conserves B12 and excretes very little of it. Most adults have at least a three-year supply of vitamin B12 stored in their liver and other tissues, and a very small number of people can go without B12 in their diet for as long as 20 years before depleting their stores and developing deficiency symptoms. On the other hand, some people can develop a deficiency within a year of not having any vitamin B12.

In fact, the most common cause of vitamin B12 deficiency isn't a lack of the vitamin in the diet — it's the diminished ability of the body to absorb the vitamin. This problem happens to a number of older adults and isn't strictly a vegetarian issue. A variety of age-related factors, including higher incidence of atrophic gastritis, a condition that reduces the body's ability to release vitamin B12 from foods, are responsible for this. For these reasons, recommended intakes of B12 are higher for people over age 50 than for younger adults.

Despite the theoretical risk, few cases of vitamin B12 deficiency in vegans have been reported. That may be due to several reasons, including the fact that folic acid can mask the anemia caused by vitamin B12 deficiency. Folic acid is found in plant foods, especially green, leafy vegetables. Vegetarians, especially vegans, tend to get a lot of folic acid in their diets, so it's possible that a vitamin B12 deficiency could go undetected.

Finding reliable sources of B12

Vitamin B12 is being manufactured all around you — and inside you, too. The vitamin is produced by *microorganisms* — bacteria in the soil, ponds, streams, rivers, and in the guts of animals, including humans. So if you were living in the wild and drinking from a mountain stream or eating vegetables pulled directly out of the ground, you'd likely have natural sources of B12 in the water and soil clinging to your food. Today, you buy your vegetables washed clean and you drink sanitized water. That's best for public health, but it does eliminate a source of B12.

If you eat any animal products — eggs, cheese, yogurt, cow's milk, or other dairy products — you're getting vitamin B12. Nonvegetarians get even more vitamin B12 from meat, poultry, and seafood.

Your intestines also produce vitamin B12, but it's produced past the site of absorption. In other words, you make vitamin B12, but it's not a reliable source.

REMEMBER

Take heed: If you eat few or no animal products, make sure you have a reliable source of B12 in your diet. It's easy to find reliable sources of vitamin B12, such as B12-fortified plant milks, fortified breakfast cereals, or even a B12 supplement. Include them in your diet regularly, just to be on the safe side.

Distinguishing between the different B12s

Just when you thought you understood — here's a twist on the B12 story.

Vitamin B12 comes in many forms. Some forms, including *cyanocobalamin,* are active in human metabolism. Other forms of vitamin B12 are known as *analogs.* The analogs are inactive in the human body.

TECHNICAL STUFF

Why would I burden you with this information? Because a considerable amount of confusion exists over which foods are reliable sources of vitamin B12, especially for vegans. In the past, sea vegetables, tempeh, miso, and nutritional yeast were touted as being good sources of vitamin B12. When those foods were tested for vitamin B12 content for purposes of labeling the food packages, the labs used a microbial assay that measured for all forms of vitamin B12 — not just specifically for active vitamin B12. So people bought the foods thinking they were getting the amount of B12 that the label listed, when, in fact, much of what was listed may have been analogs.

Scientists think that up to 94 percent of the vitamin B12 in these foods is actually in analog form. Some are concerned that analogs may compete for absorption with active vitamin B12 and promote a vitamin B12 deficiency.

TIP

Many of these food products, such as breakfast cereals and meat substitutes, are mainstream brands that you can find in any supermarket. Make it a habit to check the food labels regularly, though, because food manufacturers have been known to change the formulation of products from time to time. Other fortified products that are easy to find are soymilk and other plant milks. If you can't find them in your neighborhood supermarket, you'll find lots of choices at a natural foods store.

A product that many vegetarians — especially vegans — enjoy using is nutritional yeast. It has a savory flavor similar to that of Parmesan cheese, and many people use it the same way. You can sprinkle it over salads, baked potatoes, pasta, casseroles, cooked vegetables, and popcorn.

TIP

If you use nutritional yeast as a source of vitamin B12, be sure to buy the right kind. The regular yeast used for baking that you commonly find in the supermarket isn't what you want. Instead, look for brands such as Red Star Vegetarian Support Formula (VSF), KAL, Bob's Red Mill, Bragg Premium, and Now Foods, at your natural foods store. These all contain sources of vitamin B12 that are biologically active for humans. If the store doesn't have it, ask the manager to order some for you.

WARNING

Some vegetarians think that tempeh, miso (a fermented soy product used as a soup base or condiment), tamari (a fermented soy sauce product), bean sprouts, and sea vegetables such as kombu, kelp, nori, spirulina, and other forms of algae, are reliable sources of B12. They aren't, so be careful. These foods contain mostly inactive analogs of vitamin B12, rather than the form that the human body needs, and they can interfere with absorption of active vitamin B12. Red Star VSF, KAL, Bob's Red Mill, Bragg Premium, and Now Foods nutritional yeast are examples of products that contain the form of vitamin B12 that your body can use.

Considering vitamin supplements

For vegetarians who need a reliable source of vitamin B12, using a supplement is a foolproof way to go. You can use a supplement instead of or in addition to eating fortified foods.

TIP

If supplements are your primary source of vitamin B12, you can get what you need by taking a daily supplement containing 25 to 100 micrograms or a bigger supplement of 1,000 micrograms twice a week. Your body actually needs much less than these amounts, but these standard doses will help ensure that your body has amounts necessary to absorb what you need.

Omega-3s and Your Health

The idea that vegetarians need to pay attention to their intake of *omega-3 fatty acids* (or n-3 fatty acids) is relatively new. Research suggests that vegetarians get lots of *omega 6 fatty acids* (or n-6 fatty acids) in their diets, such as linoleic acid from corn, cottonseed, sunflower, and soybean oils. Linoleic acid is an *essential fatty acid,* a substance essential for health that your body can't produce and that you have to get from food.

Vegetarians get fewer n-3s, including alpha-linolenic acid, another essential fatty acid that's found in flaxseeds, canola oil, cooked soybeans, tofu, pumpkin seeds, walnuts and walnut oil, and other foods. For some vegetarians, lower intakes of n-3s may have a negative effect on eicosapentaenoic acid (EPA) and docosahexaenoic acid (DHA) production, n-3 fatty acids that are physiologically active and essential for humans. N-3s such as alpha-linolenic acids get converted into EPA and DHA in your body.

The nutrition science related to omega-3 fatty acids is complex. The most important thing to remember is that vegetarians should try to get good food sources of n-3 fatty acids in their diets often.

REMEMBER

If you eat fish, you have a direct source of EPA and DHA in your diet, so no conversion is necessary. (Eggs contain a small amount of DHA but no EPA, unless the chickens have been fed flaxseed.) If you don't have a direct source of EPA and DHA in your diet, you have to eat enough n-3 fatty acids to enable your body to convert them to EPA and DHA.

Spotting the best vegetarian sources of omega-3s

Sea vegetables such as nori, kelp, kombu, dulse, and others are often touted as being direct sources of EPA and DHA. You can find these vegetables at Asian markets and natural foods stores. Many vegetarians enjoy cooking with these foods. However, these foods, in fact, have undetectable amounts of DHA, and their EPA content can be quite variable.

TIP

Supplements made from *microalgae* (microscopic forms of algae) rich in DHA are also available in natural foods stores. They're made with non-gelatin capsules, so they're suitable for vegans to use. If you aren't confident that you're getting enough n-3s, consider taking a DHA supplement of 200 to 300 micrograms per day. Consult your health-care provider for individualized advice. DHA supplements made from microalgae are well-absorbed and can boost blood levels of DHA and EPA.

Other good sources of alpha-linolenic fatty acids for vegetarians include ground flaxseeds, flaxseed oil, canola and walnut oils, hempseed products (including veggie burgers and cheese made with hemp) whole or chopped walnuts, and soybeans. Some products, such as Oatly Full Fat Oatmilk Chilled, Ripple Kids Plant-based Milk, Ripple Unsweetened Original Plant-based Milk, House Foods Omega-3 Tofu, and Good Catch Plant-based Tuna, are also available fortified with DHA.

Getting the omega-3s you need

Don't worry about micromanaging your n-3 fatty acid intake. You don't have to count the grams of fat. Just stay aware of the need, follow the eating guide in Chapter 7, and think about using some of the good food sources of n-3 fatty acids more often in your diet.

Other Vitamins and Minerals

A long list of vitamins, minerals, and other substances are necessary for your health. Those I mention in this section — vitamin D, zinc, and vitamin B2 (also known as riboflavin) — merit discussion because, like other nutrients I cover in this chapter, they're generally associated with animal products. You may wonder if it's difficult for vegetarians to get enough of these.

Don't worry — just read on.

The sunshine vitamin: Vitamin D

Vitamin D is actually a hormone that regulates your body's calcium balance for proper bone mineralization. Your body is designed to make vitamin D when your skin is exposed to sunlight. Theoretically, you don't have to get any from foods.

If your skin is light, you need from 5 to 15 minutes of sunshine on your hands and face each day to make enough vitamin D. People with darker skin need more sun exposure.

Of course, that's how it works in the ideal world.

In reality, many people are at risk of vitamin D deficiency because they live in large, smog-filled northern cities where they don't have as much exposure to sunlight as they may need. Others at risk include people with very dark skin (especially those living at northern latitudes), people who are housebound and rarely see the light of day, and people who don't get regular exposure to sunlight because they cover their entire bodies with clothing or sunscreen every time they go outdoors. As you age, your ability to produce vitamin D also diminishes, so older people may also be at greater risk of deficiency.

Food sources of vitamin D

Few foods are naturally good sources of vitamin D, and most vegetarians don't eat the ones that are. Eggs are a source, and so is liver, but liver isn't recommended for anybody because of its high cholesterol content and because an animal's liver is a primary depository for environmental contaminants.

In the U.S., milk has been fortified with vitamin D for many years as a public health measure to protect people who may have inadequate sunlight exposure. If you drink milk, you get a vitamin D supplement in effect. However, you'd need to drink 5 cups of milk each day to meet the adult recommendations for vitamin D intake if you didn't have sunlight exposure or other sources of the vitamin.

Vegetarians and vegans have several potential sources of vitamin D in addition to sunshine. Some brands of plant milks are fortified with vitamin D, as are some brands of margarine and breakfast cereals. Read the food labels to be sure. Unlike cow's milk, plant milk is not required by law in the U.S. to be fortified with vitamin D. Also, just like with cow's milk, for most brands of fortified plant milk, you would need to drink 5 cups a day if your exposure to sunshine were limited.

Bottom line: It's a good idea to consider taking a vitamin D supplement if your sun exposure is limited.

TECHNICAL STUFF

Foods can be fortified with different forms of vitamin D, including vitamin D2 or vitamin D3. Vitamin D2, called *ergocalciferol*, is vegan and can be sufficient for maintaining the body's vitamin D status. It's made by irradiating provitamin D (from plants or yeast) with ultraviolet light. Vitamin D3, called *cholecalciferol*, may not be vegetarian. It's made from fish liver oils or *lanolin*, which is sheep wool fat. Usually, the food label states the form of vitamin D used. If it doesn't, you may have to check with the manufacturer to determine the source. Vegan forms of vitamin D3 are available.

Vitamin D supplements

If you get little exposure to sunlight and you aren't sure whether you're getting enough vitamin D from fortified foods, check in with your health-care provider or a registered dietitian nutritionist for advice. Most vegetarians need a vitamin D supplement to ensure that they're getting enough. I include more advice about the pros and cons of taking supplements in Chapter 4. At the end of this chapter, I provide some suggestions to help you find a registered dieting nutritionist.

For your health: Zinc

Your body needs zinc for proper growth and development. Zinc plays a role in various chemical reactions that take place in your body, as well as in the manufacturing of new proteins and blood, and it helps to protect your body's immune system.

Some vegetarians have trouble meeting recommendations for zinc intake, and the phytates in some plant foods may bind with zinc and prevent your body from absorbing it. Even so, vegetarians in North America and other Western lands are seldom found to have zinc deficiencies.

REMEMBER

Meat is high in zinc, but vegetarians can find plant sources, including dried beans and peas, mushrooms, nuts, seeds, wheat germ, whole-wheat bread, and fortified cereals. Dairy products and eggs are also good sources of zinc for vegetarians who eat those foods. Even though zinc deficiency is rare in vegetarians, you should take extra care to get plenty of zinc-rich foods in your diet.

TIP

Some methods of cooking and preparing foods may increase the availability of zinc. For example, sprouting seeds, cooking or serving foods in combination with acidic ingredients such as tomato sauce or lemon juice, and soaking and cooking legumes may make zinc more available to the body.

The other B: Riboflavin

Another name for vitamin B2 is *riboflavin*. Riboflavin has multiple functions in the body, primarily related to its role in enabling enzymes to trigger various chemical reactions.

Riboflavin is present in small amounts in many foods, and many of the foods that are the most concentrated in riboflavin come from animals. Among the richest sources are milk, cheddar cheese, and cottage cheese. Other animal sources include organ meats such as liver, other meats, and eggs.

So vegetarians who eat dairy products have options, but what about those poor vegans? Isn't it a challenge for vegans to get enough riboflavin?

REMEMBER

Nope. You'll find lots of good plant sources of riboflavin, including almonds, asparagus, avocados, bananas, beans, broccoli, some brands of fortified plant milks and breakfast cereals, kale, lentils, mushrooms, peas, seeds, sesame tahini, sweet potatoes, tempeh, tofu, and wheat germ.

Vegans haven't been found to have symptoms of riboflavin deficiency, even though some studies have shown that they have lower intakes of riboflavin than nonvegetarians.

REMEMBER

You don't have to eat mountains of broccoli to get enough riboflavin. Riboflavin is spread widely throughout the plant world, and you have many choices. As always, one of the chief strategies for ensuring that your diet is adequate is to limit the junk foods and to pack your meals with as many nutrient-dense foods as you can.

Diving in Deeper: More Information for Nutrition Techies

Nutrition science is complex, and not everybody is interested enough to get a degree in nutrition or *dietetics* to understand it. That's okay. I hit the high points in this book and tell you what you need to know to do a competent job of getting started on living vegetarian.

However, if you're the kind of person who likes to read the fine print, and you feel the urge to go a lot deeper into the science of vegetarian nutrition, there are two sources I highly recommend.

Drumroll, please.

The Dietitian's Guide to Vegetarian Diets. This is the go-to textbook for health professionals who want an up-to-date reference on vegetarian nutrition, including counseling points to give to individuals living vegetarian lifestyles. It is comprehensive and highly technical, though the writing style makes it easier to read than many similar texts. Most health professionals and others with a science background will find the content useful.

The large-style paperback published by Jones & Bartlett Learning is in its Fourth Edition and is available from online sources. The authors are Reed Mangels, Virginia Messina, and Mark Messina.

Position of the Academy of Nutrition and Dietetics: Vegetarian Diets. The Academy of Nutrition and Dietetics (AND) — formerly known as the American Dietetic Association — is the major professional organization for dietitians and nutritionists. The Academy publishes brief papers on timely topics, including this one on vegetarian nutrition.

Think of it as a vegetarian textbook in a nutshell.

You can find the paper online at www.eatrightpro.org/-/media/eatrightpro-files/practice/position-and-practice-papers/position-papers/vegetarian-diet.pdf.

Point of pride: I was the primary author of the Academy's 1988 and 1993 position papers on vegetarian diets.

Reconciling the changing nature of nutrition science

Times change, though, and the science of nutrition changes with it. What I wrote about vegetarian diets in 1988 and 1993 was the best we knew, based on the evidence we had at that time. The current position paper builds on those that came before it — and it improves on them.

As scientific evidence accumulates over time, it can change the shape and direction of the advice that results from it. At times, recommendations can take a sharp turn in a different direction. Most of the time, though, the changes are smaller or more subtle.

Diet advice is influenced by external factors, too, including new technologies that expand the range of food choices. Good examples are the number of plant milks and other plant-based food products in mainstream supermarkets today.

REMEMBER

Don't let changing dietary recommendations bother you. Vow to keep up with the science. It's the natural evolution of knowledge, and it represents a process of continual improvement in what we know about how best to take care of our health.

Finding a qualified diet coach

Sometimes it's helpful to get expert assistance in making lifestyle changes. To find a reliable source of one-on-one dietary assistance, I recommend that you ask your health-care provider for a referral to a *registered dietitian nutritionist (RDN).*

TIP

Be mindful about individuals who claim to be nutrition experts but lack education or credentials from generally recognized academic institutions. For some perspective, read the Academy of Nutrition and Dietetics' description of a registered dietitian nutritionist on their website www.eatrightpro.org/about-us/what-is-an-rdn-and-dtr/what-is-a-registered-dietitian-nutritionist. The AND maintains a searchable database that you can use to find a qualified practitioner near you. Go to: www.eatright.org/find-a-nutrition-expert.

» Taking a critical look at supplements

» Making sure you use supplements safely

» Understanding the role of herbs and probiotics

» Finding information about supplements

Chapter **4**

Supplement Smarts

I f your household is like most, you have a stash of vitamin and mineral supplements in your pantry or medicine cabinet. In fact, the supplement industry estimates that American consumers spend several billion dollars each year on nutrient-packed pills, gel tabs, and capsules. Considering the popularity of these products, what I tell you in this chapter may come as a surprise.

If you take vitamin and mineral *supplements* — concentrated doses of individual nutrients — you may think of them as little daily doses of nutritional insurance. In one sense, that idea may contain a tidbit of truth. If your diet is heavy on French fries and soft drinks, and your idea of a vegetable is a dollop of ketchup, you're probably missing out on a wide range of essential nutrients. In that case, it may not hurt — and it may even help, at least a little — to fill in some of the gaps with a tablet. Something is better than nothing, right?

Perhaps, but it's not ideal.

REMEMBER

The truth is, the best way to get the complete array of vitamins, minerals, and other essential substances you need is to get them the way they're packaged naturally — in whole foods. No single food has it all — not bananas, milk, a sandwich, an energy bar, or a smoothie. Different foods provide different constellations of the nutrients found in nature. Take them together, though, in a diet that has enough calories to meet your energy needs and a reasonable variety of whole-some foods, and the nutritional puzzle pieces typically fall into place to give you the complete complement of what you need.

Of course, exceptions happen.

Your diet may not be picture-perfect. Other times, there may be unique, physiological differences among individuals that increase the need for specific nutrients. That's why it's important to understand how best to focus your efforts on improving your diet and what role, if any, supplements should play.

In this chapter, I help you simplify your vitamin and mineral regime. I give you the latest on which supplements science says are useful and not useful, and I help you understand when and if a particular supplement makes sense for you. Most importantly, I help you stay safe if you do decide to use supplements. I also talk about dietary supplements that are relatively new to store shelves — including herbs and probiotics — and explain what they are, how to use them, and where to find reputable sources of ongoing information about all these products.

Examining What the Science Says

It may seem like a no-brainer: "If a little bit of [fill in the name of your favorite vitamin or mineral] is good for me, more must be even better." If only it were that simple.

WARNING

As it turns out, some of the vitamins and minerals you may have been taking for years may not be doing you any good, and some may even be causing you harm. A substantial body of research conducted in recent years has called into question the use of some of the most common supplements, including vitamins C and E and even beta-carotene. On the other hand, science has also shed light on the real benefits of a few select supplements — like folic acid — for some people under certain circumstances.

Sound complicated? It is and it isn't.

The science of nutrition is complex, and as the years go by, scientists learn more and more about how our amazing bodies use the nutrients we need for health. Forty years ago, that nutrient list included a few dozen vitamins and minerals. Today, scientists know that foods contain hundreds of substances — and maybe more — that support your health. Many of these substances work in synergy with one another when they're all present together in whole foods, but they act differently in your body when you take them separately in concentrated doses.

It can be frustrating sometimes when recommendations change, but that's the nature of science. Dietary recommendations are based on the best evidence available at the time, and they get better — and more accurate — as more research findings become available.

The good news is that I translate all this information into straightforward, practical advice that can help you make the most of your diet — whether you're a part-time or full-time vegetarian — taking only the supplements you actually need to support your health. Your wallet may benefit, too!

WARNING

Some people worry that vegetarians are more prone to nutritional deficiencies and, therefore, should have a greater-than-average need for supplements. Not so, and if you're considering becoming a vegetarian, the information in this chapter will help disabuse you of that worry. If you're already following a vegetarian eating style and relying on outdated information about vitamin and mineral supplements, this chapter may save you some money and improve your health.

In this section, I answer a few common questions you may have about the science of supplements.

Do supplements work?

If you're wondering whether supplements work, the answer, for the most part, is no.

That's the short answer. There are some qualified exceptions, including times when vegetarians may need a specific nutrient supplement. In general, though, vitamin and mineral supplements give most people a false sense of security. People greatly overestimate the likely benefits of supplements, and they don't recognize the potential pitfalls.

REMEMBER

Although supplements are a huge business — packing the shelves at supermarkets, drugstores, natural foods markets, and specialty shops at the mall — little, if any, evidence has shown that they're effective in lowering the risks for chronic disease for healthy adults. Despite a few exceptions — folic acid for some women of childbearing age, vitamin D, and vitamin B12 for older adults, for example — the bulk of the research on vitamin and mineral supplements generally doesn't support the exaggerated benefits claimed by the supplement industry.

TECHNICAL STUFF

A paper published in February 2009 in the *Archives of Internal Medicine*, for example, found that in a study of 160,000 older adult women, those who took vitamin and mineral supplements had no significant differences in the risk of death, heart disease, and certain forms of cancer than those who didn't take supplements. Another study, this time of more than 30,000 adults enrolled in the

National Health and Nutrition Examination Survey (NHANES), published in the *Annals of Internal Medicine* in May 2019, found no association between supplement intakes and mortality. And the National Academy of Medicine, part of the prestigious National Academies of Science, Engineering, and Medicine (NASEM), has concluded that the available evidence doesn't support the health claims for some of the most popular supplements in recent years, including vitamins C and E, selenium, and beta-carotene.

This news can be hard to accept. After all, you, like me, may have grown up taking children's chewable vitamins in the morning and feeling virtuous as an adult for dutifully downing your once-a-day nutritional insurance pill. Old ideas about health can be hard to shake, especially those that have been as entrenched as the supplement routine. Even if you can understand the issue intellectually, it can be difficult to let go emotionally. You may be familiar with the concept of insurance, but when you apply that concept to nutritional supplements, it falls short.

Can they hurt me?

It may seem hard to believe that something you need for good health can have a downside. After all, the vitamin C in a fresh orange or a plate of lightly steamed broccoli florets is an important substance in many of your body's physiological processes. If you don't get enough of this vital nutrient, you'll develop the deficiency disease scurvy.

The same is true of other vitamins, minerals, and nutrients you get from foods. If you don't get enough of these important substances, your health can suffer. That's why over the years, nutritionists have chiefly focused on problems associated with the lack of — and not the abundance of — these nutrients. After deficiency diseases were identified, nutrition scientists pushed for everyone to get enough calcium, iron, vitamins A, B, C, D, and E, and more.

And supplements came to be. Extracted from foods or produced in laboratories, supplements became the easy way to replace nutrients that were in short supply in people's diets. This seemed to make sense — most people figured that supplements couldn't hurt, and maybe they could help.

More recently, though, that way of thinking has been called into question. Science suggests that nutrients behave differently when they're not a part of the total package of a whole food. In other words, vitamin E from a gel cap may not have the same benefits as the vitamin E found in whole seeds, nuts, or leafy greens.

REMEMBER

Supplements may, in fact, cause problems under certain circumstances. Taking high doses of individual nutrients, for example, can cause nutrient imbalances that didn't exist before. If you take large amounts of supplemental zinc, for instance, you can deplete your body's copper stores. That's because the zinc and copper interact with each other. If they were present together in a whole food instead, the effects of the other nutrients in that food may provide some balance and counteract the effects of the individual minerals. So supplements lack the natural checks and balances found in foods that contain the entire spectrum of nutrients. Even multivitamin and mineral tablets aren't complete. They contain a long list of vitamins and minerals, but they don't include phytochemicals and other substances important to health, some of which probably haven't been identified yet.

Worse, some supplements once thought to provide special protection against heart disease and some forms of cancer have more recently been linked with increased health risks instead. For example, research has found that people at high risk for lung cancer — especially smokers — can actually increase their risk for lung cancer by taking beta-carotene, a supplement that was previously thought to prevent cancer. Even vitamin E, taken in high doses, has been found in some studies to increase the risk of death.

WHAT CAN I DO INSTEAD?

Looking for a great way to save money? Skip the supplements. Switch to nutrient-dense, whole foods instead.

Just a single serving of many of these nutritional powerhouses can provide you with a hefty dose of the vitamins, minerals, and other substances you need in greater quantities to support health. Good choices include:

- **Dark green, leafy vegetables:** A healthy serving provides you with a big dose of dietary fiber, folic acid, iron, vitamins A and C, potassium, and sometimes calcium. Add a fistful of baby spinach leaves to a pita pocket sandwich, or roll the fresh greens into a bean burrito. Ribbons of cooked kale add a nutritious punch to a plate of black beans and rice, and you can stir cooked, chopped collard greens or spinach into a pot of lentil soup.

- **Deep orange fruits and vegetables:** Think peaches, apricots, sweet potatoes, and orange, yellow, or red bell peppers. These foods are rich in vitamins A and C, as well as dietary fiber. Add a thick slice of a juicy, red tomato to a sandwich, or add a generous handful of grated carrots to a hummus wrap sandwich. Stir some chopped, dried apricots into a bowl of hot oatmeal.

(continued)

(continued)

- **Whole, unprocessed grains:** In addition to being the B vitamin storehouses, grains are a rich source of dietary fiber and trace minerals. You get a nice dose of all these when you reach for a bowl of shredded wheat or bran flakes cereal, a sandwich on whole-wheat bread, or a steaming bowl of seven-grain cereal.

- **Dried beans and other legumes:** Think of these as the multivitamin and mineral supplements that they are, jam-packed full of dietary fiber, protein, folic acid, manganese, iron, and a wide range of other minerals. They're versatile, too — enjoy bean or lentil soup, bean burritos and nachos, black bean dip, or a bowl of chili.

- **Seeds and nuts:** Sprinkle them here, there, and everywhere. Examples include almonds, sunflower seeds, walnuts, pecans, and pumpkin seeds. Add them to salads, hot cereal, and casseroles. I like a handful of chopped walnuts on a bowl of rice pudding. You can't beat seeds and nuts as a source of health-supporting essential fatty acids, and they're a good source of protein, dietary fiber, and many vitamins and minerals, too.

Start thinking differently about what it means to supplement your diet. Fresh, wholesome foods like these are an enjoyable — and low-cost — way to ensure that you get the nutrients you need to be well.

Recognizing When a Supplement Makes Sense

Supplements may not be the best route to good nutrition for vegetarians, but they can be a reasonable crutch to support you in times when you don't have a better option. Many vegans, in fact, need to take vitamin B12 supplements, and others may benefit from supplements of vitamin D, calcium, iodine, and possibly DHA unless they eat foods fortified with these nutrients. In this section, I help you understand how to identify the times when you may need a supplement, and I explain how to be selective in using vitamin and mineral supplements. In most cases, that means your supplement routine will be inexpensive and include just a short list of products.

WARNING

Keep in mind that supplements are only meant to fill in the nutritional gaps in your diet. If somebody tells you that you need a long list of high-cost supplements, a warning bell should go off in your head, triggering a critical examination of the recommendation and, perhaps, a second opinion from your health-care provider.

Special situations that call for a supplement

Supplements aren't ideal, but they may be worth considering if your circumstances are such that the benefits of taking a supplement outweigh the risks.

I cover those cases in Chapter 3, where I discuss the nutritional nuts and bolts of living vegetarian. Though you can easily get enough iron, calcium, omega-3 fatty acids, B vitamins, vitamin D, iodine and zinc from vegetarian diets, in some instances, a supplemental boost of one or more of these nutrients may be merited if you aren't getting enough from the foods you choose.

TECHNICAL STUFF

If you're healthy, your body should generally be able to adapt to varying dietary conditions, absorbing more of a particular nutrient when you need more and absorbing less when you need less. If you get enough calories to meet your energy needs and you eat a reasonable variety of wholesome foods but your diet alone isn't enough to keep nutrients at normal levels in your body, a more complicated problem is likely the culprit.

Another time when a nutritional supplement may be recommended is during pregnancy. I discuss the use of prenatal supplements in Chapter 19. Vegetarians aren't more likely than nonvegetarians to need prenatal supplements, but some people mistakenly think that people who don't eat meat when they're pregnant miss out on vital nutrients. This isn't so, but if you're pregnant or planning to get pregnant, your health-care provider may still recommend a prenatal vitamin and mineral supplement.

The bottom line is that, with the exception of vitamin B12 for vegans, vegetarians aren't more prone than meat eaters to develop nutritional deficiencies. Vegetarians can generally get the nutrition they need from foods. They don't need supplements unless they have reason to believe that their intake isn't sufficient or that an underlying health problem or other complication is causing a nutrient imbalance.

TIP

Not all health professionals are equally familiar with vegetarianism and qualified to counsel vegetarians about their diets. If you do need help sorting out the pros and cons of vitamin and mineral supplementation, seek out a registered dietitian nutritionist who's knowledgeable about vegetarian diets. A *registered dietitian nutritionist* is a food and nutrition expert who has met specific criteria for education and experience as set forth by the Commission on Dietetic Registration, has passed a national registration exam, and has completed continuing education requirements. Search online for a registered dietitian nutritionist who practices in your geographic area and has expertise in vegetarian nutrition by going to the Academy of Nutrition and Dietetics (AND) website at `www.eatright.org/find-a-nutrition-expert`.

In addition, the National Academies of Science, Engineering, and Medicine (NASEM) recommends that certain groups take supplements, whether they're vegetarian or not. Specifically, the NASEM recommends that all adults over the age of 50 take a vitamin B12 supplement to ensure that they're getting enough. The NASEM also recommends that women in their childbearing years take a folic acid supplement. Research suggests that folic acid supplementation may help prevent neural tube defects in babies, and many women have difficulty reaching the recommended level of 400 micrograms of folic acid per day. Vegetarian women can take a bow, though: Their food folate intakes are typically much higher than those of nonvegetarians.

Nutritional insurance

Do you need to take out a nutritional insurance policy by popping a daily multivitamin and mineral supplement? The consensus among registered dietitian nutritionists is that filling dietary gaps with supplements isn't ideal and that whole foods are best.

Still, nutritionists aren't in complete agreement about what role, if any, once-a-day supplements should play in your diet, whether you're a vegetarian or not. Some suggest taking them every so often — once or twice a week, for example — just for good measure.

No evidence exists to suggest that taking low, periodic doses of multivitamin and mineral supplements is helpful, but no evidence exists to indicate that it's a problem, either. The choice is really a personal judgment call. Some nutritionists do advocate taking a supplement during times when you feel you aren't eating particularly well.

Vitamins and minerals are necessary ingredients in your diet to help ensure that various processes in your body function normally. They don't give you energy by themselves, as some people mistakenly think. Only *macronutrients* can do that. Macronutrients are components of your diet that your body needs in relatively large quantities, including carbohydrates, proteins, and fats.

As for me, the only supplement I take is vitamin D. I rely on whole foods for all of my other nutritional needs. Of course, you and I do get some unintentional supplements in some of the foods we eat. Many ready-to-eat breakfast cereals, including the ones I buy, are *fortified* with a smattering of vitamins and minerals, and the plant milk I drink is fortified with vitamin B12.

Fortification is the practice of boosting the nutritional value of a product by adding vitamins and minerals not already present in that food.

So nutritionists don't exactly know what the value of a supplement is if you take it in small doses or infrequently. If it makes you feel better because you're taking it, then go for it — the risk of harm is small.

Using Supplements Safely

The benefits of nutritional supplements are largely unproven, and the side effects can be undesirable. If you're considering using supplements, think carefully about what you plan to take, how much the tablet or capsule contains, and how often you plan to take it.

When it comes to supplements, it's important to get individualized advice. The recommendations in this book are meant to apply to a general adult audience. Your individual needs may be somewhat different, especially if you're being treated for a disease or medical condition. In that case, be sure to follow the advice of your doctor or other health-care provider.

Daily supplements versus high-potency formulas

Most common, once-a-day multivitamin and mineral supplements supply about 100 percent of the amounts recommended on a daily basis. Some even provide less than 100 percent of some nutrients. That's okay — these are supplements, not replacements for the nutrients in foods.

Many people believe that it's a good thing when a supplement contains five or ten times the daily recommended dosage. (After all, more is better, right? Wrong!) If you want to take a multivitamin and mineral supplement, choose one that supplies *no more* than 100 percent of the amounts recommended on a daily basis. Check the bottle's label to see what the supplement includes and how much.

High-potency formulas that contain multiple times the recommended daily amounts of nutrients are sometimes marketed as special formulations for people under stress (who isn't?) or for people with other needs requiring super-high dosages. Don't fall for these marketing ploys. They play on those hard-to-shake beliefs that more must be better. If you have a problem requiring unusually high doses of certain nutrients, leave it to your health-care provider to prescribe the supplement.

Multivitamins versus individual vitamins and minerals

Ordinary, once-a-day multivitamin and mineral supplements are probably benign when they provide up to 100 percent of the recommended daily amounts of nutrients. Taken now and then — or even daily — they probably won't harm you. If you buy generic or store brand varieties, they may not cause much damage to your pocketbook, either.

Similarly, taking low doses of individual vitamins and minerals — those sold as isolated, separate nutrients — once in a while is probably harmless. However, many individual nutrients come in capsules or tablets that contain multiple times the recommended daily amount.

WARNING

You increase the chances of creating problems for yourself when you take individual vitamins and minerals instead of taking them as part of a larger grouping of the nutrients that occur in foods naturally. That's especially true when you take dosages that are many times more than what you need in a day.

REMEMBER

Remember that the best sources of nutrients are the whole foods that contain the array of nutrients in amounts and combinations found in nature. The next best option, though not ideal, is the multivitamin and mineral solution. Your last choice should be individual nutrients, unless your doctor or other health-care provider specifically recommends them.

When supplements act like drugs: Being aware of interactions

Vitamins, minerals, and other nutrients can have drug-like effects in your body when you take them in high doses. A good example is niacin, one of the B vitamins. High doses of niacin change the production of blood fats in your liver. People at risk for coronary artery disease can use a special prescription form of niacin to lower their triglyceride and LDL ("bad cholesterol") levels and raise their HDL ("good cholesterol") levels. That's a pretty powerful use of a vitamin.

WARNING

Other nutrients can have similarly potent effects when you take them in large doses. Like niacin, they can cause physiological changes in your body. High doses of vitamin C, for example, can cause your body to absorb less copper. Nutrients can also interact with one another, changing the natural balance of nutrients. High doses of zinc, for example, can deplete your copper stores. Certain vitamins and minerals in high doses can also interfere with the action of prescription drugs you may be taking and can either enhance or diminish the effects of those medications. For example, folic acid supplements may lessen the effects of phenytoin (Dilantin), a prescription medicine used to treat seizures. (Herbs may have an effect as well. I cover those in the next section.)

TIP

If you already take supplements, including herbs or other alternatives, tell your health-care provider what you're taking. Better yet, provide a written list. It will help ensure that you don't forget any individual item, and it will give your health-care provider an accurate and up-to-date picture of everything you're taking. The more information your health-care provider has about you, the more likely your provider will be able to warn you of potential side effects.

Considering Herbs and Probiotics

People who follow vegetarian diets tend to be more aware than the average eater of food and nutrition matters. As a vegetarian, you're more likely to hear messages — accurate or not — about your vitamin and mineral needs and about alternative dietary supplements.

Of course, you can supplement your diet with all sorts of things. In discussions about vegetarian diets, most people focus on vitamin and mineral supplements. But some people — vegetarian or not — add bran to their diets for a natural laxative, and others add flaxseed oil for the essential fatty acids. In the broadest sense, anything you add to your diet can be considered a supplement, including peanut butter on a cracker.

TECHNICAL
STUFF

In 1994, the U.S. Congress passed into law a similar but slightly narrower description of dietary supplements in the Dietary Supplement Health and Education Act (DSHEA). That law defines a dietary supplement as any product meant to supplement the diet with one or more dietary ingredients, taken by mouth in tablets, capsules, powders, liquids, and in other forms, and labeled as a dietary supplement.

In this section, I zero in on two specific kinds of supplements — herbs and probiotics — that have been the subject of increasing interest among vegetarians and others interested in diet and health. In both cases, the science is evolving, and the federal government is putting research dollars into studying the benefits and possible risks of each.

Understanding what they are

Herbs and probiotics are completely different things, but both are forms of dietary supplements used by many vegetarians and others interested in their potential health benefits. If you want to be a well-informed vegetarian, you should have at least a rudimentary knowledge of these two dietary embellishments.

Herbs

Herbs are plants used in small quantities for various purposes. Herbs can be grouped into two categories:

>> **Culinary herbs,** such as rosemary and sage, are used for the flavor and aroma they add to foods. These plants are considered herbs and not vegetables, simply because they're used in such tiny amounts. Vegetarians love to use herbs and spices in cooking. *Spices* are usually made from the roots, bark, and other, non-leafy parts of the plants.

>> **Medicinal herbs** are generally thought to confer health benefits, and many people use them for their potential therapeutic effects. (Some people refer to these as *botanicals,* another name for herbs.) Just as some people believe that vitamin and mineral supplements protect health by boosting immunity or preventing heart disease and cancer, some people believe that certain herbs may have similar effects.

TECHNICAL
STUFF

Some herbs are used for both medicinal and culinary purposes. Ginger is safe and effective during pregnancy, for example, in small quantities for short periods of time to relieve nausea and vomiting, according to the National Center for Complementary and Alternative Medicine, a unit of the National Institutes of Health. Ginger also happens to taste good in a variety of vegetarian dishes, including soups and stir-fry.

When I talk about herbal supplements, though, I'm generally referring to medicinal herbs taken for their therapeutic benefits, rather than culinary herbs. Herbal supplements can be composed of a single herb or a combination of two or more herbs.

Examples of popular medicinal herbs include

>> Black cohosh

>> Echinacea

>> Feverfew

>> Gingko

>> Ginseng

>> Kava

>> Red clover

>> Saint-John's-wort

>> Valerian

TIP

A comprehensive list of popular herbs, including their common names, uses, and possible side effects, is available online from the National Center for Complementary and Integrative Health at www.nccih.nih.gov/health/herbsataglance.

Probiotics

Enough about plants, though. Bugs are important, too.

In addition to herbal supplements, vegetarians often read about *probiotics,* or friendly bacteria. These are the good kind of bugs to have in your food.

The idea is that if you take these live microorganisms as supplements in capsule or powder form, or if you eat them in whole foods, they can replace or increase your body's natural supply of good bacteria.

If you take an antibiotic to fight an infection, for example, the medicine kills off the bad bacteria as well as the friendly bacteria that are naturally present in your intestines. These friendly bacteria are necessary for the normal functioning of your intestines.

You may be able to use probiotics to restore the natural supply of friendly bacteria in your intestines, though. Probiotics include yeast and a range of other microorganisms. Supplements, or yogurt with *active cultures,* such as *Lactobacillus bulgaricus* or *Streptococcus thermophilus*, may help to repopulate your intestines with these good guys.

Some scientific support also exists for the benefits of probiotics in the treatment of diarrhea and irritable bowel syndrome, the prevention and treatment of urinary tract infections, and the prevention and treatment of eczema in children. It's too early to make concrete recommendations, though. In fact, it's even possible that some benefits may be caused by a *placebo effect.* In other words, the benefits may all be in your head.

TIP

You can buy probiotics as dietary supplements in many retail stores, in addition to natural foods stores and pharmacies, or you can get them by eating whole foods. Common vegetarian foods that contain probiotics include some brands of yogurt, soymilk and other soy products such as miso and tempeh, kefir (a drinkable form of yogurt), and fermented milk (such as buttermilk). Fermented vegetables such as sauerkraut and kimchi — a traditional Korean dish made from pickled vegetables and seasonings — also contain probiotics.

Many brands of yogurt contain active cultures. Look for those words — "active cultures" — on the package to be sure that you're getting a dose of friendly bacteria when you eat that product. Other products, such as kefir, may use the word "probiotic" on the label to show that the product contains active cultures. Still others, such as buttermilk, may simply list "bacterial cultures" on the product's ingredient list.

Knowing how to use them safely

You may be surprised to discover that federal guidelines regulating the marketing and sales of nutritional supplements are quite loose. The products aren't held to the same standards as prescription drugs or over-the-counter medications. In fact, companies can start marketing nutritional supplements without having to prove that their products are safe or effective at all.

That alone should cause you to hesitate — and to do a little research of your own — before you decide to use a dietary supplement.

Herbal supplements, in particular, merit special attention. Just as with vitamin and mineral supplements, if you use herbal supplements, be sure to let your health-care provider know. Your provider understands your total care plan and may recognize when a supplement has the potential to cause a problem.

Talking to your health-care provider is especially important if you're on medications or contemplating surgery. Like high levels of vitamin or mineral supplements, some herbal supplements have the potential to interfere with medications you may be taking. Others may affect your risk for bleeding during surgery or may alter the way you react under anesthesia.

If you're pregnant or breastfeeding, it's also best to let your health-care provider know if you're taking an herbal supplement. Before giving an herbal supplement to a child, check with your child's health-care provider, too. Though you may have nothing to worry about, it's better to be safe. Most research on herbal supplements has been conducted on adults, and little if any has been conducted on pregnant or nursing people or children.

Be aware that dosages may be different between brands. Also, discrepancies are sometimes found between what's in the supplement bottle and what the label says the product contains. The plant species used or the amount of the active ingredient listed can be different from what you may think you're getting. Products may also be contaminated with pesticides, other herbs, and other substances that may not be safe to ingest.

In contrast to herbal supplements, probiotics don't seem to pose much risk, though more research is needed on their use by young people, older adults, and people with depressed immune systems. For healthy adults, the most common side effects are gas and bloating — uncomfortable, perhaps, but not serious.

Locating Reliable Sources of More Information

A great deal of research is being conducted on dietary supplements, so recommendations can change in relatively little time. That's why it's important that you know where to go for accurate, up-to-date information about their use and safety.

One first-line source of information is your health-care provider. Physicians, registered dietitian nutritionists, pharmacists, physician assistants, and other providers don't always have all the answers. They may not know, for example, where the science stands on the use of evening primrose oil or ginseng.

They do know where to go to get the information, though, and they usually have access to medical libraries or researchers and other experts who can provide reliable feedback.

TIP

I also highly recommend the following resources:

>> **The National Center for Complementary and Integrative Health:** Access this clearinghouse online at www.nccih.nih.gov for updates on research about herbal supplements and probiotics. Fact sheets and other materials are available in English and Spanish.

>> **The Office of Dietary Supplements at the National Institutes of Health:** Find it online at https://ods.od.nih.gov. Resources include comprehensive fact sheets with information about specific vitamins, minerals, and herbal supplements; advice for supplement users and tips for older adults; and background information about dietary supplements.

>> **MedlinePlus, a service of the U.S. Library of Medicine and the National Institutes of Health:** Find it online at https://medlineplus.gov. This site lets you search by the first letter of herbs and other supplements for detailed information compiled from a variety of authoritative sources. It also provides a link to the Dietary Supplements Labels Database, which you can use to

compare the ingredients in more than 125,000 labels of dietary supplement products. If you prefer, you can go to the database directly at `https://ods.od.nih.gov/Research/Dietary_Supplement_Label_Database.aspx`. You'll find links to additional publications and resources on dietary supplements on this site, too.

» **Planning the details of your dietary switch**

» **Steering clear of animal ingredients**

» **Getting started on your lifestyle change**

Chapter **5**

Making the Transition to Meat-Free

"Where are you going?" the cat asked.
"I don't know."
"Well, either road will get you there."
　　　　　　　—*LEWIS CARROLL*, ALICE'S ADVENTURES IN WONDERLAND

D on't be like Alice, who doesn't know which route to take to get where she wants to go. If you want to change your eating style, *how* you do it isn't as important as having a plan for getting there. Without a plan, you're less likely to achieve your goal.

We all have different styles of doing things. What's important is that you find a method that works for you. There's no right or wrong way of making a lifestyle change, as long as you're successful. So do what's comfortable for you. In this chapter, I cover key points to think about in formulating your plan of action as you make the switch to a vegetarian eating style.

Finding the Right Approach

In this section, I present two approaches to consider as you plan your transition to a vegetarian lifestyle. I also cover pros and cons to think about as you weigh the options for making the change.

Going cold tofu: Presto! vegetarian

One day he's chewing on a 10-ounce rib-eye at a local steakhouse, and the next day he's ordering the black bean burger at his neighborhood natural foods cafe. It's not a likely scenario, but some people do make an overnight decision to go vegetarian. They see a video or hear a lecture that inspires them, or they read a book or story about the horrors of the slaughterhouse. Suddenly, it all adds up to . . . change! It can't happen fast enough.

Instant vegetarian

The overnight transition to vegetarianism is seldom flawless, but those who do it are motivated to make the change as soon as possible. Some people just prefer to make big changes quickly as opposed to dragging them out over months or years. That's fine.

Benefits of the quick switch

Making the switch to a vegetarian diet in one leap has some benefits:

>> People who make big changes right away tend to notice the benefits quickly and enjoy the benefits sooner. That may be especially appealing if you have health concerns. For example, if you're overweight, you may notice weight loss sooner, or if you're a person with diabetes, your blood sugar level may drop.

>> You get immediate gratification. Your personality may be such that you need the satisfaction that comes with taking immediate action and reaching your goal as soon as possible.

>> You know you'll get there in this lifetime. In comparison to people who take the gradual approach (see the later section "Taking your time: The gradual approach" for details), people who make the change all at once jump one big hurdle to arrive at their goal. They don't run the risk that the others do of getting stuck in a rut along the way.

The overnight approach works best for people who:

» Have done some homework: Even a little bit of reading or talking with another vegetarian about basic nutrition questions and ideas for quick and easy meals can help immensely.

» Are surrounded by support: The overnight approach is easiest for people who live or work with other vegetarians and have someone they can emulate or question about basic nutrition and meal-planning issues.

» Are relatively free of other distractions: Making a big change overnight is easier if you don't have a new baby, a new job, or an 80-hour workweek.

WARNING

If you switch to a vegetarian diet and find yourself tired and hungry or irritable, you may not be eating enough. Some people who switch overnight haven't had time to figure out what they can eat. They end up eating only a few different types of foods, and they often don't get enough calories.

Don't fall prey to the "iceberg lettuce syndrome" — the situation where the only thing new vegetarians know they can eat is lettuce. You can eat all kinds of foods — see Part 3 for ideas.

WARNING

If you're a diabetic and you switch to a vegetarian diet, visit your health-care provider. People with diabetes who adopt a vegetarian diet frequently need less insulin or oral medication and need to have their dosages adjusted. In some cases their blood sugar levels decrease enough to allow them to discontinue their medication altogether. Don't attempt to change your medications without checking with your doctor or other health-care provider first, however.

Drawbacks of overnight vegetarianism

If you take the instant route to gratification, you'll soon find out that you have no time to develop necessary new skills and to put supports in place. It takes time to absorb the background information about nutrition and meal planning, as well as to learn how to deal with all sorts of practical issues such as eating out and handling questions from friends and family. These are some of the things that are necessary for a successful transition, and if they're not taken care of before you dive in, your entry can be a bit chaotic, or you may even do a big belly flop.

REMEMBER

If you opt for the overnight approach, use your wits to do the best you can at the outset, but come up with a plan for a smoother transition as soon as possible. Get yourself educated, get a plan, and get some support. I include plenty of tips throughout this book.

Taking your time: The gradual approach

When it comes to making a major lifestyle change, most people fare best by taking the gradual approach. You probably will, too.

Let your diet evolve at your own pace as you develop new skills and educate yourself about the new eating style. As you master each new skill, you'll become more secure and comfortable with meal planning and handling a variety of food-related situations. In Parts 2 and 4 of this book, I provide you with lots of practical information to help make the transition to a vegetarian lifestyle as easy as possible.

Benefits of the gradual approach

Advantages to making a gradual switch to vegetarianism include:

>> Your new eating habits are more likely to stick. Making changes gradually allows you to collect the information and support you need to make it work and helps you build a strong foundation.

>> The gradual approach may be less disruptive to your routine. If you have more time to adapt to each change every step of the way, you may have a better chance of sticking with it.

Drawbacks of easing in

WARNING

The gradual approach has disadvantages, too. Keep these in mind and try to avoid them:

>> Getting stuck in a rut along the way. You can get stuck anywhere along the line and never make the transition to a full-fledged vegetarian diet. Some people cut out red meat as an initial step, but they never make it any further. They're forever stuck in the chicken-and-fish rut, or they get as far as substituting cheese and eggs for meat. Their blood cholesterol levels soar because they're living on cheese omelets, macaroni and cheese, and grilled cheese sandwiches.

Don't let this happen to you. Have a plan to keep moving.

>> Procrastinating and dragging the change out too long. If you take too long to make the change, it may never happen. Don't delude yourself. If you want to adopt a vegetarian diet but it's been a year since you started, it's time to put pen to paper and develop a more structured plan with dated goals for getting there.

Smoothing the Way

Whether you choose to make the switch to a vegetarian diet overnight or gradually, you can tackle the change in a variety of ways. It's just a matter of personal preference. You may be especially interested in nutrition and devour books on the subject, or you may love to cook and find yourself experimenting with recipes long before you get around to thinking about vegetarian meals while traveling. You may like to read, or you may prefer talking to other vegetarians or attending lectures instead.

How you choose to proceed is up to you. The following guide is only one suggestion for planning a reasonably paced transition to a vegetarian eating style. Take some time to reflect, and do what's right for you.

Defining some simple steps

Have you ever had to write a major school paper or thesis? Cringe! Any large project can seem overwhelming when you look at it in its entirety.

TIP

To tackle a big project, break it up into smaller pieces, focusing on only one task at a time. Writing down the steps you plan to take and checking them off as you master each one can give you a sense of accomplishment and help keep you motivated along the way.

Draw up a weekly or monthly plan of action outlining the things on which you want to focus each step of the way. For instance, you may want to concentrate on reading several books and other written materials for the first two months. From there, you may pick up a few vegetarian cookbooks and experiment with recipes, adding a few meatless meals per week to your schedule for the next month. Step it up to five meatless days per week for the next few months, and begin attending local vegetarian society meetings.

FEEDING FURRY FAMILY MEMBERS

Dogs are naturally omnivorous and can fare well on a diet that excludes meat. Cats, on the other hand, are carnivorous and need the nutrients found in meat. Specifically, cats must have a source of the amino acid taurine in their diets, and taurine doesn't exist in the plant world. If you don't feed your cat meat, you must provide a taurine supplement. Your veterinarian may or may not be receptive to the idea of a vegetarian diet for cats and dogs, just as many human health-care providers have no training in the fundamentals of vegetarian diets for people.

Websites can also be a good source of support. The Meatless Monday website is especially helpful, asking you to make a commitment to eat meatless meals one day a week. (www.mondaycampaigns.org).

Your plan should reflect your lifestyle, your personality and preferences, and any constraints that you may have to factor in, such as cooking for a family or traveling frequently.

REMEMBER

It helps to set time goals in your plan for transitioning to a vegetarian diet. If you can keep these deadlines in your head, fine. If not, or if you find yourself dragging your feet getting to the next step, you may need more structure. Write your plan in a notebook (or in an online journal), and break it down week by week. Give yourself a reasonable amount of time to complete each task, and stick to your plan.

Educating yourself

Education is a good first step in any plan for lifestyle change. If you like to read, you're in luck, because you can find many excellent resources on vegetarian diets. It's a great idea to spend several weeks to months reading everything you can get your hands on pertaining to vegetarianism as you make the transition.

You'll find materials on all aspects of vegetarianism. Some books, magazines, and online materials may seem to cover the same subjects, but it's worth reading them all, because each author presents the information in his or her own style, and the repetition of the subject matter can help you learn and build a solid foundation for your transition.

If you don't particularly care to read, try podcasts and audio books. Seek out recorded lectures and interactive discussions about vegetarian diets and related topics online on YouTube. You may also find some offered on college campuses, at natural foods stores, and in community centers. Or drop in on meetings of local vegetarian societies where guest speakers are often featured.

WARNING

There is one caveat, however. Although many excellent resources are available, some materials contain inaccuracies or misinformation. I include references to many reliable resources in this book, including some listed in the later section "Tracking down resources for up-to-date advice."

Reducing your meat intake

TIP

While you're doing some background researching vegetarian diets, start reducing your meat intake in some easy ways:

>> Add two or three meatless main meals to your diet each week. Begin with some easy and familiar entrées, such as spaghetti with tomato sauce, vegetarian pizza, bean burritos, vegetable lasagna, and pasta primavera.

>> Try some vegetarian convenience foods, such as veggie burger patties, veggie breakfast meats, frozen vegetarian dinners, and veggie hot dogs. They're quick and convenient. Most supermarkets carry these products, and you can also find a large selection at natural foods stores. Substitute them for their meat counterparts.

>> When you do eat meat, make it a minor part of the meal rather than the focal point of the plate. Use meat as more of a minor ingredient or side dish. Keep portions small, and extend the meat by mixing it with rice, vegetables, diced mushrooms, pasta, or other plant products. For instance, rather than eat a chicken breast as an entrée, cut it up and mix it into a big vegetable stir-fry that feeds four to six people.

From there, just keep going. Add a few more meatless meals to your weekly schedule and stick with it for a month or so. Set a date beyond which you'll be eating only vegetarian meals. Mark that date with a big star on your calendar, and then cross off each day that you're meat-free after that.

REMEMBER

Be aware that interruptions in your routine, such as a vacation, holiday, or sickness, can trigger a lapse in your eating plan. In times of stress or a break in routine, it's common to fall back into familiar patterns, including old ways of eating. Give yourself a break, and then start fresh again. With time, you'll discover how to handle breaks in routine and you won't be derailed by them.

Setting your goals

After you start the switch to vegetarianism, it's all about practicing and continuing to expand your knowledge base and experience. Expect some bumps in the road, but keep going.

Experiment with recipes, new foods, and vegetarian entrées at restaurants. Invite friends and family members over to your place for meals, read some more about nutrition and meal planning, and allow yourself more time to get comfortable with your new lifestyle.

All this is easier to accomplish if you set specific goals and a timeline for achieving them. Think about steps that seem realistic for you to achieve, and estimate the length of time you think it will take to master each step. Sketch out a plan in a notebook or set up a spreadsheet or table on your computer.

Table 5-1 shows a sample schedule for making the transition to a vegetarian lifestyle. Your own transition may take more or less time. Adjust the timeline — and the specific steps — to suit your own needs and preferences.

TABLE 5-1

Twelve Months to a Vegetarian Eating Style

Time Frame	What to Do
Months 1–2	*Get educated about basic nutrition, meal planning, dealing with social situations, and other aspects of vegetarian diets.* Borrow books from the library, listen to podcasts and audio books, buy a few good resources at a bookstore, visit vegetarian organizations online for materials, attend lectures, and subscribe to vegetarian magazines. Absorb information.
Month 3	*Begin to reduce your meat intake.* Add two or three meatless meals each week, experiment with new products, make a list of all the vegetarian foods you already enjoy, and when you do eat meat, make it a minor part of the meal, rather than the focal point of the plate.
Months 4–6	*Cut back even more on your meat intake.* Plan five meatless days each week. Limit meat to use as a side dish or a minor ingredient in a dish. Plan a cutoff date after which you'll eat only vegetarian meals. Mark that date on your calendar. A week or two before that date, stop buying meat and products containing meat, such as soup with ham or bacon and baked beans with pork. Keep a food diary or log of everything you eat for several days. You'll refer to it later to gauge your progress. Be specific about the ingredients. For example, if you eat a sandwich, note the kind of bread and filling you chose.
Months 7–8	*Look into joining a local vegetarian society or attending a national vegetarian conference.* Seek out occasions when you can be surrounded by like-minded individuals. Continue reading and absorbing information. Continue experimenting with new recipes. Go out to eat and order vegetarian entrées at restaurants.
Months 9–12	Practice. Continue to seek new information. Socialize and invite friends and family members to your home for vegetarian meals. Look back over the past year and evaluate how you've handled holidays and special occasions, vacations, and breaks in your routine. Do some situations need attention, such as eating away from home or finding quick and easy meal ideas? Keep a food diary for several days and compare it to your first one (which I suggest starting in months 4–6).

Monitoring your progress

After you complete the initial steps in the transition to a vegetarian diet, keep a food diary from time to time for several days or weeks — whatever you can manage. Spot-checking your diet now and then helps you stay aware of what you're eating. Recording not only what, where, and when you eat but also how you feel and who you're with may help you become aware of behavior patterns you may want to target for change.

TIP

Keep a notebook to use as a food diary, or try an online food diary app. Some charge a monthly fee. A very simple, free online food diary form is available from the U.S. Centers for Disease Control and Prevention here: www.cdc.gov/ healthyweight/pdf/food_diary_cdc.pdf. An added bonus of maintaining your diary online is that some, such as www.myfooddiary.com, will tally your daily intake of calories and nutrients and also let you know how many calories you're burning with exercise.

Making Sure It's Meat-Free

Avoiding obvious sources of meat, fish, and poultry is relatively easy. You probably recognize a chicken leg or steak when you see one. Living vegetarian gets trickier when animal ingredients and their byproducts are added to products in small quantities that may be hard to see or taste.

In this section, I help you find those hidden ingredients.

Being wary of hidden animal ingredients

Many foods contain hidden animal ingredients. Some are present in very small amounts. Casein and whey — both derived from dairy products — are acceptable for vegetarians but not for vegans. Others, such as rennet (which comes from the stomach lining of calves and other baby animals), are typically unacceptable to all vegetarians. I include a list of hidden animal ingredients in Table 5-2. Decide for yourself what you are and aren't willing to eat.

In some cases, an ingredient may originate from either an animal or plant source, and you can't determine which from the label. You may need to contact the manufacturer and ask (see the later section "Communicating with food companies" for more info).

TIP

Many hidden animal ingredients are found in store-bought, prepackaged foods. A good way to avoid hidden animal products is by making some of these items yourself. For example, consider making your own salad dressings, refried beans, and baked goods. You have more control over the ingredients in your foods when you make them yourself at home.

TABLE 5-2   # Hidden Animal Ingredients

Ingredient	What It Is	Where You Find It
Albumin	The protein component of egg whites	As a thickener or texture additive in processed foods, such as creamy fillings and sauces, ice cream, pudding, and salad dressing
Anchovies	Small, silver-colored fish	Worcestershire sauce, Caesar salad dressing, pizza topping, Greek salads
Animal shortening	Butter, suet, lard	Packaged cookies and crackers, refried beans, flour tortillas, ready-made pie crusts
Carmine (carmine cochineal or carminic acid)	Red coloring made from ground-up cochineal insects	Bottled juices, colored pasta, some candies, frozen pops, "natural" cosmetics
Casein (caseinate)	A milk protein	As an additive in dairy products such as cheese, cream cheese, cottage cheese, and sour cream; also added to some soy cheeses, so read the label
Gelatin	Protein from bones, cartilage, tendons, and skin of animals	Marshmallows, yogurt, frosted cereals, gelatin-containing desserts
Glycerides (mono-, di-, and triglycerides)	Glycerol from animal fats or plants	Processed foods
Isinglass	Gelatin from the air bladder of sturgeon and other freshwater fish	As a clarifying agent in alcoholic beverages, some jellied desserts
Lactose (saccharum lactin, D-lactose)	Milk sugar	As a culture medium for souring milk and in processed foods such as baby formulas and sweets
Lactylic stearate	Salt of *stearic acid* (tallow, other animal fats and oils)	As a conditioner in bread dough
Lanolin	Waxy fat from sheep's wool	Chewing gum
Lard	Fat from the belly, butt or shoulder of pigs	Baked goods, refried beans
Natural flavorings, unspecified	Can be from meat or other animal products	Processed and packaged foods
Oleic acid (oleinic acid)	Animal *tallow* (solid fat of sheep and cattle separated from the membranous tissues)	Synthetic butter, cheese, vegetable fats and oils; spice flavoring for baked goods, candy, ice cream, beverages, condiments
Pepsin	Enzyme from pigs' stomachs	With rennet to make cheese
Propolis	Resinous cement collected by bees	Sold in chewing gum and as a traditional medicine in natural foods stores

Ingredient	What It Is	Where You Find It
Stearic acid (octadecanoic acid)	Tallow, other animal fats and oils	Vanilla flavoring, chewing gum, baked goods, beverages, candy
Suet	Hard white fat around kidneys and loins of animals	Margarine, mincemeat, pastries
Tallow	Solid fat of sheep and cattle separated from the membranous tissues	Margarine
Vitamin A (A1, retinol)	Vitamin obtained from vegetables, egg yolks, or fish liver oil	Vitamin supplements, fortification of foods such as breakfast cereals, low-fat and skim milk, and margarine
Vitamin B12	Vitamin produced by microorganisms and found in all animal products; synthetic form (cyanocobalamin or cobalamin on labels) is vegan	Supplements, fortified foods such as breakfast cereals, soymilk, and rice milk
Vitamin D (D1, D2, D3)	D1 is produced by humans upon exposure to sunlight; D2 (ergocalciferol) is made from plants or yeast; D3 (cholecalciferol) comes from fish liver oils or lanolin	Supplements, fortified foods such as milk, margarine, yogurt, and orange juice. (**Note:** A vegan D3 supplement is available under the brand name Vitashine.)
Whey	Watery liquid that separates from the solids in cheese-making	Crackers, breads, cakes, processed foods

Communicating with food companies

If you aren't sure whether a product is meat-free, check company websites for ingredient information. If you don't find the answers you need, check the website or package for an online chat option or a phone number you can call to speak with a customer service representative.

Some ingredient questions may be beyond the ability of a customer service representative to answer. If you sense the individual you're speaking with doesn't know the answer, ask to speak with a supervisor. Another alternative: Put your question in writing and send a more formal inquiry via email or snail mail to the company. Food companies take customer inquiries about diet matters very seriously — lawsuits have resulted from false or misleading information about ingredients being given to consumers.

It may take some digging and persistence, but you can usually get answers to your questions about the sources of ingredients in food products.

NONFOOD PRODUCTS THAT CONTAIN ANIMAL INGREDIENTS

Animal ingredients may turn up in some surprising places, including cosmetics, lotions, perfume, and household supplies such as glue and ink. Many vegans avoid such products, although it can be difficult for anyone to avoid them completely, considering the extent of their use.

Glycerides, lanolin, lecithin, oleic acid, stearic acid, tallow, and vitamin A, for example, are often used to make cosmetics. Lanolin is used in ointments and lotions, and many soaps contain oleic acid, stearic acid, or tallow. Read product labels carefully if you want to avoid these ingredients, and check with the manufacturer if you're in doubt about the source.

Tracking down resources for up-to-date advice

TIP

The Vegetarian Resource Group publishes the "Vegetarian Journal's Guide to Food Ingredients," listing the uses, sources, and definitions of hundreds of food ingredients, as well as whether ingredients are vegan, vegetarian, or nonvegetarian. You can view the guide online at www.vrg.org/ingredients.

Vegans can find information about animal-free nonfood products by visiting People for the Ethical Treatment of Animals (PETA) online at www.peta.org.

Applying More Advice for Getting Started

You're on your way! This section offers more tips to make the journey a little easier. Some people are their own worst critics. Although you don't want to delude yourself into thinking that you're making progress when you're not, you also don't want to be too harsh with yourself if you have a setback now and then. Change takes time and patience.

REMEMBER

Occasional slips are normal. If you have a lapse, pick up where you left off and start again. No one is keeping score but you.

Scouting out supermarkets

Living vegetarian doesn't require you to buy special foods or ingredients. However, after you make the switch to a meatless diet, you'll find a big world of new products you'll probably want to try, as well as new ways to put familiar ingredients together.

Now's the time to encourage creativity. Break with your usual shopping routine and visit some new stores. Walk up and down all the aisles, including the frozen foods case. You'll find dozens of vegetarian foods. Buy a few on this trip, and then try a few more next time.

REMEMBER

Whole foods — products that are as close to their natural state as possible — are the healthiest. However, prepared foods and vegetarian specialty products — such as frozen entrées, veggie burger patties, and boxed mixes — can be an acceptable convenience. They're nice to have on hand for occasions when you don't have time to cook and need something quick and easy.

TIP

When you sample new products, expect to find a few duds. Next time, try another brand of the same type of product, because different brands of the same product can vary. Veggie burger patties and soymilk are two examples of products that vary greatly in flavor and texture, depending on the brand.

After you start experimenting with new foods, you'll discover a long list of great products that will become regulars in your kitchen. I cover much more about ingredients and shopping in Chapters 6 and 7.

Scanning websites, cookbooks, magazines

Surf the web for vegetarian recipes and get lost perusing all of the delicious ideas you'll find online. Go to your local library and check out all the vegetarian cookbooks and magazines you can find. If you have friends who are vegetarians, borrow their cookbooks. Then begin to page through each one.

Read the names of the recipes. If you see one that grabs your attention, look at the list of ingredients. If the recipe inspires you, make the dish. When you find a cookbook with lots of recipes that appeal to you, go to a bookstore and buy it, or order it online. Natural foods stores also carry a good selection of popular vegetarian cookbooks. If you'd rather store, organize, and manage your recipes online, maintain a digital cookbook or recipe app for quick and easy meal planning. More on this topic is included in the section on "Assembling an online recipe box" in Chapter 8.

When you orient yourself to the options on a vegetarian diet, you may be surprised at the variety. You may also notice lots of ethnic foods from cultures that have vegetarian traditions. A vegetarian diet has more variety than a meat-centered diet. Reviewing recipes and cookbooks will help you see that.

Listing vegetarian foods you already like

If you're new to a vegetarian diet, it's helpful to make a list of the vegetarian foods you already enjoy. Make them often. You probably eat a number of meatless foods and haven't thought of them as being vegetarian until now. Here are some examples:

>> Baked potato topped with broccoli and cheese

>> Bean burritos and tacos

>> Grilled cheese sandwiches

>> Lentil soup

>> Macaroni and cheese

>> Pancakes

>> Pasta primavera

>> Peanut butter and jelly sandwiches

>> Pizza margherita and pizza with vegetable toppings

>> Spaghetti with tomato sauce

>> Vegetable stir-fry over rice

>> Vegetarian lasagna

If your favorite vegetarian foods happen to contain dairy products such as cheese or milk, gradually reduce the amount and switch to nonfat varieties. They contain less saturated fat and are healthier for you. Better yet, experiment with plant milks and cheeses made from almonds, soy, and other plant-based ingredients.

You can probably modify some of your other favorite foods to make them vegetarian. Some examples:

>> **Bean soups:** Leave out the ham or bacon. Experiment with herbs, spices and other seasonings to amp up the flavor as needed.

>> **Breakfast meats:** Use veggie versions of link sausage or sausage patties and bacon. They taste great and can replace meat at breakfast or in a BLT.

» **Burgers:** Buy veggie burger patties instead of meat.

» **Chili:** Make it with beans, tempeh, textured vegetable protein or similar plant-based, ground beef substitutes instead of meat.

» **Hot dogs and luncheon meats:** Buy veggie versions. All natural foods stores carry them, and so do many supermarkets. They look and taste like the real thing but are better for you.

» **Meatloaf:** Even this all-American food can be made with lentils, chopped nuts, grated vegetables, and other ingredients. Many vegetarian cookbooks and recipe websites include a number of delicious variations. Try the recipe for Everybody's Favorite Cheese and Nut Loaf in Chapter 15.

» **Pasta sauces:** Why add meat or meat flavorings when you have basil, oregano, mushrooms, red peppers, sun-dried tomatoes, pimentos, black olives, and scores of other delicious ingredients to add flavor to sauces? Great on cannelloni, stuffed shells, manicotti, ravioli, fettuccine, and steamed or roasted vegetables.

» **Pizza:** Think of the crust as a blank canvas for your inner artiste. Be creative! Delicious pizza toppers over a thin layer of pizza sauce include baby spinach leaves, pineapple chunks, mushroom slices, diced bell peppers, broccoli florets, chopped red onion, garlic, olives, basil leaves, jalapeno pepper slices . . . the list goes on. Just leave off the meat and go easy on the cheese, if you use it at all.

» **Sandwiches:** Load up on lettuce, tomatoes, mustard, chopped or shredded vegetables, and a little cheese if you like, but leave out the meat. Use pita pockets, tortilla wraps, hard rolls, and whole-grain breads to give sandwiches more character.

» **Stuffed cabbage:** Instead of using pork or beef, fill cabbage leaves with a mixture of seasoned rice and garbanzo beans.

2

Planning and Preparing Your Vegetarian Kitchen

Evaluate how to set up your kitchen for maximum efficiency, so that you have ready access to the most common and versatile ingredients for vegetarian meals.

Determine where to shop to get what you need, using strategies for getting the best values.

Identify the most practical equipment to have on hand for easy meal prep.

Understand the basic cooking techniques you should know to get the best results from your kitchen adventures.

Chapter **6**

Getting Familiar with Common Vegetarian Ingredients

Vegetarian meals don't have to be exotic, made with ingredients you can't pronounce or buy at your local supermarket. In fact, they can be as all-American as corn on the cob, baked beans, and veggie burgers.

But if you're interested, vegetarian cooking can be an introduction to a whole new world of flavors, textures, and aromas based on culinary traditions from around the world. Many vegetarian cookbooks and online recipe collections draw on these traditions, which contribute greatly to the diversity of foods that many vegetarians enjoy.

In this chapter, I describe useful ingredients in vegetarian cooking. You may already use some, but others may be unfamiliar to you. All are healthful, multi-purpose ingredients worth knowing about and keeping on hand. I also shed some light on the often-confusing topic of natural and organic products to help you make well-informed choices when you shop.

Building the Foundation of the Vegetarian Diet

It's important to keep on hand ingredients in a variety of forms. Fresh is best, of course, but fresh isn't always the most convenient option. So plan to keep a range of fresh, frozen, canned, and packaged foods in your kitchen.

Bringing home the beans

Before we talk about beans, let's take a moment to clear the air.

I know beans have a bad rap. It may have started with that famous campfire scene in the 1974 Mel Brooks movie, *Blazing Saddles*. Never fear — I help you understand how to get a grip on gas in Chapter 22.

But as far as nutritionists like me are concerned, beans have superpowers. It just so happens that vegetarians tend to like them, too — a lot. Beans factor big in the food traditions of many cultures around the world, forming the basis for many of the tastiest and most good-for-you foods around.

Flatulence-inducing effects aside, beans are highly nutritious and extremely versatile. You can mix several types of beans (such as garbanzos, pintos, red kidney beans, and white kidney beans) to make many-bean chili. You can mash them for dips, soups, and spreads. You can combine them with rice, pasta, or other grains to make a variety of interesting vegetarian entrées. Among others, try the following:

>> Black beans

>> Black-eyed peas

>> Cannellini beans (white kidney beans)

>> Garbanzo beans

>> Kidney beans

>> Navy beans

>> Pinto beans

Forms of beans

Beans come in several forms, all of which are useful in vegetarian cooking. Here's a rundown on the types you'll see at the store:

- >> **Canned beans:** Canned beans are one of the most nutritious and versatile convenience foods you can buy. Conventional supermarket varieties are fine, although natural foods stores carry a wide variety of organic canned beans.

Rinse canned beans in a colander before using them. Rinsing removes excess salt and the fibrous outer skins of the beans that otherwise tend to flake off and look unsightly in finished dishes.

If you have leftover canned beans, add them to a pot of soup or stir them into pasta sauce. You can also spoon them on top of a green salad or mash them with a little garlic and add them to a casserole.

- >> **Dried beans:** Beans were sold dried in bags long before canned beans were available. Some people still prefer to buy and prepare their beans from scratch. Preparing dried beans is more time-consuming, but some people prefer the flavor and texture that result.

  Dried beans are often a little firmer than canned beans. In fact, they can be too hard if you don't soak them in water long enough before cooking them. Also, dried beans don't usually contain added salt; you have to season them yourself or they'll taste bland. (The exception is bags of beans packaged with their own spice mixtures, which are often very salty.)

- >> **Frozen beans:** You can find a few types of beans, such as lima beans (also called butter beans) and black-eyed peas, in the freezer section of some supermarkets. They taste the same as fresh and are just as nutritious. Compared to canned beans, frozen beans have less sodium and may be slightly more nutritious, because nutrients can leach out of canned beans into the water in the can.

- >> **Bean flakes:** This form of dried beans is convenient and fun to use. You just shake some into a bowl, add boiling water, stir, and cover. In five minutes, you have a smooth, creamy bean paste that you can use to make nachos, burrito or taco filling, bean dip, or bean soup. The more water you add, the thinner the beans. The bean flakes themselves keep in the cupboard for months, just like dried and canned beans. After you mix the bean flakes with water, leftovers keep in the refrigerator for up to a week or in the freezer for up to six months.

  You're more likely to find bean flakes at a natural foods store than in a supermarket. Frontier Co-op and Outdoor Herbivore are two brands that make dehydrated black bean flakes and pinto bean flakes. Look for products like these in stores and online.

Whether frozen, canned, or dried, beans have approximately the same nutritional value. Convenience and flavor are the major differences.

Common dishes from around the world

Beans are used in many different cultures to make a wide range of traditional foods and dishes. Examples include:

» American navy bean soup

» Chinese stir-fried tofu and vegetables

» Ethiopian puréed lentil and bean dishes

» Greek lentil soup

» Indian curries and *dal* (Indian-style lentil soup)

» Indonesian tempeh

» Italian *pasta e fagioli* (pasta with beans)

» Mexican burritos, tacos, and nachos

» Middle Eastern hummus and *falafel* (small, round, fried cakes made from mashed garbanzo beans and spices)

» Spanish black bean soup

TIP

You can substitute many types of beans for others in recipes. For example, you can easily substitute black beans for pinto beans in tacos, burritos, nachos, and bean dip. The dark color often makes a striking contrast to other components of the meal, such as chopped tomatoes, salsa, or greens.

Eating more vegetables and fruits

The best vegetables and fruits are locally grown, in season, and fresh. Most of them are packed with vitamins, minerals, and phytochemicals. Frozen foods run a close second in terms of nutrition, and they're a perfectly acceptable alternative to fresh.

However, canned vegetables and fruits are sometimes more convenient or less expensive than fresh or frozen. Because heat destroys some vitamins, and time on the shelf can allow some nutrients to leach into the water used in packing, canned vegetables and fruits tend to be less nutritious than fresh or frozen. However, that doesn't mean they're worthless! On the contrary, canned produce can make a sizable nutritional contribution.

Varying your vegetables

Vegetarian cooking incorporates many kinds of vegetables, but some of the more popular recipe ingredients include white potatoes, sweet potatoes, onions, bell peppers, tomatoes, greens, broccoli, and many varieties of squash. Ethnic dishes make use of such less common vegetables as bok choy (in stir-fries), kohlrabi (in stews and casseroles), and arugula (steamed or in salads). I include recipes incorporating some of these in Part 3.

TIP

When you use canned vegetables, you can save vitamins and minerals that may have leached out by incorporating the liquid from the can into the dish you're making. For example, if you're making soup or sautéed vegetables to serve over rice or pasta, dump the entire contents of the can into the pot. The packing liquid may contain salt, but you can compensate by leaving out any additional salt that's called for in the recipe. Low salt and low sodium varieties of some canned vegetables may also be available in your local market.

REMEMBER

Some vegetables are worth extra attention because of their superior nutritional value. Deep yellow and orange vegetables, for instance, are particularly rich in beta-carotene, which your body converts into vitamin A. Sweet potatoes, acorn squash, tomatoes, red peppers, and pumpkin are examples. Other vegetables are potent sources of vitamin C, including white potatoes, green bell peppers, broccoli, cauliflower, cabbage, and tomatoes.

Cruciferous vegetables are another example of *super vegetables*. They contain cancer-fighting substances as well as copious amounts of vitamins and minerals. Following are a few popular examples from this group:

>> **Arugula** (pronounced a-*roo*-guh-la) is a leafy green vegetable that's distinctive for its sharp, peppery flavor. It grows wild throughout southern Europe and is native to the Mediterranean. You eat arugula raw, and you can mix it with other salad greens or let it stand alone. I include a recipe for arugula salad in Chapter 11.

>> **Daikon** (or Chinese radish) is a large, white, Asian radish. In contrast to the small red radishes that we know in North America, daikon is usually eaten cooked. However, it's sometimes used raw in salads.

>> **Kale, Swiss chard, and bok choy** (also known as Chinese cabbage) are thick, green, leafy vegetables that are best when cut or torn into strips and steamed, sautéed, or stir-fried. Many vegetarians add a little olive oil and minced garlic to these cooked greens. You can eat them plain or mix them into casseroles, soups, and other dishes.

>> **Kohlrabi** is a white, turnip-shaped vegetable commonly eaten in Eastern Europe. Like other cruciferous vegetables, it's full of potentially cancer-preventing phytochemicals and is very nutritious and flavorful. Kohlrabi is usually diced, boiled, and eaten cooked or added to stews.

Canned *jackfruit* is a versatile alternative to beef or pork for BBQ sandwiches, sliders, and other foods in which the large, tropical fruit mimics shredded meat in texture. The unripe variety is bland and picks up the flavor of seasonings and other ingredients that are cooked in the same dish.

Picking fruits

You can use fruits in vegetarian meals in many creative ways — to make cold soups, warm cobblers, pies, and quick breads, for instance. I like to add bits of fruit — mandarin oranges, strawberries, and chunks of apple and pear — to green salads. Many of the dessert recipes in Chapter 14 call for fruit, which cuts the calories and adds important nutrients to sweet treats.

Strawberries and grapes often contain substantial amounts of pesticides, and sometimes people don't wash them well before eating them. Wash all fruits under running water, rubbing with your hand or a soft cloth, or brush the fruit to remove pesticide residues, especially if you're going to eat the skin. In addition, although you may not eat the peel, be sure to wash the outsides of such fruits as melons, grapefruit, and oranges before setting them on your cutting board to slice them. If you don't, you may contaminate your cutting board surface. You may also drag any bacteria or contaminants present on the fruit's surface into the edible inner portion.

Choose plenty of deeply colored fruits to get the benefit of their rich nutritional content. Apricots, peaches, papayas, and mangoes, for example, are densely packed with many important vitamins and minerals. Watermelon, cantaloupe, oranges, and grapefruits are also super healthful.

Choosing breads and cereals

Grains are versatile — you can eat them by themselves or combine them with other ingredients to make a seemingly endless collection of dishes. Grains can be an accompaniment to a meal, such as a slice of bread or a couscous salad, or they can be the foundation of an entrée, such as rice pilaf or a plate of spaghetti. Around the world, grains are familiar ingredients in soups, salads, baked goods, main dishes, side dishes, desserts, and other foods. Examples include:

>> Chinese vegetable stir-fry with steamed white rice

>> Ethiopian *injera* (flatbread made from teff flour)

>> Indian saffron rice with vegetables

>> Indonesian *tempeh* (made with whole soybeans and a grain such as rice)

» Irish porridge (oatmeal)

» Italian *polenta* (typically made with cornmeal, baked or pan-fried, and often served with a sauce on top)

» Mexican enchiladas made with corn tortillas

» Middle Eastern couscous with cooked vegetables

» Middle Eastern *tabbouleh* (wheat salad)

» Russian or Eastern European *kasha* (toasted buckwheat) with bowtie pasta and cooked mushrooms

» Spanish rice

» Thai jasmine rice with curried vegetables

Grains come in two forms: whole and processed. Both forms are indispensable in vegetarian cooking.

REMEMBER

Whole grains are grains that have had only the outer hull removed, leaving a small, round kernel, often called a *berry.* The major advantage to using whole grains in cooking is that they're slightly more nutritious than processed grains, *and* they taste better. After you get used to the flavor of whole-wheat bread, for example, you'll probably prefer it to soft, white bread.

The major drawback to whole grains is that they take more time to cook than processed grains. Whole-grain hot cereal, for example, may take ten minutes to cook, compared to the one or two minutes it takes to make instant hot cereals.

You can find many types of grains at most supermarkets and natural foods stores. Some may be new to you. Here are some examples of how they're used:

» **Amaranth:** An ancient grain eaten for centuries in Central and South America. You can cook it and eat it as a side dish or hot cereal, or use it to make casseroles, baked goods, crackers, pancakes, and pasta. Use it as you'd use rice in recipes. Amaranth flour is also available.

» **Barley:** Barley comes in two forms: hulled and pearl.

  • Hulled barley is the more natural, more nutritious, unrefined form, having only its outermost husks removed. Not surprisingly, hulled barley is brown in color. You can use it in soups, casseroles, and stews.

  • Pearl barley is more processed than hulled barley. In addition to having the inedible outer hull removed, pearl barley also has the outer bran layer removed. Pearl barley is less nutritious than hulled barley, but it cooks faster.

» **Corn:** Corn kernels are actually the seeds of a cereal grass. You can use corn in cornbread, corn tortillas, and polenta.

» **Kamut:** An ancient type of wheat used in Europe for centuries, usually in baked goods.

» **Millet:** Tiny, beadlike seeds that come from a cereal grass. You use millet in baked goods and as a cooked cereal.

» **Oats:** Oats come from cereal grasses. Use oats as a hot cereal and in baked goods, veggie burger patties, and loaves.

» **Quinoa** (pronounced *keen*-wah): An ancient grain eaten for centuries in Central and South America. You can cook quinoa and eat it as a side dish or hot cereal, or you can use it to make casseroles, salads, a side dish with cooked vegetables, or pilaf. Use it as you'd use rice in recipes.

WARNING

Quinoa has to be processed to remove the seed coat, which contains saponin and is toxic. Before you cook quinoa, rinse it several times with water to remove any remaining saponin. The saponin is soapy; you'll know that you've rinsed the quinoa well enough when you no longer see suds. Packaged quinoa is often pre-rinsed and needs only minimal rinsing. Quinoa purchased from bulk bins often is not pre-rinsed.

» **Rice:** Rice has been grown for centuries in warm climates, where the seeds are harvested from cereal grasses that grow in wet areas called *rice paddies*. If you're a diehard white rice eater, that's fine. However, brown rice has a slightly better nutritional profile, and many people like its hearty flavor. Several quick-cooking brown rice varieties are on the market; you can find them at regular supermarkets and natural foods stores.

Supermarkets also carry many specialty rice varieties, such as aromatic jasmine rice, basmati rice, and *arborio rice* (a medium-grain rice used to make the Italian dish risotto). Jasmine and basmati rice are available in white or brown form; the brown form is slightly less refined. You can use these various forms of rice in casseroles, baked goods, puddings, and side dishes.

TECHNICAL STUFF

Rice is one of the least allergenic and most easily digestible foods. That's why rice cereal has long been one of the first solid foods introduced to infants. People who are allergic to wheat and other grains can use rice flour to make baked goods such as breads and cookies. However, rice may contain high levels of arsenic, a natural element found in the environment and linked to health problems, including some forms of cancer. Though rice manufacturers are working to lower the arsenic levels in rice, it's best for babies, young children and even adults to vary the types of grains they eat. Variety in the diet helps to protect against concentrated intakes of any ingredients that may be harmful to health.

>> **Rye:** A form of cereal grass grown for its seeds, which are ground to make flour. You use rye in baked goods, such as bread and rolls.

>> **Spelt:** An ancient type of wheat that has been used in Europe in baked goods for centuries.

>> **Teff:** One of the oldest cultivated grains in the world, teff is used in Ethiopia to make *injera,* a flat, spongy bread that's a staple food there. You can also use it in baked goods, soups, and stews.

>> **Wheat:** Wheat is grown around the world as a cereal grass and used in baked goods and pasta.

>> **Wheat berries:** Whole-wheat grains that have had only the outer hull removed. Use wheat berries in baked goods and as a hot cereal.

TIP

When you make a pot of rice (or any grain), make more than you need for one meal. You can store the leftovers in an airtight container in the refrigerator for up to two weeks. Cooked rice can also be kept in the freezer in storage bags or airtight containers for three to six months until you want to use it. You can reheat leftover rice quickly in the microwave oven. Add a splash of water and heat the rice on high for 20 to 30 seconds, longer as needed, until it is hot. Serve it with steamed vegetables, bean burritos, or tacos; top it with vegetarian chili; add it to a filling for cabbage rolls; or use it to make rice pudding. Rinsing rice before cooking is mostly a matter of personal preference. Rinsing removes some of the outer starch layer, resulting in grains that are more separate when cooked. Rice that is not rinsed before cooking tends to be creamier and stickier. Your choice depends on the result you prefer.

Selecting seeds and nuts

Seeds and nuts are excellent additions to many vegetarian dishes because they're rich in protein and other nutrients, including health-supporting phytochemicals. A handful of chopped walnuts or almonds or a sprinkling of toasted sunflower seeds makes a nice addition to a casserole, salad, or bowl of hot cereal.

Here are a couple of products made from seeds and nuts that are common in vegetarian cooking:

>> **Tahini:** *Tahini* is a smooth, rich paste made from sesame seeds. It's a traditional Middle Eastern ingredient in *hummus* — a spread made with garbanzo beans, garlic, lemon juice, and olive oil — and you can also use it to flavor salad dressings, sauces, dips, and other foods. Tahini is sold in cans or bottles. A layer of sesame oil usually floats at the top of the container; you have to stir it in each time you use the product.

WARNING

>> **Nut butters:** Don't stop with peanut butter. Cashew butter and almond butter are equally, if not more, nutritious, and they're just as delicious. You can use them in all the same ways that you use peanut butter — for sandwiches, cookies, and in cooking.

If you buy a jar of natural peanut butter, you'll notice a layer of oil at the top. Don't make the mistake of pouring the oil off, thinking that you'll reduce the fat content. If you do, you'll need a pickax to get the dry nut butter out. Storing the jar upside down to keep the oil dispersed is also risky — the oil may ooze out onto the shelf. Instead, just stir the oil back into the nut butter when you're ready to use it.

Fitting in Specialty Foods and Products

Living vegetarian can be extraordinarily simple. No fancy equipment or special food products are necessary — unless you want them.

Several specialized products do exist that many vegetarians find especially convenient. All these products are nutritious, and many are much better for your health than their animal-product counterparts. You can find most of the products I mention in this section in your neighborhood supermarket; you can find them all in a natural foods store.

Introducing soy foods and their variations

Soy foods come in dozens of forms and can take the place of meat, cheese, eggs, milk, and other animal products in recipes. Nutritionally, soy products are far superior to their meat counterparts because they're cholesterol-free, low in saturated fat, and usually lower in sodium. They're also free of *nitrates* and *nitrites*, preservatives that are commonly found in processed meat products and that may cause cancer.

Table 6-1 lists several types of soy products that are available and ways you can use them.

REMEMBER

You can use different styles of tofu in different recipes. For instance, soft tofu works well for making dips and sauces because it's easy to blend. Firm tofu works well in baked goods and as an egg replacer in many recipes. Extra-firm tofu is the style of choice for making stir-fries because the cubes can hold up when they're jostled around in the pan. Unlike cheese, tofu is never coagulated with rennet, an enzyme taken from the stomach linings of baby animals. It's always safe for consumption by vegetarians and vegans alike.

TABLE 6-1	**Soy Foods and Their Uses**
Product	Description and Uses
Meat substitutes	Meat substitutes are made from soy protein, tofu, and vegetables. Some are made to resemble traditional cold cuts, hot dogs, sausage, and bacon in appearance, texture, flavor, and aroma. You can use them in the same ways as their meat counterparts.
Miso	A rich, salty, East Asian condiment used to flavor soups, sauces, entrées, salad dressings, marinades, and other foods. This savory paste is made from soybeans, a grain (usually rice), and salt. It's combined with a mold culture and aged for at least one year. It doesn't have much nutritional value and is high in sodium, so, like most condiments, you should use it sparingly.
Soy cheese	A substitute for dairy cheese that comes in many different forms, such as mozzarella style, jack style, American style, and cream cheese style. You can use it to make sandwiches, pizza, casseroles, and spreads.
Soy margarine	Find it in natural foods stores. It's free of casein and other dairy byproducts that other brands of margarine usually contain, so it's vegan-friendly.
Soy mayonnaise	Several brands are available at natural foods stores. Use soy mayonnaise in all the ways you use regular mayonnaise.
Soymilk	A beverage made from soaked, ground, and strained soybeans. You can use it cup for cup in place of cow's milk in recipes, or drink it as a beverage.
Soy sauce	A rich, salty, dark brown liquid condiment made from fermented soybeans. Use it to add punch to stir-fried vegetables or as a dip for dumplings and egg rolls.
Soy yogurt	Made from soymilk, it often contains active cultures and is available in many flavors. Use it as a substitute for dairy yogurt.
Tamari	A type of soy sauce and byproduct of the production of miso (see above). It has a rich flavor.
Tempeh	A traditional Indonesian soy food made from whole soybeans mixed with a grain and a mold culture, fermented, and pressed into a block or cake. You can grill it and serve it as an entrée or use it in sandwich and burrito fillings, casseroles, chili, and other foods.
Textured soy protein (TSP) or textured vegetable protein (TVP)	A product made from textured soy flour that's usually sold in chunks or granules. It takes on a chewy, meatlike texture when rehydrated and is used in such foods as vegetarian chili, vegetarian sloppy Joes, veggie burgers, and other meat substitutes.
Tofu	Soybean curd that's made in a process similar to cheese making, using soymilk and a coagulant. It's bland-tasting and is available in a variety of textures and densities. You can use it in numerous ways: cubed and added to a stir-fry, marinated and baked, as a substitute for eggs and cheese, as a sandwich filling, and as an ingredient in dips, sauces, desserts, cream soups, and many other foods.

WARNING

Like cheese, eggs, meat, and other high–protein foods, tofu and tempeh can spoil if left unrefrigerated. Don't leave out foods made with tofu and tempeh at room temperature for more than two hours. After a meal, cover the leftovers and put them back in the refrigerator as soon as possible.

Making the most of milk substitutes

In addition to the soymilk, soy cheese, and soy yogurt listed in Table 6-1, you may also be interested in rice, almond, coconut, oat, hemp and other plant-based milks packaged in *aseptic* (shelf-stable) packages. These plant milks are also sold in conventional milk cartons in the dairy section in most supermarkets. People who are allergic to soy often use these alternatives.

You can buy some plant milks in powdered form in natural foods stores and online. Some soymilk is still sold in powdered form, too. In the 1960s and 1970s, before plant-based milks became mainstream, this was the form in which soymilk and most milk alternatives were sold, including some made from potatoes and oats. Fluid soymilk is more palatable and much more convenient, though. It's also easier to find these days! Try soy, rice, coconut, and other frozen desserts and plant-based coffee creamers, too.

REMEMBER

Soymilk is generally more nutritious than any of the other milk alternatives, such as rice milk, coconut milk and almond milk. Fortified soymilk has extra calcium and vitamins A, D, and B12. If you use substantial amounts of a milk alternative, fortified soymilk is usually the best choice in terms of nutrition. (Pea protein-based milk has a similar nutritional profile to soymilk as well.)

If you try unsweetened soymilk for the first time and don't care for it, give it a second chance and try another brand. Soymilk varies in flavor considerably from one brand to the next. You may have to taste three or four before you find your favorite. Most of the soymilk sold in the United States and Canada is made from whole soybeans, so it has a bit of a beany aftertaste, which some people find pleasant but others don't like. If you object to the mild bean flavor, you may prefer a vanilla-flavored soymilk to unsweetened. Soymilk does grow on you — if you use it for a while, you'll probably grow to love it.

WARNING

If you do include dairy products such as cheese, milk, and ice cream in your diet, buy the nonfat varieties. Even the so-called low-fat items are too high in fat. The problem with dairy fat is that two-thirds of it is saturated, so the fat in dairy products is a real artery-clogger.

Incorporating egg replacers

Powdered vegetarian egg replacer is an egg substitute made from a mixture of vegetable starches. You just mix a teaspoon and a half of the powder with two tablespoons of water to replace one egg in virtually any recipe. It keeps on a shelf in your cupboard almost indefinitely and is always on hand when you need it. It's free of saturated fat and cholesterol and doesn't pose a salmonella risk. Ener-G Egg Replacer is a common brand that you can find in most natural foods stores.

Considering meatless burgers, dogs, sausages, and cold cuts

Some vegetarian burger patties are made from soy (see Table 6-1), and some are grain- or vegetable-based. A wide variety is available, and they all taste different, so you need to experiment to find your favorites.

TECHNICAL STUFF

At the time of writing, food companies are experimenting with growing meat in laboratories from animal cells. A few restaurants have started selling foods made from these products. Cultured meats such as these are not considered to be vegan, and vegetarians have mixed reactions. The technology is new, and discussion and reflection on the ethical, environmental, and health implications will take some time.

Some vegetarian meat alternatives are meant to look and taste like meat, while others don't look or taste anything like meat. Vegetarian hot dogs are typically made of soy, and they taste and look like the real thing. You can cook meat substitutes on a grill and serve them the same way that their meat counterparts are served.

TIP

One of the advantages of these products is that you can take them to picnics and cookouts and join in on the food fun with all the nonvegetarians. One note: Vegetarians will want to reserve one side of the grill — or an entire grill — to themselves so that their veggie burgers and dogs aren't cooked on the same surfaces as meat. Call it a "meat-free" zone!

Meatless sausages and cold cuts are also versatile. Let these fakes stand in for their meat counterparts in sausage biscuits, sandwiches, on top of pizza, and in other creative ways. The nutritional advantage of these foods is that they're low in saturated fat, they're cholesterol-free, and many even contain a good dose of dietary fiber if they are made with whole-food ingredients such as beans, whole grains, and chopped vegetables. They're quick, convenient, and good tasting, and they work well as transition foods for people making the switch to a vegetarian diet.

Including other vegetarian convenience foods

Seitan (pronounced *say*-tan) is a chewy food made from wheat *gluten*, or wheat protein. You can buy mixes for seitan at natural foods stores, but most people find it far more convenient to buy it ready-made. Look for it in the refrigerated sections in supermarkets.

TIP

One of the best ways to sample seitan is at a Chinese or Thai restaurant, where you can try it prepared in different ways. It's often served in chunks or strips in a stir-fry.

Seitan dishes are absolutely scrumptious. Don't be surprised if you get hooked on the stuff. But because seitan is relatively unfamiliar to most Westerners, you aren't likely to find it in small-town or even medium-sized-city restaurants. You'll usually see it in vegan restaurants or big-city Asian restaurants where the menu is fairly extensive.

After you've been living vegetarian for a while, you'll discover many more interesting and delicious vegetarian specialty products.

Exploring Natural and Organic Alternatives

Living vegetarian doesn't necessarily mean that you have to buy and eat natural or organic foods. If you *are* a vegetarian, though, or if you're just interested in eating healthfully, you probably want to know something about these distinctions. In this section, I help you understand what these terms mean and how to assess their importance.

Going au naturel

No legal definition exists for the term *natural foods,* but the term is generally understood to mean that a food has been minimally processed and is free of artificial flavors, colors, preservatives, and any other additives that don't occur naturally in the food.

Assessing the benefits of natural foods

Natural foods are frequently better choices than their mainstream counterparts because they lack the undesirable ingredients of many commercially processed foods and they contain more nutritious ingredients.

For instance, natural breakfast cereals, baking mixes, and bread products are usually made with whole grains, so they contain more dietary fiber, vitamins, and minerals than products made with refined grains.

Natural foods are usually minimally sweetened, and when they are sweetened, less sweetener is used. Fruit juice is frequently used as a sweetener in lieu of refined sugar. Natural foods also typically contain less sodium than other foods, and they contain no monosodium glutamate or nitrites. The ingredients used in natural foods products are often organically grown, too.

Knowing when natural isn't enough

WARNING

Just because a food is natural doesn't mean it's nutritious. Believe it or not, natural junk foods *do* exist. Many natural sweets, candies, and snack foods have little nutritional value, just like their conventional counterparts. Even though they're natural, you should limit your consumption of them. Don't let these foods displace more nutritious foods in your diet.

Finding natural foods

Even within a particular category of food products, you usually find more healthful choices in a natural foods store than in a regular supermarket. For instance, in a regular supermarket you may find several types of whole-grain pasta. In a natural foods store, you're likely to find an entire shelf of them. The same is often true of breakfast cereals and many other product categories. Larger supermarkets may have large natural foods sections or natural foods products mixed in with conventional products.

Opting for organic

REMEMBER

The word *organic* applies to foods that are grown without persistent or toxic fertilizers and pesticides, using farming methods that are ecologically sound and earth-friendly. Organic foods must be produced and processed without the use of antibiotics, synthetic hormones, genetic engineering, sewage sludge, or irradiation.

The widest variety of organic products is available at natural foods stores, but most conventional grocery stores now also stock organic produce and organic processed and packaged foods. Natural foods stores in particular often carry seasonal organic produce from local farmers. Buying locally supports small farmers in the community and helps ensure the freshness of the products.

TIP

If you don't have access to a big natural foods store with a good supply of organic produce, seek out local farmers at roadside stands or at farmer's markets where you can buy locally grown fruits and vegetables in season. Ask the farmer if any synthetic fertilizers and pesticides were used. Some small farmers don't go to the hassle and expense of applying for organic certification of their crops, even though they use sustainable farming methods and their products may, in fact, be organic. Get to know your farmer, and ask.

REMEMBER

Organically grown fruits and vegetables generally have the same nutritional value as conventionally grown produce, but they're often not as pretty as those grown with chemical fertilizers and pesticides. They may have small blemishes, and they won't be glossy like their nonorganic counterparts, which often have a waxy coating added. Don't let the appearance of organically grown foods deter you from buying them.

Deciphering organic labels

For decades, the natural foods industry self-regulated and adhered to its own high standards for organic farming and food processing practices. In recent years, though, the market for organic foods has grown dramatically. As more commercial interests entered the organic foods market, longstanding organic standards became threatened.

TECHNICAL STUFF

In conjunction with the 1990 Farm Bill, the U.S. Congress passed the Organic Foods Production Act. Years of public discussion and debate followed, including considerable debate and disagreement between longstanding organic foods advocates and commercial newcomers who wanted to loosen the standards. In 2002, the U.S. Department of Agriculture (USDA) implemented a final rule establishing national organic standards. The rule maintains the high standards originally established by the old-guard natural product industry.

Organic growers and food manufacturers can have their products certified as "USDA Organic" through third-party state and private agencies accredited by the USDA. Labeling regulations permit products to be labeled "100 Percent Organic" if all ingredients meet the organic standards. Both these products and those containing at least 95 percent organic ingredients (the remaining 5 percent must also be approved for use in organic products) may display the "USDA Organic" label.

Products that contain at least 70 percent organic ingredients may be labeled as such on the package ingredient lists.

Weighing the choice: Organic versus conventional produce

I'll convey the most important point first: Eat more fruits and vegetables, whether they're organic or conventional. Most of us need to increase our intake of produce substantially, and that's easier to do for vegetarians than meat-eaters.

After you've done that, you can think about whether you want to eat organic or conventional produce.

Very few studies have looked at the potential health effects of long-term exposure to low doses of pesticides, herbicides, and other contaminants, but it makes sense to avoid unnecessary exposure when possible. You may never know whether your diet ultimately delayed or prevented illness, but it seems prudent to err on the side of safety. It's also important to consider the health risk to farmworkers who have much higher exposures to pesticides and herbicides.

On the other hand, organic foods have disadvantages, too: cost and access. Not everyone can afford to pay extra for organic. And despite the growth in sales of organic foods, not everyone lives in neighborhoods where supermarkets stock a big supply of them.

REMEMBER

If you don't have access to organic produce or can't afford it, cheer up. If you eat a diet that's high in fruits, vegetables, and whole grains, the fiber content of your diet will help remove environmental contaminants from your body. Roughage binds with contaminants and helps move waste through your system faster, leaving contaminants less time to be in contact with the lining of your intestines.

TIP

You can also take a practical approach to organics and avoid the dirty dozen — the 12 fruits and vegetables that are most likely to be contaminated, according to the Environmental Working Group. Avoid the conventional versions of these items if you can and instead buy organic: strawberries, spinach, kale, collard, and mustard greens, nectarines, apples, grapes, cherries, peaches, pears, bell and hot peppers, celery, and tomatoes. Stay up-to-date about the dirty dozen list online at www. ewg.org/foodnews/dirty-dozen.php. Download a smart phone app or get pocket food guides online from EWG www.ewg.org/areas-focus/food-water.

Chapter **7**

Shopping and Stocking Your Vegetarian Pantry

Much of the challenge of eating well on a vegetarian diet is having the staple ingredients on hand when you need them. Shopping for these supplies can be a rewarding adventure, partly because living vegetarian can open you to culinary options you may never have considered.

This chapter is devoted to helping you understand how to go about the task of getting the right supplies into your house — at the right price. I encourage you to go beyond your neighborhood supermarket to explore places you may never have set foot in to search for good foods. I also cover some important shopping strategies, including ways to save money without sacrificing quality or nutritional value.

Figuring Out What You Need

Before you head to the store, you should have a concrete plan for what you want to buy. You'll be more likely to end up having the range and types of foods you need to build healthy meals at home, and you'll be less likely to come home with impulsive, less-than-ideal purchases, or to forget to buy a key ingredient.

The first step in creating a plan is to look at your overall nutritional goals. From there, you draft a shopping list.

TIP

As you compile your shopping list, consider what's fresh and available locally. Search the Internet for a list of seasonal produce. Locally grown, in-season fruits and vegetables are especially nutritious and flavorful. They have not had to be picked before they are fully ripened or shipped long distances to market.

Sketching out your meal plans

In Chapter 3, I cover the basics of vegetarian nutrition and provide background information about meeting your needs for vitamins, minerals, protein, and other components of a health-supporting diet.

This nutrition information is shown in the quick-reference guide in Table 7-1. Use this information to help you think about the foods that belong on your plate and on your shopping list.

TABLE 7-1   **Food Guide for North American Vegetarians**

Food Groups	Foods and Serving sizes	Sources of Calcium
Vegetables 5 or more servings per day	½ cup cooked or 1 cup raw vegetables	Cruciferous vegetables: bok choy, broccoli, collards, mustard greens, turnip greens
Grains and starchy vegetables 4 or more servings per day (Choose more whole grains than refined.)	1 slice bread, 1 medium corn or flour tortilla, 1-ounce dry cereal, ½ cup cooked cereal, rice, quinoa, pasta, or other grains, ½ cup potatoes or sweet potatoes	Calcium-fortified cereals, some brands of English muffins and corn tortillas
Legumes, dairy products, and eggs 3 or more servings per day	½ cooked beans, tofu, tempeh, textured vegetable protein (TVP) 1 cup soymilk, pea protein milk, cow's milk 1-ounce hard cheese, 1 cup low-fat soy or cow's milk yogurt 3 ounces veggie meats ¼ cup peanuts or soy nuts 2 tablespoons peanut butter 1 egg	Calcium-set tofu, calcium-fortified soymilk and pea protein milks, cow's milk, cheese, white beans

Food Groups	Foods and Serving sizes	Sources of Calcium
Fruits 3 or more servings per day	1 medium piece of fruit, ½ cup fruit, ½ cup fruit juice, ½ cup dried fruit	Calcium-fortified fruit juices, figs, navel oranges
Nuts and seeds 1 or more servings per day (Include a daily source of alpha-linolenic acid such as walnuts, ground flaxseeds, chia seeds, hempseeds; or canola, flaxseed, hempseed, or walnut oil.)	¼ cup nuts, 2 tablespoons seeds, 2 tablespoons nut or seed butter	Almonds, almond butter
Healthy fats Limit when lower calorie intake is desired	1 teaspoon oil, butter, margarine, mayonnaise	
Plant milks made from tree nuts, flaxseeds, hempseeds, rice, and oats Servings per day as desired. (Although they make important nutritional contributions to diets, these milks are low in protein and can't replace pea protein or soy/cow's milk in the protein group.)	1 cup	All milks fortified with calcium

Adapted from The Dietitian's Guide to Vegetarian Diets: Issues and Applications, 4th Edition by Reed Mangels, PhD, RD; Virginia Messina, MPH, RD; and Mark Messina, PhD, MS, 2021. (Jones & Bartlett Learning).

TIP

Use the following tips in conjunction with Table 7–1 to help you sketch out your meal plans:

>> Eat a variety of foods, and get enough servings to meet your energy needs.

>> Eat six to eight servings of calcium-rich foods from the food guide in Table 7-1. These foods can pull double-duty and count as servings from other food groups at the same time. For example, a serving of calcium-fortified orange juice also counts as a serving from the fruit group.

>> Every day, include two servings of foods that contain omega 3 fatty acids (n-3 fats). Find these foods in the nuts and seed group and in the healthy fats group. Examples of one serving of these foods include the following:

- 1 teaspoon (5 milliliters) of flaxseed oil

- 3 teaspoons (15 milliliters) of canola or soybean oil

- 1 tablespoon (15 milliliters) of ground flaxseed

- ¼ cup (60 milliliters) of walnuts

Use primarily canola oil and olive oil for cooking to help ensure an optimal balance of fatty acids in your diet.

>> Be sure to get enough vitamin D through sun exposure, eating fortified foods, or taking a supplement.

>> Get at least three reliable food sources of vitamin B12 in your diet every day. One serving is equal to the following:

- 1 tablespoon (15 milliliters) of nutritional yeast including such brands as Red Star Vegetarian Support Formula (VSF), KAL, Bob's Red Mill, Bragg Premium, and Now Foods

- 1 cup (250 milliliters) fortified plant milk

- ½ cup (125 milliliters) cow's milk

- ¾ cup (185 milliliters) yogurt

- 1 ounce (28 grams) of fortified breakfast cereal

If you don't consistently get enough vitamin B12 from food sources, take a B12 supplement. Aim for 25 to 100 micrograms (mcg) daily or 1000 mcg twice weekly.

>> Keep your intake of sweets and alcohol to a minimum to help ensure that you have enough room in your diet for the nutritious foods listed in the food guide.

Keeping a grocery list

People have different shopping styles, just as they have different personalities. Some people like to plan their week's meals, draw up a corresponding shopping list, and buy only what they need to make the meals they've planned. Other people prefer the casual approach — walk up and down the aisles, and put whatever strikes their fancy into their basket. At home, they decide what they're having for dinner based on what they feel like making and the supplies they have on hand.

REMEMBER

Do what works for you. However, be aware that maintaining a list does have its advantages, especially when you've made a change in your eating habits and are developing new eating skills. Planning ahead gives you more control over your meals.

The grocery lists that follow are only suggestions of what you may want to buy to stock your vegetarian kitchen. You can adapt them to suit your individual preferences. If you like them just the way they are, you may want to photocopy them and make enough copies to last a few months. Tape a fresh list to the door of your refrigerator after each shopping trip. Check off items that you need and add any that aren't listed. I provide separate lists for items that you buy weekly and items that you buy less often.

Shopping by the week

You have to purchase the foods on this list fairly frequently because they're perishable and will keep in the refrigerator for only a week or two before spoiling. Use the list to help you decide which foods you want to buy this week. Vary your choices depending on seasonal availability of fruits and vegetables or just to help ensure you get a good mix of nutrients in your diet. I include tips for keeping fruits and vegetables fresh longer in Chapter 8.

Fresh Fruits (especially locally grown)

Apples

Apricots

Bananas

Blueberries

Cantaloupe

Cranberries

Grapefruit

Grapes

Honeydew

Kiwi

Lemons

Limes

Mangoes

Nectarines

Oranges

Peaches

Pears

Pineapples

Plums

Strawberries

Watermelon

Other _____

Prepared Fresh Fruits

Bottled mango or papaya slices

Cut fruits

Fresh juices — orange, grapefruit, apple cider

Packaged fruit salad

Other _____

Fresh Vegetables (especially locally grown)

Asparagus

Bean sprouts

Beets

Bell peppers

Bok choy

Broccoli

Brussels sprouts

Cabbage

Carrots

Celery

Collard greens

Corn

Cucumbers

Kale

Leeks

Mustard greens

Onions

Potatoes

Spinach

Sweet potatoes or yams

Tomatoes

Other _____

Prepared Fresh Vegetables

Fresh juices — beet, carrot, carrot/spinach

Packaged fresh herbs — basil, dill, mint, rosemary, others

Packaged cut vegetables and mixed greens

Other _____

Fresh Deli Items

Four-bean salad

Fresh marinara (seasoned tomato) sauce

Fresh pasta salad

Fresh pizza (with veggie toppings; try cheeseless)

Fresh salsa

Hummus

Other _____

Dairy/Dairy Replacers, Eggs/Egg Replacers, and Tofu

Eggs (or vegetarian egg replacer)

Nonfat cheese or plant-based cheese

Nonfat yogurt or plant-based yogurt

Skim milk or plant milk

Tofu (fresh or aseptically packaged)

Other _____

Breads and Other Grain Products (especially whole grain)

Bagels (eggless for vegans and lacto vegetarians)

Bread loaves

Breadsticks or rolls

English muffins

Pita pockets

Pizza crusts, ready-to-bake

Taco shells

Tortillas

Other _____

Meat Substitutes

Meatless crumbles (for chili and taco filling)

Meatless deli slices

Meatless hot dogs

Veggie burger patties

Other _____

Shopping by the month

Some items keep for a long time in a cupboard, refrigerator, or freezer, so you can shop for them fairly infrequently. The following list suggests items you may want to buy on a monthly basis. You may be able to buy many of these nonperishables in large quantities to save money.

CUPBOARD STAPLES

Canned Goods

Applesauce

Artichoke hearts

Beans — vegetarian baked beans, garbanzo, black, pinto, kidney, navy, split (Look for reduced sodium varieties)

Bean salad

Fruits — any fruits, cranberry sauce, fruit cocktail (Look for water- or juice-packed varieties)

Pasta sauce

Peas — green peas, lentils, black-eyed peas

Pumpkin and fruit pie fillings

Soups — lentil, tomato, vegetarian split pea

Tomato sauce and paste

Vegetables — asparagus, carrots, corn, green beans, peas, tomatoes (Look for reduced sodium varieties)

Vegetarian refried beans

Other _____

Snacks and Treats

Baked potato chips and baked tortilla chips

Bean dip

Flatbreads (including matzo) and breadsticks

Granola bars

Popcorn (bag kernels or microwave)

Rice cakes and popcorn cakes

Whole-grain cookies

Whole-grain crackers

Other _____

Herbs and Spices

Basil, dried

Bay leaves, whole

Black pepper, cracked or ground

Cinnamon, ground

Cumin, ground

Curry powder, ground

Dill, dried

Garlic, powder or flakes

Ginger, dried

Oregano, dried

Paprika, ground

Salt, iodized table salt

Vegetable bouillon

Other _____

Beverages

Bottled fruit juice

Juices — beet, carrot, or tomato

Plain or flavored mineral water or seltzer water

Plant milks – soy, cashew, almond, others (aseptically packaged)

Sparkling cider or grape juice

Other _____

Dry Goods

Beans and bean flakes

Coffee and tea

Cold cereal (whole-grain) — raisin bran, shredded wheat, bran flakes, others

Couscous (whole-grain, if available)

Grains — barley, millet, bulgur wheat, kasha, amaranth, spelt, teff, quinoa, kamut, others

Hot cereal (whole-grain) — oatmeal, whole-wheat, mixed grain

Pasta (eggless for vegans and lacto vegetarians)

Rice — basmati, jasmine, brown, wild, arborio, others

Soup mixes or cups

Textured vegetable protein (TVP)

Tofu (aseptically packaged)

Vegetable oil spray

Vegetarian egg replacer

Whole-grain bread, pancake, and all-purpose mixes

Whole-wheat flour, other flours

Other _____

Condiments

Basil pesto

Chutney

Fruit spreads, jams, jellies and preserves

Honey (for nonvegans)

Horseradish, marinades, BBQ sauce

Ketchup

Mustard

Olives

Pickles and pickle relish

Salad dressing

Salsa

Soy or avocado oil mayonnaise

Stir-fry sauce

Sun-dried tomatoes

Syrups and molasses, including agave and maple syrups

Vinegar — balsamic, herbed, fruited, malt, rice, others

Other _____

Dried Fruits

Apples

Apricots

Blueberries

Cherries

Currants

Dates

Figs

Mixed fruits

Prunes (also known today as "dried plums")

Raisins

Other _____

FREEZER STAPLES

Frozen bagels (eggless for vegans and lacto vegetarians)

Frozen entrées

Frozen fruit and juice bars

Frozen fruit juice

Frozen pasta (eggless for vegans and lacto vegetarians)

Frozen bags of cooked rice and other cooked grains

Frozen vegetables

Frozen waffles and pancakes

Italian ices and popsicles

Meatless bacon

Meatless burger patties (veggie burgers)

Meatless crumbles (for chili and taco filling)

Meatless hotdogs

Meatless sausage links and patties

Muffins and dinner rolls

Nondairy ice cream

Nonfat frozen yogurt

Sorbet

Other _____

Let's Go Shopping! Considering the Options

Many people — especially vegetarians — find that they purchase certain items at one store and others at another store. For instance, you may shop at a natural foods store to buy frozen vegetarian entrées, specialty baking mixes, whole-grain pastas and breakfast cereals, and your favorite brand of plant milk by the case. Then perhaps you shop at a conventional supermarket for such items as toilet paper, fresh produce, and toothpaste.

It all depends on your personal preferences. This section includes a quick run-down of your options, listed generally in order of most to least common.

Your neighborhood supermarket

Conventional supermarkets have undergone a transformation during the past twenty years because of the rapid expansion of the natural foods and organic foods markets. In years past, your neighborhood supermarket may have had a special aisle for "health foods" where the soymilk and vegetarian specialty items were shelved. Today, these foods are more likely to be integrated with all the other foods in the store.

Your neighborhood supermarket also probably carries a much wider variety of natural products, organic foods, and vegetarian specialty items than it did in the past. Depending on the store, the selection may be comprehensive enough that you can do most of your shopping in one stop.

Warehouse stores

WARNING

Buying in volume can be economical, but it isn't always the best approach. Think carefully before you buy a giant jar of pickles, a huge bottle of ketchup, or a 20-pound bag of rice! Not only can storage space be a challenge, but some foods may spoil before you can reasonably use them up.

An extra-large bottle of vegetable oil, for example, may go rancid before you can use it all. Buy too many croutons, and they may become stale before you get to the bag's bottom.

On the other hand, warehouse stores can be a good place to find excellent values on such vegetarian staples as canned beans, fresh fruits and vegetables, prepared soups and ready-to-eat, fresh or frozen vegetarian entrees, tubs of hummus, veggie burger patties, and other meatless specialty items.

Natural foods stores

If you've never set foot in a natural foods store, now's the time to do it. You may not shop there for all your groceries and supplies, but you should take a look at the many vegetarian specialty items and other great choices available. Natural foods stores include large national chains such as Whole Foods Market, Wild Oats Market, and Sprouts Farmers Market, as well as many regional and independent, locally owned stores.

Some people buy everything they need at natural foods stores, including non-food items, because natural foods stores often carry a wider selection of environmentally-friendly cleaning supplies and paper goods than other stores. Big natural foods stores are common in large, metropolitan areas, and prices may be better and the variety greater than in cities that have only small stores.

Farmer's markets and CSA farms

Many communities have farmer's markets where locally grown, seasonal fruits and vegetables are sold. You can often find locally produced honey, jams and jellies, and baked goods at the farmer's market, too.

REMEMBER

Not all sellers who grow and produce their foods organically pay to have their foods certified as organic, so ask your local farmers for details about their approach. That's an advantage to buying from local farmers — you can establish a relationship with these people over time and grow to know and trust their food.

WARNING

Be careful, though. Some farmer's markets permit large wholesalers to sell out-of-state products. Ask questions about the source of the produce you see to make sure you're getting locally grown food, if that's important to you.

An alternative or supplement to seasonal produce from the farmer's market is food from a *CSA* farm. CSA stands for *community-supported agriculture*. Residents of a community pay a local farmer a predetermined amount of money upfront. In return, they get a portion of the harvest throughout the growing season. If you subscribe to a CSA farm, expect to pick up your food at a centrally agreed-upon location. In some cases, home delivery may also be available.

REMEMBER

The advantages to getting your food from farmer's markets and CSA farms are that foods are more likely to be fresh and at their peak of nutritional value, and you support your local farmers by giving them your business.

Ethnic food markets

Shopping at ethnic supermarkets can be an entertaining and enjoyable experience. Go with an open mind and be ready to experiment with a few foods you've never tried before.

You're more likely to find these markets in medium-sized or larger metropolitan areas and in communities with large concentrations of immigrants from different countries. In some cities, you'll find many different types of ethnic grocery stores — Indian, Asian, Mexican, Middle Eastern, kosher, and many more. Each one carries foods and ingredients that are commonly eaten in those cultures but are frequently difficult to find in mainstream North American stores.

In Indian grocery stores, for instance, you'll be amazed to see the many types of lentils that you can buy — red, orange, yellow, brown, and so on. You may find small, skillet-sized pressure cookers used in India to quick-cook dried beans and lentils. You'll also find unusual spices and a variety of Indian breads.

TIP

You may see the same products — Indian heat-and-serve, single-serving entrées, for example — at conventional supermarkets at substantially higher prices. Go with a list, especially if you have to drive a distance to get to the store.

In Asian grocery stores, you'll find vegetables such as some Chinese greens that are shipped to the store from overseas but that aren't typically found in U.S. stores. You'll find unusual condiments as well.

In all these ethnic food stores, you'll see a wide range of traditional foods, many of which are vegetarian or just different, and you can incorporate them into your vegetarian menus at home. More than anything, a trip to one of these stores may inspire you to sample foods of another culture and to expand your own culinary repertoire.

Food cooperatives

Many communities also have food cooperatives, or co-ops. A *co-op* is a group that purchases foods in volume for distribution to its members, usually at a reduced cost. The costs are reduced because of the power of the group to buy in volume, so larger groups may be able to get better prices than smaller groups. Co-ops frequently emphasize natural foods products, and the arrangement can be especially helpful in small towns and rural areas, where people don't have access to large natural foods stores with good variety and competitive prices.

Membership rules vary from one co-op to another. Some co-ops ask their members to contribute a certain number of hours each month to help unload trucks and bag or distribute groceries. Others don't require that you work, but they may give an additional discount to those who donate their time.

Gourmet stores and gift shops

Upscale or gourmet foods stores are a fun place to look for interesting specialty items such as jams and preserves, other condiments, canned soups, pasta sauce, and a wide variety of packaged foods, often produced locally or from boutique producers or international sources. Many of these products are appropriate for vegetarians. The downside: They're often expensive. Gourmet stores can be a good place to shop, though, if you need a special gift for the vegetarian on your list.

Online sources

A good alternative for people who don't have time to shop or can't find certain food items in their local stores is to shop online. Ordering through Instacart and Amazon are two of the simplest options.

There are many other good online sources for vegetarian and vegan products, too. A few examples include BESTIES Vegan Paradise at `https://bestiesvegan paradise.com/`, The Vegetarian Site at `https://store.thevegetariansite.com/index.php?route=common/home`, PlantX at `https://plantx.com/`, and many others.

Other places to try

Bargain stores such as Grocery Outlet are good places to check for deeply discounted vegetarian specialty products. Inventories change frequently, so you may not be able to find a specific item if you need it. If you're open to surprises, though, you may find some good buys.

TIP

Specialty grocery stores such as Trader Joe's often carry a sizable selection of vegetarian foods at competitive prices. Look for name brands here, as well as products such as plant milks sold under the store's private label.

Making the Most of Your Shopping Adventure

Regardless of where you shop, a few more tips and suggestions may help ensure that you have a good supply of nutritious ingredients on hand at home. The ideas I include in this section have worked for me and for many other vegetarian shoppers.

Slowing down to see what's new

Every now and then, spend a little more time than usual roaming up and down each aisle of your favorite grocery store to find out what's new. It's a good way to notice products you may like but didn't know were available in your area.

That's especially true in the produce department. Many people make a beeline for the iceberg lettuce and tomatoes and don't notice much else. Take an extra ten minutes to peruse the piles of colorful fruits and vegetables, and pick up something you've never tried before.

Experimenting with new foods and products

Speaking of trying foods that are new to you . . .

Expect to find a few duds. Along the way, though, you're also likely to find some new favorite foods. Unless you take a risk and try something new, you may never know what you're missing!

That's the way I discovered — and grew to love — mangoes and papayas. I didn't like the flavor of mango the first time I tasted it, but I tried it again. By the second or third try, I was hooked.

If you haven't tried soymilk or almond milk, plant-based yogurt, meatless hot dogs, or meatless crumbles (for tacos, burritos, chili, and spaghetti sauce), I recommend them, if only to help you become aware of the options. If you've never eaten an arugula salad or fresh kale, let the recipes in Chapters 11 and 12 be your introductions.

Don't see what you need? Ask the manager

If you want to buy a specific product but you don't see it in your favorite store, ask to speak with the manager. Chances are good that they can place a special order for you.

TIP

Store managers can often arrange for you to purchase certain foods such as plant milks and canned or bottled foods by the case at a discount. If the demand is high enough, the store may even begin to stock that product regularly.

Keeping Your Costs Under Control

Living vegetarian can be a very cost-effective lifestyle. Diets that include little or no meat, eggs, cheese, or other dairy products tend to be built around foods that are relatively inexpensive, such as beans, pasta, rice, and vegetables.

WARNING

The economy of a vegetarian diet can be lost, though, if you find yourself depending on too many specialty products and ready-made foods. To hold down the cost of your meals, keep the suggestions in this section in mind.

Collecting the building blocks to keep on hand

It's important to keep a good supply of basic ingredients on hand so that you can whip up a meal in a relatively short amount of time. The most practical ingredients are shelf-stable — you can leave them in your pantry for several months before using them. Good examples include pasta, canned soups, several varieties of canned beans and canned tomatoes, rice, dry cereal, hot cereal, and condiments. Most of these items are inexpensive.

Good freezer basics include several types of frozen vegetables, veggie burger patties, whole-grain rolls and bread, and frozen fruits such as mixed berries (for a quick dessert, see the Berry Cobbler recipe in Chapter 14).

Buying in volume — or not

REMEMBER

Buying in volume isn't always the most economical way to shop. If food spoils before you can use it, you may end up spending more than you otherwise would have spent on a smaller quantity of food. If you shop at a warehouse store, you may also want to factor in the membership cost in addition to the cost of the food itself when evaluating whether buying in large quantities makes sense economically.

TIP

One remedy: Consider saving by buying in volume and splitting the item with a friend. For example, you may buy a case of oranges or a large container of prewashed salad greens and each take half.

Perusing private labels and store brands

Compare prices among brands. Private label and store brand products — including breakfast cereals, canned goods, plant milk, peanut butter, and many other foods — can cost significantly less than similar brand-name products. The quality is often indistinguishable from one brand to the next, too. You won't know until you try!

Scaling back on specialty items

Expensive specialty items — gourmet condiments, frozen entrées licensed by famous chefs, and many boutique-brand packaged foods — can take a big bite out of your food budget. Give them as gifts now and then, and enjoy the champagne raspberry preserves when a jar comes your way. In general, though, these foods are too costly to be staples for most of us. Scale back on these items if you're working on keeping your costs under control.

TIP

Similarly, many specialty products in natural foods stores can be pricey. One way to save money at natural foods stores is to buy staples — beans, rice, lentils, granola, seeds, and nuts — from bulk food bins. You won't pay for unnecessary packaging, and you can take only the amount you need.

Getting the best value — nutritiously

Sometimes, the best value isn't the least expensive option.

For example, a standard bag of carrots from your supermarket may remain in your refrigerator so long that the veggies turn to rubber. You can pay more for a bag of prepeeled carrots (or any prewashed, preprepared vegetable), and if the added convenience helps ensure that you eat your veggies, the extra cost may be worth it.

On the other hand, junk foods — such as many packaged cookies, cakes, and other desserts — are also relatively expensive. If you have them in your house, you're very likely to eat them. By keeping them out of the house in the first place, you not only save money but also protect the nutritional quality of your diet, too.

Preparing meals at home

The typical American spends about 40 percent of their food budget on meals eaten away from home. That means that eating more meals at home can potentially save you a lot of money.

Establish the habit of making simple meals at home. This does not have to be time-consuming, nor does it require you to have top-chef cooking skills. The information I cover in Parts 2 and 3 in this book — as well as in Chapter 16 — can help you get started.

TIP

Consider growing some of your own ingredients, too. Tomatoes, bell peppers, lettuce, and herbs such as basil and parsley are easy and fun to grow, even in small spaces. You'll save money, and fresh ingredients for your homecooked meals will be right outside your back door. Countertop hydroponic gardens such as the Aero-Garden brand are another convenient option.

» Knowing the fundamentals of vegetarian cooking

» Giving new life to old recipes

» Building your vegetarian recipe library

Chapter **8**

Cooking Tools and Techniques

Adopting a vegetarian diet is a good reason to brush up on basic cooking skills. If you understand how to use simple tools and techniques in the kitchen, you'll be able to enjoy more healthful, good-tasting vegetarian meals in your own home.

That's important.

The more meals you eat at home instead of away, the more money you save, and the more control you have over the ingredients in the food. Preparing your own meals gives you the flexibility to adapt traditional recipes by removing the meat and other animal ingredients. It's also a good way to improve the overall quality of your diet, because you can cut back on added sodium and sugar at the same time that you limit artery-clogging saturated fat and cholesterol from meat, eggs, cheese, and other dairy products.

TIP

Anticipate potential problems to minimize the chances for cross-contamination from meat and other animal products if you order foods at a nonvegetarian or nonvegan restaurant. Ask the waitstaff about how foods are prepared. For example, inquire about whether the spinach salad is topped with bacon bits, or whether veggie burger patties are cooked on the same surface as meat burgers. Adjust your order as needed.

Cooking your own vegetarian meals at home from scratch or by using some convenient shortcuts also gives you an opportunity to be creative. After you develop confidence in your cooking skills, you'll be able to experiment with new and delicious combinations of basic ingredients — vegetables, rice, pasta, beans, and fruit. You'll be less likely to get into a rut and more likely to be the mealtime destination of choice among your family and friends.

In this chapter, I introduce the tools you need to fix simple vegetarian meals. I cover the ins and outs of cooking with some common vegetarian ingredients and convenience products, as well as how to modify your favorite nonvegetarian family recipes to make them veg-compatible. The emphasis is on simple and practical ways to be your own vegetarian chef.

Tools You Really Need

The world is full of kitchen gadgets and appliances that make the work easier and save you time. You can do without them, but having them makes cooking more enjoyable.

Then there are the true necessities, the tools without which it would be very difficult to cook from scratch. In this section, I outline the equipment you need to outfit a basic vegetarian kitchen.

TIP

Use the lists I provide to do a quick inventory of your own kitchen. Consider what's missing and what you need to buy. Yard sales and kitchen supply outlets are great places to pick up inexpensive but serviceable pieces. If you do buy second-hand items, however, examine them carefully to ensure you understand what you are buying. If you have an induction cooktop on your stove, for example, you'll need stainless steel, not aluminum, cookware.

Target and Ikea are good options for beginner cooks because those inexpensive items will give you an idea of what works best for you before you spend a lot of money on higher priced items. Target sells high-quality Lodge cast-iron skillets.

REMEMBER

Spend the time to make sure you have the equipment you need for a fully functional kitchen. If you don't have what you need, you may find it frustrating — and even unsafe — to perform simple cooking tasks. Using a serrated knife instead of a paring knife to peel an apple, for example, is a good way to do a poor job and cut your finger while you're at it.

Pots and pans

You don't need a large collection and they don't have to be top-of-the-line, but you do need several good-quality pots and pans in various sizes. Invest now and you'll use these to make a lifetime's worth of health-supporting vegetarian meals.

TIP

Stainless steel is clean, safe to use, and a good choice for most pots and pans. Consider buying pots and pans in a set if your budget allows. Sets are usually cheaper than buying individually, and they often include lids.

Choose four to six of the following to handle most of your cooking needs, from pasta sauce and potatoes to chili and soup:

>> 1-quart saucepan

>> 2-quart saucepan

>> 3-quart saucepan

>> 4-quart saucepan

>> 4½-quart pot

>> 6-quart pot or larger (such as a stock pot or stew pot), if you cook for a crowd or for batch cooking or freezer meals.

REMEMBER

A skillet is also invaluable. You'll use it for everything from cooking pancakes and grilling sandwiches to sautéing onions and mushrooms. Choose a heavy-duty, 10-inch, pre-seasoned cast-iron skillet from a company with a reputation for making such high-quality products, like Lodge (www.lodgemfg.com). Stainless steel is fine, too. I also recommend getting one or more of the following:

>> 7-inch skillet

>> 9-inch skillet

>> 12-inch skillet

TIP

Try to get at least one skillet lid — it comes in handy for steaming greens and other times when you need to hold the heat in with what you're cooking. If you buy the same brand of pots, pans, and skillets, it's likely that one or more of the lids that come with some of the pieces will fit other pieces as well.

Knives

You may have noticed the large wooden knife blocks that some people keep in their kitchens, filled with an assortment of scary-looking blades that have figured prominently in several bad movies.

Vegetarians have no need for all those meat-piercing utensils.

REMEMBER

All you need is four different kinds of knives, and only one looks like it could play a role in an action flick (Figure 8-1 shows you what some of these knives look like):

>> **6-inch, serrated knife.** Use it for cutting fruits and vegetables, especially tomatoes. You'll use this knife more than any other.

>> **Paring knife.** This is for cutting certain fruits like apples and pears, peeling potatoes, and similar tasks. The blade is short — 3 or 4 inches — so it's easy to maneuver.

>> **10-inch, serrated bread knife.** Use this for cutting cakes and similar foods.

>> **10-inch chef's knife.** This one has a long blade that's widest near the handle, gradually tapering to a point at the end. Holding the point on the cutting board, you rock the blade up and down from the handle to chop salad greens, fresh vegetables, fruits, and other ingredients.

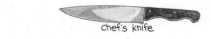

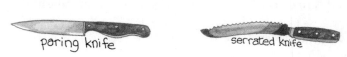

FIGURE 8-1: The basic knives you need for vegetarian cooking.

Illustration by Elizabeth Kurtzman

Assorted extras

Most vegetarian cooks need some baking supplies, including pans, sheets, measuring cups, and utensils. At a minimum, you need:

>> Two baking sheets

>> Muffin pan for baking cupcakes and muffins

>> 8-inch square baking pan

- 9-x-13-inch baking pan

- Two standard loaf pans

- Two 9-inch pie pans (cake pans aren't as useful, so they're optional)

- Set of two or three stainless steel mixing bowls

- At least one set of dry measuring cups (for the most accurate measurement of dry ingredients such as flour and sugar)

- At least one set of measuring spoons

- 2-cup liquid measuring cup (for the most accurate measurement of liquids such as water, oil, and plant milk)

You may be able to whip a yogurt dressing with a fork and spread hummus into a serving bowl with the flat side of a paring knife. However, having the proper utensils for certain uses in the kitchen gives you better results and may be easier to use. The following items are so practical that I deem them necessary for a complete vegetarian kitchen:

- Three or four wooden spoons in various shapes and sizes

- Two or three silicone spatulas

- Set of silicone pot lids in varied diameters (great as splash guards in the microwave oven and for holding in the heat on serving bowls of cooked foods)

- Stainless steel spatula for flipping pancakes and veggie burgers or removing cookies from a cookie sheet

- Soup ladle

- Stainless steel colander

- Pizza cutter

- Pastry brush

- Pastry blender

- Pasta fork

- Two stainless steel whisks, one small, one larger

- Hand-held bean or potato masher

- Large, stainless steel, slotted spoon

REMEMBER

A well-equipped kitchen also includes attractive and functional serving bowls and plates, as well as at least a few clean, attractive tablecloths, placemats, cloth napkins, and decorative hot pads or trivets to place under hot dishes on the table.

These features are important, because the way in which you present food can influence how well others receive the food. If it looks appealing, people are more likely to expect it to taste good.

Handy Appliances You May Actually Use

If you're like many people, you have an appliance graveyard lurking in the back of a kitchen cupboard or pantry. Those bread machines and waffle irons that seemed like a good idea at the time are collecting cobwebs in dark corners around the house.

TIP

One key to positioning yourself to cook your own vegetarian food at home is to clear some space. If your countertop and drawers are jammed with appliances and gadgets that you seldom use, get rid of them. Donate them or pack them away, but remove them from your kitchen. Make room so that you have easy access to the few appliances you may actually use to make daily meal prep easier and faster.

Which tools you need depends on the kinds of foods you like best and how you feel about performing certain kitchen tasks. For example, I like using an old-fashioned, crank-style can opener that I keep in a kitchen drawer. An advantage is that I don't have an electric can opener taking up space on my countertop.

And not everybody needs a large, countertop mixer. A hand-held mixer may work just fine for your needs, or maybe all you need is a simple whisk. Think about your equipment needs and remove what you don't need to free up precious kitchen space.

In the following sections, I tell you about several appliances that many vegetarians find particularly handy.

High-speed blenders

Blenders are useful for whipping up fresh fruit smoothies and fresh vegetable blends. An advantage of a high-speed blender over a juicer — another popular appliance — is that it preserves the dietary fiber in fruits and vegetables and may be easier to clean.

WARNING

Ordinary kitchen blenders are inexpensive, but their motors tend to overheat easily when the blender is used to process thick mixtures such as hummus (see the recipe in Chapter 10) and some smoothies (Chapter 9 includes two smoothie recipes). A heavy-duty, restaurant-quality blender such as the

Vita-Mix (www.vita-mix.com) holds an advantage over ordinary blenders because it has a larger capacity and stronger motor. The trade-off is that the Vita-Mix is much more expensive.

TIP

Make cold melon soup by placing fresh cantaloupe or honeydew chunks, nonfat unflavored yogurt, and a few teaspoons of honey in a blender and processing until creamy. For thinner soup, add orange or apple juice by the tablespoon until the soup reaches the right consistency. Serve in a rimmed soup bowl with a dash of cinnamon or nutmeg and a sprig of fresh mint on top. Make a vegan version easily using plant-based yogurt and maple syrup or agave syrup as sweeteners.

Food processors

Mini food processors — those with only a one- or two-cup capacity — can be a great help in grating, mincing, and chopping small amounts quickly. I use mine to grate carrots or a small chunk of red cabbage for color in a salad, or when I don't feel like chopping an onion by hand.

Larger, full-capacity food processors are a must-have in many vegetarian households. They make quick work of larger chopping jobs, and the results are often more consistent than when you chop by hand.

TIP

It's amazingly simple and quick to make fresh *gazpacho* — a cold, traditional Spanish soup made with fresh vegetables — using a food processor. You'll find many variations, but most include one or more of the following ingredients, blended until smooth: fresh, uncooked tomatoes, onions, cucumbers, bell peppers, celery, olive oil, chives, minced garlic, red wine vinegar, and lemon juice. I include a recipe for Classic Gazpacho in Chapter 11.

Rice cookers

One of the pitfalls of cooking rice the traditional way — in a pot on the stovetop — is that if you don't watch it carefully, the rice can quickly boil over and make a mess. Enter the rice lover's best friend: the rice cooker.

Some people swear by their rice cooker for that reason: It lets you make perfectly steamed rice while you're out of the kitchen doing something other than watching the stove. Rice is also a mainstay of many ethnic vegetarian meals — as an accompaniment to Indian and Asian entrées as well as with a variety of bean dishes. You can find several recipes in Chapter 12.

A great way to store leftover cooked rice is to portion it into airtight plastic bags and place them in the freezer. The rice will keep for three to six months that way. When you're ready to use it, transfer the frozen rice onto a plate or into a bowl and reheat it in a microwave oven. Eat it with leftover chili, stew, stir-fry, or Indian entrées.

Pressure cookers

Name a gadget that can cook a two-hour meal in ten minutes. Nope, it's not a magic wand — it's a *pressure cooker*. A pressure cooker enables you to cook a vegetarian casserole, stew, or bean dish in the time it takes to set the table.

The way a pressure cooker works is simple. You place foods such as beans, rice, lentils, or root vegetables in the cooker with water or another liquid. You tightly seal the pot and set it over high heat on the stove. As the steam inside the pot builds, the pressure inside the pot increases, raising the temperature to 250 degrees — far above the boiling point of 212 degrees. Under these conditions, foods get soft and cook faster than they would by other means.

Some people remember their mother's — or grandmother's — old jiggle-top pressure cooker from 30 years ago or more. Those old-fashioned pressure cookers hissed, rattled, and clanged so violently that at times they seemed as if they were about to blow a hole through the ceiling.

Newer jiggle-top pressure cookers from companies such as Mirro and Presto are much easier and safer to use and include features that prevent too much pressure from building up.

European companies such as Kuhn Rikon, Magefesa, and Zepter make pressure cookers with stationary pressure regulators instead of the old jiggle-top variety. Stationary regulators don't clog as easily, making it safer to leave the kitchen while the cooker is in use. These newer pressure cookers are quieter and may require less water to reach high pressure. After the food is done, you can release the pressure on the stovetop, in contrast to old models that had to be set in the sink and doused in cold water to bring the pressure down.

You can find a variety of pressure cookers in specialty stores, as well as some good buys online. You may even find some sold in Indian food markets, including short, squatty, pressure frying pans. Pressure cookers are a standard tool in Indian cooking because they're so useful in shortening the cooking time for lentils, rice, and many of the dried beans used in Indian dishes.

Pressure cookers come in several shapes and sizes. If you want only one, a 6- or 8-quart cooker is the most practical size to buy. It may look big, but when you use a pressure cooker, you fill it from only one-half to three-quarters full. The remainder of the space is needed for the steam that builds up inside the pot.

REMEMBER

Note that European models designate the volume of the pot in liters rather than quarts. A 6-liter pressure cooker is roughly equivalent to a 6.5-quart cooker; a 7-liter cooker is about the same size as a 7.5-quart cooker. Prices vary widely by make and model.

TIP

If you want to try your hand at using a pressure cooker, a good resource is *Great Vegetarian Cooking Under Pressure* by pressure cooker guru Lorna J. Sass (William Morrow Cookbooks). Another good resource is registered dietitian Jill Nussinow, "The Veggie Queen." Visit her website at www.theveggiequeen.com/pressure-cooking.

Slow cookers

A '70s-era kitchen aid that's still being used by many is the *slow cooker,* a removable stoneware crock with a lid set into a heating element. Slow cookers allow you to dump ingredients into a pot, turn on the heat, and walk away. At the end of the day, you come home to the smell of dinner, wafting through your home, ready to serve.

Newer models include timer and temperature controls, whereas the original model had only a few settings. Slow cookers come in various sizes, from very small — good for singles and couples — to family-sized models. Others are made with locking lids, carrying handles, and travel bags for people who want to cook and carry a dish to get-togethers with family and friends.

TIP

Slow cookers work well for making vegetarian-style meals with combinations of vegetables, beans, lentils, and grains such as rice, oatmeal, bulgur wheat, and others. For example, you can use a slow cooker to make the recipes for Fruited Oatmeal (see Chapter 9), Lentil Soup (see Chapter 11), Cashew Chili (see Chapter 11), and Cuban Black Beans (see Chapter 12).

Multicookers

Many people swear by a multicooker, which combines the functions of a pressure cooker, slow cooker, and rice cooker all in one. These days, more people buy multicookers than stand-alone pressure cookers.

The Instant Pot is the most recognizable example, but Ninja and Breville are two other examples, of many. Multicookers can even be used to make your own yogurt.

One of these all-in-one appliances can save counter space and help to keep your kitchen more clutter-free.

Many food websites have instructions for converting slow cooker recipes to the Instant Pot. There are also a number of cookbooks on the market that are dedicated to vegetarian and vegan multicooker recipes.

Electric tea kettles

Electric tea kettles are relatively inexpensive — under $40, or about the cost of a common coffee maker — and they can save you time. Just add hot water and flip the switch. You get boiling water in less time than it takes to heat water on the stovetop.

It's a quick and very convenient way to have hot water in a hurry when you want to make a single serving of oatmeal, a soup cup, or a hot drink. It's also useful for rehydrating bean flakes and instant couscous used in some vegetarian dishes, and for giving a jump-start to a pot of hot water for cooking pasta or rice.

Vegetarian Cooking Basics

You don't have to be a professional chef to fix good vegetarian meals. You don't even have to impress your friends. All you have to do is satisfy yourself (and your family — maybe).

If you're already an accomplished cook, you probably need no reassurance that you'll be adept at fixing vegetarian masterpieces after you figure out what you want to make. That won't take long, because you're already skilled and creative.

On the other hand, if you're like most people, you're no pro, but you somehow manage to put together reasonably appealing meals most of the time. Usually, that means whipping dinner together in a half hour or less, with the emphasis on less.

Vegetarian cooking can be as simple or as complicated as you want it to be. In this section, I cover some of the basic skills that any beginning vegetarian needs.

Mastering simple cooking skills

Becoming comfortable and confident in the kitchen takes time and practice. Like driving a car or knitting a sweater, you get better at it over time.

Each of the cooking techniques I describe requires hands-on experience. If you're a beginning cook, consider asking an experienced friend or family member to guide you at the start, or look into taking a cooking class at your local natural foods store or community college.

Baking

You'll use your oven to make many vegetarian foods, including casseroles, baked potatoes, breads and rolls, pies, winter squash, and more. A few key points are important to follow when you bake:

REMEMBER

>> **Preheat the oven.** Set the oven to the temperature called for in the recipe. Give the oven at least 10 or 15 minutes to reach the correct temperature before putting the dish in.

>> **Use the timer.** Don't rely on your nose to tell you the food is ready. Set the oven timer, or use a free-standing timer. Many people use the timer on their smart phone or smart speaker device. Make sure that you're in a place in the house where you'll hear the timer going off when the food is ready.

>> **Measure precisely.** Think of dry ingredients in cakes, breads, rolls, and other baked goods like a science experiment. You have to add the flour, baking soda, and baking powder in the right proportions for the ingredients to react together properly. Use measuring spoons and cups to measure amounts accurately.

TIP

A digital kitchen scale can also work well for making accurate measurements of dry ingredients such as bread flour. If you need to convert dry ingredient measures in cups, ounces, or grams, an Internet search for the conversions is often the easiest way to do it.

>> **Check for doneness.** Poke a toothpick or knife into the center of the baked good to see whether it's ready to come out. If the toothpick or knife comes out clean, the food is probably done. If not, check again in another few minutes.

Boiling

You need to know how to boil water on the stovetop for cooking grains, dried beans, pasta, rice, and a number of other foods. In most cases, this entails bringing a pot or saucepan of water to a boil over medium heat, adding the food, and then turning the heat down to let the food simmer for a period.

When cooking some foods, such as a pot of rice, you need a lid to keep the steam inside the pot. You can cook other foods, such as pasta, without a lid to help ensure the water doesn't boil over the sides.

Setting a timer is helpful so that you know when a food should be done cooking. Be careful not to overcook some foods, such as pasta, which can become mushy if it's left in the water too long.

Steaming

Steaming vegetables such as broccoli, cauliflower, and cabbage by cooking them for a short time in a small amount of water is a great way to preserve their nutrients. It takes only minutes to steam most vegetables so that they're tender enough to eat while retaining their color and crispness.

The microwave oven is the quickest and easiest way to steam foods. Set the food in a glass container and add a few tablespoons of water. Cover with a paper towel or a silicone pot lid and heat. A medium-sized baking potato needs six to eight minutes to cook, while a small serving of broccoli may need only a few minutes on high.

Steaming foods on the stovetop is also easy and quick. To steam fresh broccoli, for example, cover the bottom of a pan with about an inch of water and heat it to boiling. Add the broccoli, cover with a lid, reduce the heat to low, and let the broccoli steam for as long as desired or until tender when pierced with a fork. When the food is done, remove the pot from the stove and drain the excess water into the kitchen sink.

Be careful when you drain the water after steaming foods, whether you cook the food in a microwave oven or on the stovetop. When you remove the lid or cover, hold the pot or bowl away from your face so that escaping steam doesn't burn you.

If you're looking for kitchen gadgets specifically for steaming, consider trying one of the following:

>> **Bamboo or stainless-steel steamer baskets:** You set them into a pot with boiling water, and they hold the food just above the bottom of the pan. A lid is placed on top. The advantage in using these baskets is that they help fragile foods such as dumplings or tiny vegetables stay intact better and prevent nutrients from being leached into the cooking water.

>> **A free-standing, electric steamer:** These small appliances are inexpensive and simple to operate and clean. You can find them in most discount and home stores.

CARING FOR CAST-IRON COOKWARE

TIP

Follow the manufacturer's recommendations for pre-seasoning new skillets as needed, and cleaning and regularly seasoning cast-iron pots, pans, griddles, and other cookware. Instructions may vary from one brand to the next, depending on how the cookware is made. In general, though, you should clean cast-iron cookware by using nothing but a stiff, nylon brush or a sponge and hot water. After removing food residue, use a clean towel to dry your cookware. Air-drying can cause cookware to rust. Use a paper towel to rub the cooking surface with a light coat of vegetable oil, and then store the cookware in a cool, dry place. Place a piece of newspaper or a paper towel between pots and their lids to promote air circulation and prevent rust formation.

Sautéing

Many vegetarian recipes begin by asking you to sauté onions, garlic, celery, or bell peppers before adding other ingredients. To *sauté* is to fry foods in a small amount of fat — usually vegetable oil — over high heat.

Begin by adding a tablespoon or two of olive oil or another vegetable oil to a skillet to keep food from sticking and to help distribute the flavors. When the skillet is hot, add the food and stir frequently to prevent sticking. Onions are done when they're translucent. Garlic may brown a bit, and celery and peppers become soft when done.

You can also try stir-steaming your food, by using a little bit of water in the bottom of the pan instead of oil to sauté.

Stewing

Soups, stews, and chili are examples of foods that are often left to *stew* or simmer on low heat on the stovetop for an hour or more before serving. They have to be stirred every so often with a long-handled spoon to keep food from sticking to the bottom of the pot.

A deep stew pot or stockpot is ideal for making large batches of foods like these, which tend to splatter if the heat is too high or the pot is too full. A lid — tipped to let steam escape — can help keep your stovetop and burners clean.

Prepping fruits and vegetables

The first step in preparing most fruits and vegetables is to wash them thoroughly, even if you're using organic produce. Harmful bacteria can be present on any produce, and you need to take precautions to be safe.

Using your hands or a soft brush, rub fruits and vegetables as you hold them under fast-running water for several seconds, removing all visible traces of dirt and debris. Soap isn't necessary, and research has found little or no advantage to commercial fruit and vegetable rinses.

For fruits and vegetables such as broccoli and strawberries that have lots of crevices, soak them in a pan or sink full of water, swishing to help dislodge tiny bits of debris, and then rinse them well.

REMEMBER

Even if you don't plan to eat the peel, it's important to wash the outsides of foods like watermelon, cantaloupe, and oranges before setting them on a cutting board or slicing them. If you don't, bacteria on the outside of the food could contaminate the cutting board's surface and anything you set on it afterward. Cutting unwashed foods can also permit bacteria to get into the part of the food that you're going to eat.

The right knives can make peeling, chopping, and cutting much easier. Use a paring knife to peel and cut apples, pears, peaches, cucumbers, bell peppers, and radishes. A chef's knife is useful for chopping romaine lettuce, herbs, greens, and pineapple. Use a serrated knife to slice soft fruits and vegetables such as tomatoes and kiwi fruit. (For more information and an illustration of these knives, refer to Figure 8-1 and the earlier section on knives.)

TIP

Save time fixing meals by pre-preparing fruits and vegetables. Take a half hour when you return from shopping to wash and cut up produce. Store precut fruits and vegetables in airtight containers in the refrigerator so that they're ready when you start fixing a meal.

TIP

Look for ways to be efficient when you prepare fresh fruits and vegetables. Chop several bell peppers or onions at a time, for example, and store the extra in ¼-cup portions in airtight plastic bags in the freezer. Do the same thing with fruit. You can cut up peaches and strawberries, freeze them, and use them later to make smoothies or to serve for dessert with ice cream.

Cooking extra now for later

Batch cooking is a great way to save you time and effort in the kitchen. It means making a larger amount of a recipe and setting part of it aside for later. For little additional effort, you can have enough food for two or more meals in the time it takes you to prepare one.

Batch cooking works best for foods that you can store in the refrigerator for at least a few days or in the freezer for several weeks. For example, you can serve a big pot of chili for dinner one day and store the remainder in the refrigerator and use it for lunches for the next couple of days. Or you can freeze part of a large lasagna and reheat it for a quick meal another day.

Some salads even store well for days in the refrigerator. Pasta salad, bean salad, and other marinated vegetable salads, for example, can keep in the refrigerator for up to several days.

Discovering a few tricks for cooking with tofu and tempeh

People often talk about tofu and tempeh as if they're bookends and go together like a matching pair. The fact is, they look and taste very different, and their functions in recipes vary, too. Another common misconception is that if you're a vegetarian, you probably eat a lot of tofu. (Most nonvegetarians have never heard of tempeh.) It's not necessary to eat tofu and tempeh to be a full-fledged vegetarian, but you can certainly make some good-tasting dishes with these nutritious soy foods. If you are unfamiliar with tempeh, or you would like more information about tofu, see Table 6-1 in Chapter 6.

TIP

If you do care to experiment with tofu and tempeh, here are a few tips to make the most of these ingredients:

>> When you use tofu as a meat substitute, you usually cut it up into cubes and stir-fry it (extra-firm tofu works best for this), or you marinate it and cook it in slabs or chunks. If it's frozen first and then thawed, tofu develops a chewy texture that resembles that of meat.

>> Try using tofu to make cream soup without milk or cream. Just purée some soft tofu with vegetable broth and mix it into the soup.

>> You can use tempeh in ways that meats are more traditionally used. For instance, you can grill, barbecue, bake, or broil strips or blocks of tempeh. You can use chunks of tempeh with vegetable pieces for shish kebabs or to make stews, casseroles, and other combination dishes.

Adapting Traditional Recipes

When I think about adapting traditional recipes to make them suitable for vegetarians, I can't help but remember a 1970s TV show that left a lifelong impression on Boomers like me. That show — *Gilligan's Island* — was all about a group of castaways from a tourist boat, stranded on a deserted tropical island.

Living off the land, this group somehow managed to bake the most luscious-looking coconut cream and banana cream pies. As a kid with a mother who baked, I was mesmerized — and confounded — by the idea that they could do this without milk, eggs, or butter.

"Well, they had coconut milk," I thought. But no eggs or butter. And those pies looked so good.

The show was fictional, but the idea that plant-based ingredients can perform just as well in recipes as animal ingredients is the truth. You'll be surprised to discover how easy it is to cook the vegetarian way, and you may be equally as pleased to know that you don't have to throw away your old family favorites!

REMEMBER

When you substitute plant-based ingredients for animal ingredients in recipes, anticipate that the characteristics of the finished products may be at least somewhat different from the qualities of foods made with animal products.

WARNING

I encourage you to try substituting plant-based ingredients for animal products in your favorite nonvegetarian recipes. If you do, however, one caution is in order: Expect to experiment before you get it right. If you don't use a vegetarian cookbook in which the recipes have already been tested, you'll have to fiddle around with traditional, nonvegetarian recipes until you hit on the ingredient substitutions and proper amounts that work best.

In the following sections, I show you how to make many of your favorite foods without using any animal products whatsoever. That way, you'll be prepared to adapt recipes for any kind of vegetarian diet. Of course, if you're a vegetarian who eats dairy products and eggs, you may not care to work those ingredients out of your recipes. However, if you're a vegan or you just want to lower your intake of saturated fat and cholesterol, the information is very useful.

In many cases, you can use any of several different foods as a substitute for an animal product in a recipe. Experiment to find the one that gives you the best result. Figure 8-2 shows some common substitutions.

TIP

When you modify a recipe, use a pencil to note on the original recipe the substitutions you made and how much of each ingredient you used, or update the recipe online right away on your app or online recipe. When the product is finished, jot down suggestions for improvements or any minor adjustments that you want to make next time. Whenever you make an adjustment, erase and update your written notes on the recipe and be sure to make the changes on any electronic files or apps that you use.

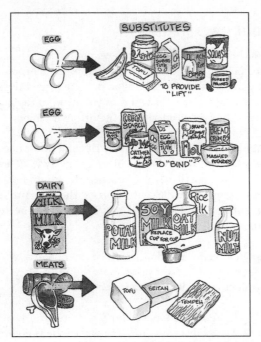

FIGURE 8-2: Common vegetarian substitutes.

Illustration by Elizabeth Kurtzman

Replacing eggs

How many times have you wanted to bake a batch of cookies, only to find that you were missing a vital ingredient, such as eggs?

Bet you didn't know that those eggs aren't so vital. If you had known that you could substitute any of several other foods for the eggs in your recipes, you wouldn't have had to waste a minute running to the store.

Eggs perform a number of functions in recipes, including binding ingredients, leavening, affecting texture, and affecting color (such as in a sponge cake or French toast). So your choice of a substitute depends on how well it can perform the necessary function. In some cases, the egg's effect in the recipe is so slight that you can leave it out altogether, not replace it with anything else, and not even notice that it's missing.

In this section, I look at some of the foods that you can use to replace eggs in recipes.

Baking without eggs

In baked goods, you usually use eggs for *leavening*, or lightness, and to act as a binder. In some recipes, eggs are beaten or whipped, incorporating air into the product and decreasing its density. The type of baked good determines whether you can leave out the egg entirely, or whether you need to replace it with another ingredient to perform the egg's function in the original recipe.

For example, in baked goods that are relatively flat and don't need a lot of leavening, such as cookies and pancakes, you can often get away with leaving out the egg and not replacing it. That's particularly true when the original recipe calls for only one or two eggs. In recipes that call for more eggs, the eggs probably play a much greater role in leavening or binding, and you'll find that the recipe fails if you don't replace them.

TIP

If you omit the eggs in a recipe and don't replace them, add a tablespoon or two of additional liquid — plant milk, fruit juice, water, and so on — for each egg you omit to help the product retain its original moisture content.

In baked goods that are light and have a fluffy texture, you want to replace eggs with an ingredient that provides some lift. Try any of the following to replace one whole egg in a recipe:

REMEMBER

>> Half of a ripe mashed banana. This works well in recipes in which you wouldn't mind a banana flavor, including muffins, cookies, pancakes, and quick breads.

>> ¼ cup of any kind of tofu, blended with the liquid ingredients in the recipe — soft or silken tofu works especially well.

>> 1½ teaspoons commercial vegetarian egg replacer, such as EnerG Egg Replacer, mixed with 2 tablespoons of water. This product is a combination of vegetable starches and works wonderfully in virtually any recipe that calls for eggs. Natural foods stores usually sell this in a 1-pound box.

>> ¼ cup applesauce, canned pumpkin, canned squash, or puréed prunes. These fruit and vegetable purées may add a hint of flavor to foods. If you want a lighter product, also add an extra ½ teaspoon of baking powder to the recipe, because using fruit purées to replace eggs can make the finished product somewhat denser than the original recipe.

>> 1 heaping tablespoon soy flour or bean flour mixed with 1 tablespoon water. This combination thickens and adds lift.

>> 2 tablespoons cornstarch beaten with 2 tablespoons water. This mix also thickens and adds some lift.

>> 1 tablespoon finely ground flaxseeds whipped with ¼ cup water. This blend also thickens and adds some lift.

Holding ingredients together without using eggs

In foods where the ingredients need to stick together, such as vegetable and grain casseroles, lentil loaves, and vegetarian burger patties, you need an ingredient that acts as a binder. Eggs traditionally serve that function in nonvegetarian foods like meatballs, meatloaf, hamburgers, and many casseroles, but you can find plenty of alternatives if you want to omit the eggs.

REMEMBER

Moist foods such as casseroles or some vegetarian loaves may not require any additional moisture when you're removing or replacing eggs. In these cases, you'll need to experiment to determine whether the finished dish is moist enough without extra liquid to compensate for the eggs you've left out.

TIP

With the following substitutions, you'll probably find that you have to experiment a bit to determine just the right amount of an ingredient to serve the purpose in a specific recipe. A good starting point with most recipes is 2 or 3 tablespoons of any of these ingredients, or a combination of them, to replace one whole egg. If the original recipe calls for two eggs, start with 4 to 6 tablespoons of egg substitute.

Try any of the following to replace eggs in a recipe where eggs are used to bind food:

>> Arrowroot starch

>> Cornstarch

>> Finely crushed breadcrumbs, cracker meal, or matzo meal

>> Mashed potatoes, mashed sweet potatoes, or instant potato flakes

>> Potato starch

>> Quick-cooking rolled oats or cooked oatmeal

>> Tomato paste

>> Whole-wheat, unbleached, oat, or bean flour

TIP

When working with dry ingredients such as arrowroot or cornstarch, some recipes may work best if you mix the dry ingredients with water, vegetable broth, or another liquid (about 1½ teaspoons of dry ingredient to 2 tablespoons of liquid) first, and then add the mixture to the recipe in place of the egg.

Some of the egg substitutes may affect the flavor of the finished product, too, so you should consider that when you decide which ingredients to use. For instance, if you add sweet potato to a burger patty, you may be able to taste it in the finished product, whereas if you mix some sweet potato into a casserole, its flavor may be more disguised by the other ingredients. On the other hand, the extra flavor that some of these ingredients add may be a pleasant surprise.

TIP

If you're looking for another substitution, try replacing one whole egg with ¼ cup of any kind of tofu blended with 1 tablespoon of flour. (See the nearby sidebar "Imitating egg with tofu" for more information on tofu as an egg substitute.)

For an egg white substitute, boil whole flaxseeds in water, straining and discarding the flaxseeds. Allow the mixture to cool until a gel forms. Since there are no flaxseeds in the final product, it looks like egg whites.

Cooking with dairy substitutes

Replacing dairy products in recipes is incredibly easy. The dairy products you're most likely to find in recipes are milk, yogurt, sour cream, butter, and cheese. You can easily substitute good nondairy alternatives for any of these products.

Getting the cow's milk out

You can replace cow's milk in recipes by using soymilk, rice milk, almond milk, oat milk — really any plant milk. Just try it. Substitute any of these alternatives cup for cup for cow's milk. Most plant milks come in sweetened or unsweetened varieties. Use unsweetened plant milk in savory recipes. Either sweetened or unsweetened varieties work fine in most desserts and smoothies.

IMITATING EGG WITH TOFU

Tofu can stand in for eggs in all sorts of recipes. Usually it's invisible as an ingredient, but sometimes it works as an egg imposter. Here are some examples:

- Use chopped firm tofu or extra-firm tofu in place of egg in recipes for egg salad sandwich filling. Just make your favorite egg salad recipe, but use chopped tofu instead of hard-boiled eggs. You can even use egg-free or vegan mayonnaise instead of regular mayonnaise for a vegan version. See the recipe for Tofu Salad in Chapter 11.

- Add chopped firm tofu to mixed green salads or spinach salad in place of chopped hard-boiled eggs. You can also add chopped or minced tofu to bowls of Chinese hot and sour soup.

- Make scrambled tofu instead of scrambled eggs. Vegetarian cookbooks often include recipes for making scrambled tofu. The recipes usually include turmeric to give the tofu a yellow color, similar to that of scrambled eggs. Try the recipe for Scrambled Tofu in Chapter 9. Use scrambled tofu to fill pita pockets or as a sandwich filling on hoagie rolls.

Unsweetened and vanilla flavors are the most versatile varieties of plant milk because the mild flavors blend in with just about any recipe. You can try unsweetened plant milks in savory recipes such as some main dish sauces and soups. Use vanilla soymilk in sweeter dishes, such as puddings and custards, and on cereal, in baking, and for smoothies.

TIP

Make your own version of nondairy buttermilk by adding 2 teaspoons of lemon juice or vinegar to 1 cup of plant milk.

Removing sour cream and yogurt

You can use plant-based yogurts and sour cream in most of the same ways that you use the dairy versions, including baking, making sauces and dips, and eating as is. Because these substitutes sometimes separate when they're heated on the stove, they may or may not work in certain sauce recipes. Most of the time, however, you'll find that you have no problems substituting them for dairy yogurt and sour cream.

Choosing cheesy alternatives

Nondairy cheese alternatives of the past did not melt as well as regular, full-fat dairy cheeses, though they generally melted better than nonfat dairy cheeses. That's partly because of their high vegetable fat content. Newer products on the market today, however, melt quite well.

Experiment with cheese replacers to find the brands you like the best and the varieties that work best in your recipes.

TIP

Make your own nondairy substitute for ricotta cheese or cottage cheese by mashing a block of tofu with a fork and mixing in a few teaspoons of lemon juice. You can use this "tofu cheese" to replace ricotta cheese or cottage cheese in lasagna, stuffed shells, manicotti, Danish pastries, cheese blintzes, and many other recipes. Nutritional yeast works well as a substitute for Parmesan cheese on casseroles, salads, baked potatoes, popcorn, and pasta. It has a savory, cheesy flavor. You'll find it in natural foods stores as well as conventional supermarkets.

Making better butter choices

You can use stick-style, nondairy margarine in recipes in place of regular margarine or butter, but it's not ideal. That's because any kind of regular, stick-style margarine still contains saturated fat, which may promote coronary artery disease.

Soft, tub-style margarines such as Earth Balance and Canoleo generally contain less saturated fat than harder, stick-style varieties. Read the labels and look for those containing as little saturated fat per serving as possible. Experiment with these in recipes, because the soft nature of the product may cause it to perform differently in different recipes.

TIP

You can also use liquid vegetable oil to replace butter in some recipes. Use about 14 tablespoons, or ¾ cup plus 2 tablespoons, of vegetable oil to replace 1 cup of butter. This substitution may not work as well in recipes for baked goods as it does in other recipes, so experiment to find the amount that works best.

Using meat substitutes

Some vegetarian dishes are originals — they've been meatless from the start, and they don't cry out for a meat-like ingredient. Examples include falafel (deep-fried Middle Eastern chickpea balls), spinach pie, ratatouille (a spicy vegetable dish), and pasta primavera.

Other dishes were created with a meat-like ingredient in mind. Without meat — or a suitable substitute — they lack something. Examples include burgers (a burger without the burger is just a bun), sloppy Joes, and recipes that call for chunks of meat, such as stews and stir-fries.

Some meat products are stand-alone traditions — hot dogs, sausage, cold cuts, and bacon, for instance. Believe it or not, you can find some very good imposters to replace even these items. Whatever the recipe, you have lots of choices when it comes to replacing the meat. Consider the following, which I've generally listed in order of their popularity:

>> **Meatless strips, slices, nuggets, crumbles and patties:** Soy- and other plant-based substitutes that resemble chicken and beef strips, chicken nuggets, burger, ground meat, sausages, deli slices, chicken patties, and similar products are sold in the refrigerator and freezer sections in supermarkets and natural foods stores. Use them in stir-fry recipes, over rice, in casseroles, sauces, and chili, in sandwiches, and in other creative ways.

>> **Mushrooms:** Grilled or marinated, baked portobello mushroom caps are a frequent find on restaurant menus as a substitute for a burger patty. These large mushroom tops are about the same size as a typical burger patty, and they have a chewy, meaty texture and flavor. In general, mushrooms in many varieties add a rich, savory flavor to pasta sauces, stir-frys, pizzas, and other recipes.

>> **Tofu:** Tofu is a smooth, creamy food that has very little flavor or odor. It picks up the flavor of whatever it's cooked with. It can be seasoned with herbs, spices, and sauces and can be baked, fried, or sautéed and used like meat as a main dish or as an ingredient in other dishes, such as the Vegetable Stir-Fry recipe I include in Chapter 12.

>> **Tempeh:** Tempeh can be crumbled and used to make such foods as tempeh sloppy Joes, tempeh mock chicken salad, and tempeh chili.

>> **Seitan:** This chewy, meaty food is made from wheat gluten, the protein-rich mass that is left when the starch is rinsed out of wheat dough. Seitan is a popular ingredient in many Asian dishes. Its versatility makes it a convenient ingredient in cooked foods such as stews and stir-frys, but it can also be served cold, shredded or in slices, for sandwich fillings. It's sold in varied forms, included shredded, strips, slices, and chunks in natural foods stores and supermarkets.

>> **Textured vegetable protein (TVP):** This product can replace the ground meat in taco and burrito fillings, sloppy Joe filling, and spaghetti sauce. If you toss a handful into a pot of chili, people won't likely be able to tell the difference between the TVP and ground meat. You can find dry TVP in natural foods stores and through mail order catalogs, though it's largely being replaced by newer products, such as the meatless ground "beef" products sold in the refrigerator and freezer cases in supermarkets and natural foods stores.

>> **Bulgur wheat:** Bulgur wheat has a nutty flavor, and you can use it in some of the same ways that TVP is used. For example, you can toss a handful of bulgur wheat into a pot of chili and get much the same effect as you would if you used TVP. It absorbs the liquid in whatever it's cooked with, and it has the appearance of ground meat and a chewy texture.

>> **Jackfruit.** Find this fleshy, fibrous fruit in natural foods stores and supermarkets, usually sold canned or ready-to-eat as an ingredient in a wide range of dishes, including curries, stews, stir-frys, and sandwich fillings.

Factoring in other replacements for animal ingredients

Don't let any animal ingredient stand in your way of enjoying a favorite recipe.

Replace beef and chicken broths in soup with vegetable broth, available in a variety of flavors and forms. For convenience and flavor, brands that are packaged in aseptic, shelf-stable boxes and sold in many supermarkets and natural foods stores work well. Plain vegetable broth works well in most soup recipes, but consider tomato and red pepper, ginger carrot, and other variations, too. You can also use bouillon cubes, powders, and canned vegetable broths.

And if you think being vegetarian means an end to molded gelatin salads, consider this: Vegetarian sources of plain and fruit-flavored gelatin are available. They're made from sea vegetables and are sold in natural foods stores. Agar is one form, and it's made from red algae. You can use these products in the same ways that nonvegetarian gelatin is used.

REMEMBER

If you use vegetarian gelatin in recipes in which regular gelatin is usually liquefied and then added to cold ingredients, you may need to change the process a bit. Vegetarian gelatin may begin to set immediately, so you need to add the rest of the recipe's ingredients right away. If a recipe doesn't turn out well when you use the original preparation method, try blending the vegetarian gelatin into cold liquid first, and then bringing the liquid to a boil.

Selecting Vegetarian Recipes

If you are new to living vegetarian, you may find yourself wondering from time to time, "What can I make for dinner tonight?" That's understandable. If you're like most people, old ways take time to change. You need time and support to establish new habits. You need ideas to help you begin.

That's where vegetarian recipes come in.

When it comes to finding inspiration from good vegetarian recipes, you have lots of options. Use the information that follows to help you get started.

Curating cookbook classics

Though you can modify traditional nonvegetarian recipes to remove the animal ingredients, it can help to have a few vegetarian cookbooks on hand as well.

Vegetarian cookbooks are useful for a couple of reasons. They provide explicit instructions for making recipes that may be new to you. You can even use a recipe as a starting point and modify it to make the dish uniquely your own.

And some people like to peruse cookbooks just for the ideas they can inspire. If you find yourself in a rut, thumbing through a favorite cookbook may remind you of something you haven't made in a while.

Countless excellent vegetarian cookbooks are available, ranging from vegan to lacto ovo vegetarian and including cuisines from many different cultures. I'm not going to attempt to list them here. However, you should realize that it's common to find one or two favorite cookbooks that you return to over and over again. Other cookbooks may contain only one or two recipes that you make now and then.

As you shop for vegetarian cookbooks, be especially attuned to the complexity of the recipes and the number and type of ingredients used. In my experience, the most practical cookbooks for home cooks are those with simple recipes requiring only basic cooking skills and equipment. Ingredient lists should be short and be relatively free of exotic ingredients that you aren't likely to use often or that may be expensive or hard to find.

In fact, I'm a strong advocate of learning to cook using no recipes at all. After you develop confidence in cooking, you should be able to freestyle it. Put together foods that taste good — like the ingredients in a veggie burrito or a pot of vegetarian chili — without the need to measure. That's culinary freedom!

You do have to use precise measurements in baking, which requires that certain ingredients be present in exact proportions. For most other simple recipes, though — fruit salad, a batch of hummus, or veggie lasagna, for instance — you can use a little more or less of this or that and everything will turn out just fine.

Assembling an online recipe box

If you prefer a minimalist approach, forget about cookbooks. Simply save, store, and organize your favorite recipes on your electronic device — computer, cellphone, or tablet. The benefits are many.

At its simplest, a digital recipe box can be nothing more than a folder where you keep all of your recipes or bookmarks in one place. Separate recipes into subfolders the way old time recipe boxes were arranged, with separate sections for appetizers, salads, soups, breads, entrees, desserts, holiday favorites — whatever categories make sense for you.

If your collection becomes big enough, though, it can get tiresome to search for a recipe, especially if you forget the name of the dish. Bookmarked recipes can also be lost if the website link changes or disappears over time.

Step it up a notch by using one of the many recipe apps on a smart device or an online recipe organizer. Some are free and others require a subscription, such as my favorite NYT Cooking, which includes thousands of recipes, video instructions, and a personal recipe box. The New York Times cooking app includes many vegetarian recipes.

The advantages to most recipe apps or online recipe organizers are that they let you search and quickly review recipes, decide what you want to make, and even create shopping lists. You can also share your favorite recipes more easily if you store them electronically.

3

Meals Made Easy: Recipes for Everyone

Practice some of the starter recipes. They cover the range of food categories. Many may become regular additions to your table.

Examine the short ingredient lists and simple preparation instructions, understanding that preparing vegetarian meals can be quick and easy, requiring only basic cooking skills.

Adapt recipes to suit your own needs and tastes. Modify them to add or subtract animal ingredients (like butter, milk, and eggs) using information in Chapter 8 and throughout the book.

Assess recipes to determine what you liked, what you didn't like, and ideas for changes you'd like to try the next time you make them.

Chapter 9

Beyond Cereal and Toast: Whipping Up Breakfast Basics

Although breakfast for many people is a bagel or glass of juice as they run out the door, eating a nutritious meal in the morning doesn't have to take a lot of planning or preparation. That's fortunate, because breakfast is important. It gives you an energy lift as you start your day and helps you stay alert and perform your best.

Some good vegetarian and fuss-free options include a bowl of cereal with milk, a piece of fruit, a cup of yogurt, or toast and jam. When you do have more time to prepare a meal in the morning, making something a little more substantial can be fun. You can make most breakfast classics, including breakfast breads and egg dishes, in a variety of ways to include as many or as few animal ingredients as you care to eat.

I include several examples in this chapter to get you started.

Cucumber Lemon Infused Water

INGREDIENTS

1 medium cucumber

1 large lemon

32 ounces (one quart) of cold, filtered water

DIRECTIONS

1 Rinse the lemon and unpeeled cucumber under running water. Leaving skins and peels on, slice each into ¼ inch rounds. Set aside 4 or 5 slices each of lemons and cucumbers, removing and discarding any large lemon seeds that may be loose and ready to fall out.

2 Place lemon and cucumber slices into the bottom of the carafe or pitcher. Fill with water up to within 1 to 2 inches of the top. Measurements do not have to be precise; using more or fewer lemon or cucumber slices, or more or less water, does not substantially change the quality of the result.

3 Chill for at least one hour before serving. Water can be kept fresh in the refrigerator for about one day.

PER SERVING: *Calories 6 (From Fat 1); Fat 0g (Saturated 0g); Cholesterol 0mg; Sodium 1mg; Carbohydrate 3g (Dietary Fiber 1g); Protein 0g.*

TIP: Fill a clear glass carafe or pitcher with this freshly flavored water for an inviting beverage that complements most any meal, any time of day. Set it out on the table, chilled, and consider keeping extra on hand in the refrigerator to encourage healthful, calorie-free hydration throughout the day.

VARY IT! Add several sprigs of fresh mint leaves, or substitute lime slices in lieu of cucumbers. Don't be afraid to experiment. Try fresh strawberries, rosemary sprigs, freshly grated ginger, orange slices, kiwi slices, fresh cranberries or blueberries . . .

GETTING OFF TO A SMOOTHIE START

Unlike their cousin the milkshake, smoothies made with fresh fruit and either nonfat milk or plant alternatives are low in calories and saturated fat and contain no cholesterol. They take only minutes to make in a blender and make a refreshing and convenient take-and-go breakfast alternative. I include two examples here — use your imagination to create other variations.

TIP

Vegans can replace frozen yogurt with plant-based alternatives available in natural foods stores. Ice cubes, crushed in blending, improve the mouth feel or texture of smoothies, making them frostier.

Very Berry Smoothie

INGREDIENTS

1 cup vanilla soymilk or other plant milk

½ ripe banana

1 cup frozen mixed berries (strawberries, blackberries, blueberries, and raspberries)

2 tablespoons pure maple syrup

DIRECTIONS

1 Place all the ingredients in a blender.

2 Blend on high speed for about 1 minute or until smooth, stopping every 15 seconds to scrape the sides of the blender with a spatula and to push the solid ingredients down to the bottom of the blender.

3 Pour into a tall (16-ounce) tumbler or two smaller (8-ounce) glasses and serve immediately with a long-handled spoon and a straw.

PER SERVING: *Calories 190 (From Fat 27); Fat 3g (Saturated 0g); Cholesterol 0mg; Sodium 63mg; Carbohydrate 39g (Dietary Fiber 3g); Protein 4g.*

TIP: Rich purple jewel tones dotted with tiny black flecks create a light, attractive refreshment. Serve this smoothie in a clear glass to show off the pretty colors. This one's a crowd-pleaser, so if you have company, plan to multiply the recipe.

Orange Juice Smoothie

INGREDIENTS

1 cup orange juice

2 cups frozen nonfat vanilla yogurt or plant-based yogurt

½ cup fresh orange sections (remove every bit of peel and white membrane — see Figure 9-1 for instructions)

1 teaspoon pure vanilla extract

5 or 6 ice cubes

Sprig of fresh mint, for garnish (optional)

DIRECTIONS

1 Place all the ingredients in a blender.

2 Blend on high speed for about 1 minute or until smooth, stopping every 15 seconds to scrape the sides of the blender with a spatula and to push the solid ingredients down to the bottom of the blender. Thin the mixture as needed with a little more orange juice until it reaches the desired consistency.

3 Pour into two tall (16-ounce) tumblers and garnish with fresh mint (if desired). Serve immediately with long-handled spoons and straws.

PER SERVING: *Calories 304 (From Fat 0); Fat 0g (Saturated 0g); Cholesterol 0mg; Sodium 132mg; Carbohydrate 65g (Dietary Fiber 1g); Protein 9g.*

NOTE: This delicious drink is reminiscent of the orange Creamsicles some of us enjoyed in summers past.

VARY IT! The fresh orange tastes great in this recipe, but you can leave it out if it's too much work or if you happen to be out of oranges.

Sectioning an Orange to Eliminate Membranes

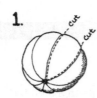

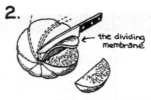

1.

2.

cut

cut

the dividing
membrane

FIGURE 9-1:
The easy way to
remove the white
membranes of
an orange.

Illustration by Elizabeth Kurtzman

On the Light Side

If you prefer to scoop and munch your breakfast instead of drinking it, you can still keep it light and quick with fresh fruit and yogurt. Here I suggest a sweet, hydrating cut fruit salad with the pleasing aroma of fresh mint. Pair it with a layered yogurt parfait or try a little cross-over action: Add a dollop of yogurt to a dish of fruit salad or add a scoop of fruit salad to your yogurt parfait. It's morning, and you are in command of the day.

Minty Melon and Berry Salad

INGREDIENTS

1 cup cubed honeydew melon

1 cup cubed watermelon

1 cup cubed cantaloupe

1 cup mixture of blueberries, raspberries, and blackberries

3 or 4 fresh mint leaves, torn into small pieces

DIRECTIONS

1 Dump the melon and berries into a medium-sized bowl. Add the mint.

2 Stir gently with a wooden spoon or rubber spatula to distribute and mix the fruit and mint leaves.

3 Cover and chill for at least two hours before serving.

PER SERVING: *Calories 64 (From Fat 3); Fat 0g (Saturated 0g); Cholesterol 0mg; Sodium 16mg; Carbohydrate 16g (Dietary Fiber 2g); Protein 1g.*

NOTE: If you make this salad the night before, the fresh mint leaves infuse the fruit with their sweetness and delicious aroma.

TIP: This simple salad is good any time of day as a side dish with a sandwich, tossed into a green salad, or as a light dessert. Eat a bowlful or add a scoop to a bowl of cereal or yogurt for breakfast. Pack leftovers for a mid-morning snack at work or school.

TIP: If you can't find fresh mint off season, check to see if there is an Indian food market in your neighborhood. Indian grocers often stock mint year-round in bulk.

Yogurt Parfait

INGREDIENTS

¾ cup low-fat vanilla yogurt or plant-based yogurt, divided

½ cup mixed berries, divided

⅓ cup granola

Dash of ground cinnamon

DIRECTIONS

1 Spoon about ¼ cup of yogurt into the bottom of a 12-ounce clear glass goblet, jar, or bowl. Add half of the berries on top of the yogurt, then top the berries with half of the granola. Don't worry about smoothing out the layers.

2 Add another ¼ cup of yogurt on top of the berry and granola layers. Top this with the last half of the berries, followed by the last half of the granola.

3 Spoon the remaining yogurt on top, and sprinkle with a dash of cinnamon. Eat immediately or chill overnight.

PER SERVING: *Calories 314 (From Fat 46); Fat 5g (Saturated 1g); Cholesterol 0mg; Sodium 112mg; Carbohydrate 63g (Dietary Fiber 5g); Protein 8g.*

TIP: For this easy breakfast alternative, layer yogurt, fruit, and granola in a clear glass container to make a visually appealing and convenient one-dish meal. If you assemble it the night before, the granola will soften and the flavors will blend together — morning comfort food!

VARY IT! Free-style it and use whatever ingredients, including fresh, seasonal fruit, you have on hand to create variations. Unsweetened, unflavored or coconut yogurt work as well as vanilla. Consider adding sliced almonds. A dash of nutmeg or cardamon is a tasty alternative to cinnamon.

CHOOSING YOGURT

Supermarkets carry an eye-popping range of yogurt choices. What to buy is largely a matter of personal preference. There are many plant-based varieties available made from coconut milk, soymilk, and other plant milks. Dairy varieties may be fat-free, low-fat, or made from whole milk. Greek style yogurt is strained and contains less water, so the yogurt is denser in consistency compared to regular varieties.

Of course, you can also make your own yogurt very simply at home. Check online or in kitchen or electronics stores for electric yogurt makers. They range in price from about $25 to $50 and generally are convenient, easy to use, and make delicious homemade yogurt. You actually can make homemade yogurt quite easily without any special equipment. Search the Internet, and you'll find plenty of easy-to-follow recipes.

WARNING

Be aware that some brands of yogurt contain gelatin, an animal-derived ingredient that vegetarians avoid. Read labels carefully. Some yogurts are thickened using agar-agar or pectin instead, which are plant-based and serve the same purpose as gelatin in yogurt.

REMEMBER

Most varieties of yogurt work well in cold dishes such as yogurt parfaits or cold, creamy soups made with yogurt. However, if you plan to heat the yogurt to make a sauce, experiment first. Some varieties of yogurt, especially those made from plant milk and nonfat cow's milk, may separate when heated.

Using Tofu to Take the Place of Eggs

A big surprise to many people who are new to vegetarianism is that tofu works wonderfully as a stand-in for eggs in certain recipes. Although it can't take the place of an egg fried sunny side up, tofu can hold its own as an egg substitute in many other ways.

You can mix tofu with spices and fry it in a skillet with sliced onions and bell peppers to make a tasty variation of traditional scrambled eggs. With toast and hash browns, it makes a hearty and healthful breakfast alternative. Tofu also works wonderfully as an egg substitute in quiche.

Scrambled Tofu

INGREDIENTS

2 tablespoons olive oil

1 medium onion, chopped

2 teaspoons minced garlic

2 cups bell pepper strips
(green, red, yellow, or mixed)

2 (12-ounce) firm tofu bricks

½ teaspoon black pepper

1 teaspoon turmeric

1 tablespoon soy sauce

Salt to taste

DIRECTIONS

1 Heat the olive oil in a large skillet. Over medium heat, cook the onion, garlic, and bell peppers, stirring occasionally, until the onions are translucent and the peppers are soft — about 8 minutes.

2 Crumble the tofu into the onion–bell peppers mixture. Add the black pepper, turmeric, and soy sauce, and mix everything together with a wooden spoon or spatula. Heat thoroughly for about 2 minutes, mixing and scrambling the ingredients continuously.

PER SERVING: *Calories 149 (From Fat 90); Fat 10g (Saturated 1g); Cholesterol 0mg; Sodium 547mg; Carbohydrate 11g (Dietary Fiber 3g); Protein 8g.*

NOTE: Tofu picks up the flavors with which it's cooked, so this dish tastes very much like its egg counterpart — a savory blend of onions, bell peppers, and spices. Turmeric gives the dish its yellow hue and helps the tofu stand in for eggs.

TIP: Serve this dish hot with Seasoned Home Fries (see Chapter 11), whole-grain toast, and juice. You can also serve it hot or cold as a sandwich filling in a pita pocket or on a kaiser roll.

Putting a Vegetarian Spin on Breakfast Favorites

Pancakes, French toast, hot cereal, fresh cinnamon rolls, and other breakfast staples have always been vegetarian, but you can give these everyday foods a twist that most nonvegetarians don't. Health-conscious vegetarians often prefer to use whole grains, add such extras as dried fruit and nuts, and substitute nondairy alternatives for fatty dairy products to cut down on saturated fat, cholesterol, and animal protein. Taste for yourself.

Mom's Healthy Pancakes

PREP TIME: 10 MINUTES	COOK TIME: 5 MINUTES PER BATCH	YIELD: 6 SERVINGS (ABOUT TWELVE 5-INCH PANCAKES)

INGREDIENTS

1 cup whole-wheat flour

½ cup white flour

⅓ cup wheat germ

1 teaspoon baking soda

1 teaspoon cinnamon

1 tablespoon baking powder

½ teaspoon salt

1¾ cups skim milk or plant milk

¼ cup vegetable oil plus 1 or 2 tablespoons to grease the skillet

1 egg

2 egg whites, beaten stiff (see tip)

DIRECTIONS

1 Measure the dry ingredients into a medium-sized bowl.

2 Add the milk, oil, and whole egg, and stir well using a whisk. Break up any remaining chunks of flour by using the back of a spoon.

3 Fold in the beaten egg whites with a wooden spoon or rubber spatula. The batter will be thick but light and somewhat foamy.

4 Generously oil a griddle and heat it until a drop of water spatters when flicked onto the pan.

5 Pour the batter by ⅓-cup measures onto the hot, oiled skillet. When the pancakes are bubbly all over and the edges are browned, turn them over and cook for about 30 seconds, or until the undersides are browned. Serve immediately.

PER SERVING: Calories 253 (From Fat 99); Fat 11g (Saturated 2g); Cholesterol 37mg; Sodium 461mg; Carbohydrate 30g (Dietary Fiber 4g); Protein 10g.

TIP: Egg whites are beaten stiff when they've thickened enough to form a peak when you pull the beaters out of the bowl. If you keep beating egg whites past this point, they can collapse and become thin again. The key is to stop beating when you notice that the whites are forming soft peaks that can stand up on their own.

TIP: These pancakes are fluffy yet hearty. As kids, my siblings and I simply called them "Healthies," and we'd beg my mother to make a batch on weekend mornings. Make these pancakes as soon as possible after mixing the batter, because the leavening action of the baking powder begins as soon as it mixes with the liquid ingredients. Batter left too long will begin to lose its leavening power and can result in flat, dense pancakes. Leftover pancakes keep well in the refrigerator or freezer, and you can reheat them in the microwave oven.

Fruited Oatmeal

| PREP TIME: 5 MINUTES | COOK TIME: 5 MINUTES | YIELD: 2 SERVINGS (1 CUP EACH) |

INGREDIENTS

1¾ cup water

1 cup quick-cooking rolled oats

½ Granny Smith apple, peeled and finely diced

2 tablespoons chopped walnuts or pecans

1 teaspoon cinnamon, plus extra for dusting

2 tablespoons brown sugar, divided

DIRECTIONS

1 Bring the water to a boil in a medium-sized saucepan.

2 Add the oats and boil for 1 minute, stirring constantly.

3 Add the apple, nuts, and cinnamon, and cook on low heat for an additional 2 to 3 minutes, or until heated through. The mixture will be thick and creamy.

4 Remove from the heat and ladle into serving bowls. Top each serving with a dusting of cinnamon and 1 tablespoon of brown sugar.

PER SERVING: *Calories 273 (From Fat 72); Fat 8g (Saturated 1g); Cholesterol 0mg; Sodium 13mg; Carbohydrate 48g (Dietary Fiber 6g); Protein 6g.*

TIP: For softer apples, add the apples with the water in Step 1. Then add the oats and the remaining ingredients and cook as directed.

TIP: This recipe is very simple, but the tartness of the Granny Smith apples makes it special. Expect an oatmeal-like texture with a bit of crunch from the nuts and some sweetness added by the apples and brown sugar. You can eat this oatmeal as is, but it's delicious served with vanilla soymilk on top.

Favorite Cinnamon Rolls

PREP TIME: 45 MINUTES, PLUS 1 HOUR AND 45 MINUTES FOR DOUGH TO RISE	COOK TIME: 20 MINUTES	YIELD: 24 ROLLS

INGREDIENTS

Rolls:

1 cup whole-wheat flour

3 cups unbleached all-purpose flour, divided

1 package (¼ ounce) active dry yeast

1 cup unsweetened plant milk or nonfat milk

¾ cup sugar, divided

¼ cup vegetable oil

1 teaspoon salt

4 egg whites

¼ cup margarine

2 teaspoons cinnamon

Glaze:

1 cup powdered sugar

½ teaspoon pure vanilla extract

2 tablespoons plant milk or nonfat milk, divided

DIRECTIONS

1   In a large mixing bowl, combine the whole-wheat flour, 1 cup of the all-purpose flour, and the yeast. Set aside.

2   Combine the milk, ¼ cup of the sugar, the oil, and the salt in a saucepan and heat on low until warm (no more than 110 degrees, or just warm to the touch). Stir to blend, and then add to the flour and yeast mixture. Whisk in the egg whites.

3   Beat on high speed for about 4 minutes, stopping occasionally to scrape down the sides.

4   Stir in enough (most) of the remaining all-purpose flour to make a stiff dough.

5   Remove the dough from the mixing bowl and set it on a floured surface. Knead the dough for about 10 minutes, adding more flour by the tablespoon as needed to prevent sticking. When you're finished kneading, the dough should be smooth and elastic.

6   Set the dough in an oiled bowl, and then turn it to oil the top of the dough ball. Cover with a towel or waxed paper and let it rise in a warm place until doubled in size — about 1 hour.

7   After the dough has doubled, punch it down and divide it into two pieces. Roll each piece of dough into a rectangle about ¼-inch-thick.

8   Melt the margarine and brush it onto each rectangle of dough. In a small cup, mix the cinnamon and the remaining ½ cup of sugar, and sprinkle the mixture evenly over both rectangles of dough.

(continued)

9 Roll up the rectangles, starting at the widest ends. Pinch the ends shut with your fingers and press the seams into the dough (see Figure 9-2).

10 Cut the rolls into 1-inch pieces, and place the pieces cut side down in two oiled baking dishes or 9-inch round nonstick pans. Cover each dish with a towel or waxed paper, and let the rolls rise in a warm place until doubled in size — about 45 minutes. Preheat the oven to 375 degrees.

11 Bake for 20 minutes, or until the rolls are slightly browned. Don't overcook.

12 While the rolls are baking, prepare the glaze by mixing the confectioner's sugar, vanilla, and 1 tablespoon of the milk. Add additional milk in increments of 1 teaspoon until the glaze is thick but pourable. Drizzle the glaze over the warm rolls and serve.

PER SERVING: *Calories 164 (From Fat 41); Fat 5g (Saturated 1g); Cholesterol 0mg; Sodium 131mg; Carbohydrate 28g (Dietary Fiber 1g); Protein 3g.*

TIP: These rolls are soft, chewy, and sweet and will fill your home with the welcoming fragrance of cinnamon and freshly baked bread. Egg whites replace whole eggs in this version to reduce saturated fat and cholesterol without sacrificing flavor.

VARY IT! Add ½ cup chopped walnuts, raisins, or currants to the filling in Step 8.

ASSEMBLING FAVORITE CINNAMON ROLLS

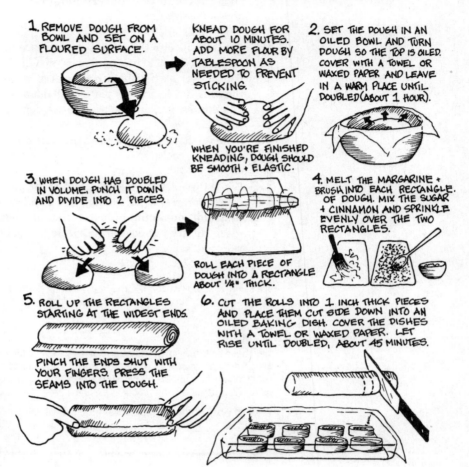

1. REMOVE DOUGH FROM BOWL AND SET ON A FLOURED SURFACE.

KNEAD DOUGH FOR ABOUT 10 MINUTES. ADD MORE FLOUR BY TABLESPOON AS NEEDED TO PREVENT STICKING.

WHEN YOU'RE FINISHED KNEADING, DOUGH SHOULD BE SMOOTH + ELASTIC.

2. SET THE DOUGH IN AN OILED BOWL AND TURN DOUGH SO THE TOP IS OILED. COVER WITH A TOWEL OR WAXED PAPER AND LEAVE IN A WARM PLACE UNTIL DOUBLED (ABOUT 1 HOUR).

3. WHEN DOUGH HAS DOUBLED IN VOLUME, PUNCH IT DOWN AND DIVIDE INTO 2 PIECES.

ROLL EACH PIECE OF DOUGH INTO A RECTANGLE ABOUT ¼" THICK.

4. MELT THE MARGARINE + BRUSH INTO EACH RECTANGLE OF DOUGH. MIX THE SUGAR + CINNAMON AND SPRINKLE EVENLY OVER THE TWO RECTANGLES.

5. ROLL UP THE RECTANGLES STARTING AT THE WIDEST ENDS.

PINCH THE ENDS SHUT WITH YOUR FINGERS. PRESS THE SEAMS INTO THE DOUGH.

6. CUT THE ROLLS INTO 1 INCH THICK PIECES AND PLACE THEM CUT SIDE DOWN INTO AN OILED BAKING DISH. COVER THE DISHES WITH A TOWEL OR WAXED PAPER. LET RISE UNTIL DOUBLED, ABOUT 45 MINUTES.

FIGURE 9-2: Favorite Cinnamon Rolls are worth the extra effort they require (and they really aren't that difficult to make!).

Illustration by Elizabeth Kurtzman

Vegan French Toast

PREP TIME: 10 MINUTES	COOK TIME: 5 MINUTES PER BATCH	YIELD: 4 SERVINGS

INGREDIENTS

2 large ripe bananas

1 cup unflavored or vanilla plant milk

¼ teaspoon nutmeg

½ teaspoon pure vanilla extract (go ahead and use it even if you're using vanilla plant milk)

1 or 2 tablespoons of vegetable oil to grease the skillet

8 slices multigrain or whole-wheat bread

Powdered sugar

Maple syrup

Sliced kiwi fruit and strawberry halves, for garnish (optional)

DIRECTIONS

1   In a blender or food processor, purée the bananas, plant milk, nutmeg, and vanilla. Pour the mixture into a shallow pan such as a pie tin, cake pan, or 8-x-8-inch baking pan.

2   Generously oil a griddle and heat it until a drop of water spatters when flicked onto the pan.

3   Dip both sides of each slice of bread into the milk mixture, and transfer each slice to the griddle. The first side will take about 2 minutes to brown. Turn gently and carefully, because the bread tends to stick to the griddle. Cook the second side for about 3 minutes.

4   Carefully remove the French toast from the griddle and turn it so that the brown side is face up. Dust each slice with powdered sugar, and serve with a pitcher of warm maple syrup. Garnish with thin slices of kiwi fruit and strawberry halves (if desired).

PER SERVING: *Calories 245 (From Fat 27); Fat 3g (Saturated 0g); Cholesterol 0mg; Sodium 229mg; Carbohydrate 48g (Dietary Fiber 5g); Protein 7g.*

TIP: Bananas and plant milk take the place of eggs in this version of French toast. Don't expect this to look or taste exactly like traditional French toast, but it's an interesting adaptation that's flavorful and nutritious.

Starting Your Day the Miso Way

Miso is a fermented soy condiment — a rich, salty, savory paste — that's a key ingredient in many East Asian dishes, including soups, sauces, gravies, and salad dressings. You can find it in natural foods stores and Asian markets. Although you may not think of using miso at breakfast time, it's a common sight on breakfast tables in Japan, where miso soup is the traditional way to start the day. I provide more information about miso in Chapter 6.

Morning Miso Soup

PREP TIME: LESS THAN 10 MINUTES	COOK TIME: 5 MINUTES	YIELD: 4 SERVINGS

INGREDIENTS

2 cups vegetable broth

2 cups hot water, divided

4 tablespoons miso

1 teaspoon fresh ginger root, grated (optional)

½ cup thinly sliced mushrooms (see Figure 9-3)

½ cup diced firm tofu

3 tablespoons thinly sliced scallion greens

DIRECTIONS

1 Pour the vegetable broth and 1 cup of the hot water into a medium saucepan.

2 In a bowl, dissolve the miso in the remaining 1 cup of hot water. Mix well, and then add to the contents of the saucepan.

3 Add the ginger root (if desired) and mushrooms and heat until simmering — about 5 minutes.

4 Remove from the heat and stir in the tofu and scallion greens. Serve in a mug or bowl.

PER SERVING: Calories 76 (From Fat 27); Fat 3g (Saturated 0g); Cholesterol 0mg; Sodium 1217mg; Carbohydrate 9g (Dietary Fiber 2g); Protein 6g.

TIP: This simple recipe for miso soup takes only minutes to make — quick enough for even the most harried of mornings. A big mugful is comforting at breakfast, but you can eat this soup as a snack or as part of a meal anytime.

How to Trim and Slice Mushrooms

FIGURE 9-3:
Sliced mushrooms are a key ingredient in Morning Miso Soup.

1. 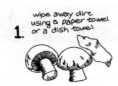 wipe away dirt using a paper towel or a dish towel

2. Cut off stem

3.  slice

Illustration by Elizabeth Kurtzman

Chapter **10**

Serving Simple Starters

Appetizers are versatile. You can eat dips and spreads now or as sandwich fillings tomorrow. You can pack leftover hors d'oeuvres in a bag lunch, or reheat them and serve them with a salad for a quick lunch.

You can also assemble several appetizers on a platter for a sophisticated — and often lighter — alternative to an entrée for dinner. The samples I include in this chapter are tasty, easy to make, and good for you, too.

Making Dips and Spreads

Recipes in this section borrow flavors from around the world. The first, hummus, is perhaps the most popular vegetarian dip. You'll find it on the menu at every Middle Eastern restaurant, and most vegetarian restaurants as well. Many variations exist, but the basic dip is made with garbanzo beans and olive oil, and it's very easy to make.

TIP

Beans, a popular ingredient in many cultures, are a staple in most vegetarian diets. They make great dips because you can purée them to a creamy texture and flavor them with a variety of ingredients. For more information about beans as ingredients in vegetarian cuisine, see Chapter 6.

The other recipes in this section are also tasty and versatile. From the cooling cucumber and dill yogurt dip and guacamole to zippy mango salsa and flavorful roasted garlic spread, these dips and spreads have wide appeal among vegetarians and meat-eaters alike. Use them to add color, flavor, and pleasing texture to your meals.

Basic Hummus with Toasted Pita Points

PREP TIME: ABOUT 10 MINUTES	COOK TIME: 15 MINUTES	YIELD: 8 SERVINGS (¼ CUP EACH)

INGREDIENTS

2 pieces of whole-wheat pita bread, each cut into 12 wedges

1 tablespoon plus 2 teaspoons olive oil, divided

1 (15-ounce) can garbanzo beans, rinsed (about 1¾ cups)

¼ cup water

1 large clove garlic, minced

¼ cup tahini

Juice of 1 large, fresh lemon (about ¼ cup)

¼ teaspoon cumin

½ fresh lemon

Paprika

DIRECTIONS

1 Preheat the oven to 350 degrees. Brush 1 tablespoon of olive oil onto the pita wedges using a pastry brush. Arrange them on a baking sheet and place into the oven.

2 While the pita wedges are browning in the oven, place the garbanzo beans, water, garlic, tahini, lemon juice, and cumin in a blender or food processor and process until smooth and creamy. Scoop into a shallow bowl.

3 Drizzle the remaining olive oil over the hummus, followed by a squeeze of fresh lemon juice and a dusting of paprika.

4 Remove the pita wedges from the oven after about 15 minutes, or when the bread is lightly browned and toasted. (If you prefer warm and chewy pita wedges, start checking the bread after 7 to 10 minutes and remove it sooner.) Arrange the pita wedges around the bowl of hummus for dipping, or serve separately in a small basket or bowl.

PER SERVING: *Calories 146 (From Fat 69); Fat 8g (Saturated 1g); Cholesterol 0mg; Sodium 155mg; Carbohydrate 17g (Dietary Fiber 3g); Protein 5g.*

NOTE: Hummus is a smooth, creamy, garlicky dip or spread made primarily from garbanzo beans, also known as chickpeas or chi chi beans. This healthful dish is popular throughout the Middle East and is typically served in a shallow bowl, drizzled with a few teaspoons of olive oil and fresh lemon juice, with warm wedges of pita bread for dipping.

TIP: You can also serve hummus as a dip for raw vegetables and as a pita pocket filling.

VARY IT! Add 1 roasted red bell pepper or 1 tablespoon chopped fresh dill in Step 1. Increase garlic by 1 or 2 cloves for a greater garlicky punch.

Spicy Black Bean Dip

PREP TIME: 10 MINUTES	COOK TIME: 10 MINUTES	YIELD: 8 SERVINGS (¼ CUP EACH)

INGREDIENTS

1 (15-ounce) can black beans, rinsed

½ cup warm water

½ small onion, minced

2 teaspoons minced garlic

¼ cup mild salsa (optional)

DIRECTIONS

1 Combine the beans and water in a 2-quart saucepan. Cook over medium heat for 2 to 3 minutes, or until the beans are hot.

2 Remove from the heat and mash the beans well with a potato masher or fork. Add the onion and garlic and stir well.

3 Return the mixture to the stovetop and heat on low for 5 minutes, stirring constantly.

4 Stir in the salsa (if desired) and heat until the beans are hot and bubbly. Add more water by the tablespoon, if necessary, until the dip reaches the desired consistency.

5 Remove from the heat and serve.

PER SERVING: Calories 55 (From Fat 9); Fat 1g (Saturated 0g); Cholesterol 0mg; Sodium 218mg; Carbohydrate 10g (Dietary Fiber 4g); Protein 4g.

TIP: This dip has a mild flavor and a smooth, creamy texture. With the salsa added, it works well as a dip for tortilla chips and for raw vegetable pieces such as broccoli and cauliflower florets, baby carrot sticks, and bell pepper strips. Depending on what you have on hand, you can garnish the dip with parsley sprigs, minced green onions or tomatoes, grated cheddar or Jack cheese, a dollop of sour cream or mashed avocado, or any combination of these ingredients. If the dip sets for about 30 minutes, it thickens enough to be used as a filling for burritos or tacos. If you plan to use this as a filling or spread, the salsa is optional.

VARY IT! In this recipe, the onions remain crunchy. If you prefer the onions cooked, sauté them for a few minutes in a teaspoon of olive oil before adding them to the beans in Step 2.

TAHINI

Tahini is a paste made from ground sesame seeds. It has a mild sesame flavor and is used as an ingredient in some dips and salad dressings. You can find tahini at natural foods stores, Middle Eastern and specialty stores, and some supermarkets. It's often sold in a can with a plastic lid or in a jar, like natural peanut butter, with a layer of oil floating on top. Stir in the oil before scooping out the tahini.

Guacamole

INGREDIENTS

1 medium avocado

¼ cup finely diced sweet onion (such as Vidalia)

1 teaspoon minced garlic

2 tablespoons lime juice

2 tablespoons salsa (optional)

DIRECTIONS

1 Cut the avocado in half, remove the seed and peel, and place the meat in a small bowl (see Figure 10-1 for peeling and seeding instructions). Mash the avocado with a potato masher or fork until it's fairly smooth.

2 Add the remaining ingredients and mix well by hand. For a much smoother result, you can purée everything in a blender or food processor. If you do so, however, stir in the salsa by hand after processing.

PER SERVING: *Calories 94 (From Fat 63); Fat 7g (Saturated 1g); Cholesterol 0mg; Sodium 66mg; Carbohydrate 9g (Dietary Fiber 4g); Protein 2g.*

TIP: Enjoy this rich, mildly flavored dip with tortilla chips, spread a layer on a sandwich, or fold some into a burrito. Avocado has a buttery consistency whether you mix the dip by hand or make it smooth in a blender or food processor. Note that you should use this recipe soon after preparation; the dip will turn dark on the surface. You can delay the discoloration by covering the surface of the dip with plastic wrap and keeping it chilled.

How to Pit and Peel an Avocado

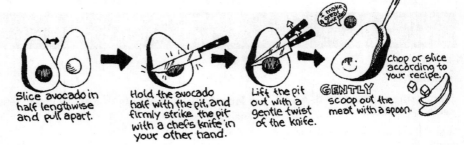

FIGURE 10-1:
Extracting the
meat of an
avocado for
blending into
Guacamole.

Slice avocado in half lengthwise and pull apart.

Hold the avocado half with the pit, and firmly strike the pit with a chef's knife in your other hand.

Lift the pit out with a gentle twist of the knife.

GENTLY scoop out the meat with a spoon.

Chop or slice according to your recipe.

Illustration by Elizabeth Kurtzman

Mango Salsa

PREP TIME: 15 MINUTES (PLUS CHILL TIME)

YIELD: 6 SERVINGS (½ CUP EACH; MAY VARY DEPENDING ON SIZE OF PRODUCE USED)

INGREDIENTS

1 large, ripe mango, pitted, peeled, and diced

½ small cucumber, peeled and finely diced

1 large ripe tomato, seeded and diced

¼ green bell pepper, seeded and chopped

¼ red bell pepper, seeded and chopped

¼ red onion, minced

1 tablespoon finely chopped jalapeño pepper

Juice of 1 large lime

3 tablespoons olive oil

2 tablespoons chopped cilantro (optional)

Salt and pepper

DIRECTIONS

1 Mix all the ingredients in a small bowl. Season to taste with salt and pepper.

2 Cover and chill for at least an hour, and stir before serving.

PER SERVING: *Calories 97 (From Fat 63); Fat 7g (Saturated 1g); Cholesterol 0mg; Sodium 101mg; Carbohydrate 9g (Dietary Fiber 1g); Protein 1g.*

TIP: You may be in the habit of buying bottled salsa from the store, but salsa is quick, easy, and inexpensive to make at home, and you can vary the flavors depending on the ingredients you have on hand. Serve this salsa with black bean burritos, as a relish on veggie burgers, or with your favorite tortilla chips.

VARY IT! Add sliced avocado or fresh pineapple chunks. Adjust the amount of jalapeño peppers to accommodate preferences for mild, medium, or hot salsa.

Cucumber and Dill Yogurt Dip

| PREP TIME: 10 MINUTES (PLUS CHILL TIME) | YIELD: 6 SERVINGS (¼ CUP EACH) |

INGREDIENTS

½ medium cucumber, peeled and finely chopped (see Figure 10-2)

1 large clove garlic, minced

1 tablespoon fresh dill, chopped

1 (8-ounce) carton nonfat, unflavored yogurt

DIRECTIONS

1 Scoop the yogurt into a small bowl. Add the cucumbers, garlic, and dill, and stir to mix the ingredients.

2 Cover and chill for at least an hour before serving.

PER SERVING: *Calories 24 (From Fat 1); Fat 0g (Saturated 0g); Cholesterol 1mg; Sodium 30mg; Carbohydrate 4g (Dietary Fiber 0g); Protein 2g.*

TIP: You serve this dip cold with whole-grain crackers, toasted pita bread points, or fresh vegetable sticks. It's similar to Greek tzatziki sauce or Indian raita — both yogurt-based dips — so it makes a good accompaniment to spinach pie (Greek spanakopita) and spicy Indian entrees. You can also use it to top a bean burrito or a baked potato!

VARY IT! Get creative. Instead of dill, try using fresh cilantro and a dash of cumin, or omit the garlic and substitute fresh mint for dill. Adding salt and pepper to taste or a squeeze of fresh lemon are also good options.

CHOPPING A CUCUMBER

1. WASH AND PEEL THE CUCUMBER USING A VEGETABLE PEELER (OPTIONAL).

2. SLICE OFF ABOUT ½" OF THE ENDS OF THE CUCUMBER

3. FOR CUCUMBER ROUNDS, MAKE EVEN, ⅛" SLICES WITH A FRENCH KNIFE.

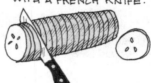

4. TO CHOP CUCUMBER INTO SMALLER PIECES, FIRST CUT LENGTHWISE. SLICE EACH HALF INTO SEVERAL LONG STRIPS, THEN SLICE THE STRIPS INTO PIECES.

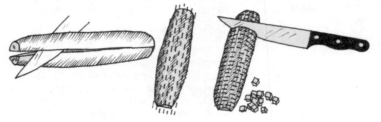

FIGURE 10-2: Chop the cucumber into small pieces.

Illustration by Elizabeth Kurtzman

Roasted Garlic Spread

PREP TIME: 1 MINUTE	COOK TIME: 1 HOUR	YIELD: 4 SERVINGS

INGREDIENTS

1 large garlic bulb

2 teaspoons olive oil

DIRECTIONS

1 Preheat the oven to 350 degrees.

2 Pull the outer, loose layers of tissue off the garlic bulb, leaving enough so that the cloves remain intact.

3 With a sharp knife, cut off the top of the bulb (about ¼ inch of the top — see Figure 10-3) to expose the tops of the cloves inside. Drizzle the tops of the cloves with the olive oil.

4 Wrap the bulb loosely in aluminum foil, seal the foil completely, and place in the hot oven.

5 Bake for about 1 hour, or until the cloves are soft. Remove from the oven.

6 Place the garlic bulb on a small serving dish. Lift the cloves out of the bulb with a dinner knife and smear the softened garlic on French bread rounds or homemade rolls. If the cloves are hard to spread, squeeze the bulb to loosen them.

PER SERVING: *Calories 20 (From Fat 9); Fat 1g (Saturated 0g); Cholesterol 0mg; Sodium 1mg; Carbohydrate 2g (Dietary Fiber 0g); Protein 0g.*

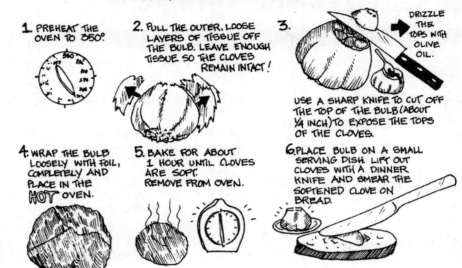

PREPARING ROASTED GARLIC

1. PREHEAT THE OVEN TO 350°.

2. PULL THE OUTER, LOOSE LAYERS OF TISSUE OFF THE BULB. LEAVE ENOUGH TISSUE SO THE CLOVES REMAIN INTACT!

3. DRIZZLE THE TOPS WITH OLIVE OIL.

USE A SHARP KNIFE TO CUT OFF THE TOP OF THE BULB (ABOUT ¼ INCH) TO EXPOSE THE TOPS OF THE CLOVES.

4. WRAP THE BULB LOOSELY WITH FOIL, COMPLETELY AND PLACE IN THE HOT OVEN.

5. BAKE FOR ABOUT 1 HOUR UNTIL CLOVES ARE SOFT. REMOVE FROM OVEN.

6. PLACE BULB ON A SMALL SERVING DISH. LIFT OUT CLOVES WITH A DINNER KNIFE AND SMEAR THE SOFTENED CLOVE ON BREAD.

FIGURE 10-3:
Roasted Garlic Spread is easy to prepare and fun to serve.

Illustration by Elizabeth Kurtzman

Creating Other Easy Appetizers

Bite-sized portions of many foods — pizza, sandwiches, and spinach pie, for example — lend themselves to serving as hors d'oeuvres or simple starters before a meal. Following are five more examples of meatless appetizers with widespread appeal.

Bruschetta with Fresh Basil and Tomatoes

PREP TIME: 10 MINUTES	COOK TIME: 8 MINUTES	YIELD: 6 SERVINGS

INGREDIENTS

6 chunky, half-inch-thick oval slices of rustic white bread

3 medium, ripe tomatoes, chopped (discard any clumps of seeds)

¼ cup high-quality, extra-virgin olive oil

8 to 10 fresh basil leaves, torn into small pieces

Coarsely ground salt and coarsely ground pepper

1 clove garlic, peeled and sliced in half

Freshly grated or shaved Parmesan cheese

DIRECTIONS

1 Preheat the oven to 400 degrees. Arrange bread slices on an ungreased baking tray.

2 Toast the bread in the oven for 3 to 4 minutes or until just lightly browned. Using kitchen tongs, turn the bread slices and toast them on the other side for another 3 to 4 minutes, until just lightly browned. While the bread is toasting, prepare the other ingredients.

3 Toss the tomatoes, olive oil, and basil in a medium-sized bowl, adding salt and pepper to taste. Set aside.

4 Remove the bread from the oven. Rub the fronts and backs of the bread slices with fresh garlic.

5 Arrange bread slices on a serving platter. Spoon tomato mixture evenly over the bread. Don't worry if some of the tomato falls between the bread slices.

6 Sprinkle lightly with Parmesan cheese or additional salt or pepper to taste.

PER SERVING: *Calories 444 (From Fat 208); Fat 23g (Saturated 7g); Cholesterol 21mg; Sodium 665mg; Carbohydrate 45g (Dietary Fiber 4g); Protein 15g.*

TIP: At its simplest, bruschetta is a quick, light, flavorful and healthful appetizer that adds color and the intoxicating aroma of fresh basil to the table. It is meant to be an informal assembly of a very few, fresh ingredients. No recipe needed; no need to be precise. Use this recipe as a guide, but by all means experiment with your own variations.

VARY IT! Add 1 teaspoon of black olive tapenade or sun-dried tomatoes to tops of the slices.

Grilled Vegetable Quesadilla

PREP TIME: 15 MINUTES	COOK TIME: 15 MINUTES	YIELD: 4 SERVINGS AS AN APPETIZER, OR 2 SERVINGS AS A LIGHT MEAL

INGREDIENTS

½ cup chopped broccoli florets

¼ cup grated carrots

¼ cup chopped onion

½ cup chopped zucchini squash

¼ cup red or yellow bell peppers, seeded and chopped

Salt and pepper (optional)

4 tablespoons olive oil, divided

2 (10-inch) whole-wheat flour tortillas

¾ cup grated, reduced-fat Jack cheese or cheddar and Jack cheese mixture, divided

Salsa; unflavored, nonfat yogurt; or reduced-fat sour cream and sliced black olives, for garnish (optional)

DIRECTIONS

1 Place the broccoli, carrots, onions, zucchini, and bell peppers in a glass bowl. Add 2 teaspoons of water, cover, and heat in a microwave oven for 3 to 5 minutes, until tender. Drain and set aside. Salt and pepper to taste (if desired).

2 Smear 2 tablespoons of olive oil on the bottom of a large skillet. Place a flour tortilla into the skillet.

3 Sprinkle half the cheese evenly on top of the flour tortilla, and then distribute steamed vegetables evenly on top of the cheese. Top the vegetables with the remaining cheese.

4 Top with second flour tortilla. Brush the top of the second tortilla with remaining olive oil.

5 Cook on medium heat. After several minutes, lift the edge of the bottom quesadilla with a spatula to check for doneness. When the bottom tortilla appears lightly browned and the cheese is melted (about 5 to 7 minutes), carefully turn the quesadilla over and cook for an additional 2 or 3 minutes, until the other side is lightly browned.

6 Remove from the heat and cut into wedges for serving. Top with a scoop of salsa, a dollop of yogurt or sour cream, and sliced black olives.

PER SERVING: *Calories 263 (From Fat 176); Fat 20g (Saturated 5g); Cholesterol 15mg; Sodium 91mg; Carbohydrate 15g (Dietary Fiber 2g); Protein 8g. Analyzed for 4.*

TIP: Cut quesadilla into wedges and serve as an appetizer with Mango Salsa (see the recipe earlier in this chapter). These also make a quick meal that kids love. Serve half of a large quesadilla with a small green salad for a light lunch or supper.

VARY IT! Substitute ¾ cup cooked, drained, chopped spinach for the vegetables to make a spinach quesadilla.

Stuffed Mushrooms

PREP TIME: 15 MINUTES	COOK TIME: 25 MINUTES	YIELD: 6 SERVINGS (3 MUSHROOMS EACH)

INGREDIENTS

18 medium white mushrooms (about 1 pound)

2 tablespoons olive oil

1 small onion, minced (about ½ cup)

2 cloves garlic, minced

½ cup breadcrumbs

1 teaspoon dried oregano

¼ cup chopped fresh parsley

¼ cup grated Parmesan cheese (optional)

Salt and black pepper

Fresh rosemary or basil sprigs, for garnish

DIRECTIONS

1 Preheat the oven to 375 degrees.

2 Rinse and pat the mushrooms to dry them. Trim off the bottoms of stems. Separate the stems from the mushroom caps to create a small crater in the bottom of each cap. Chop the stems finely and set aside.

3 In a medium skillet, add olive oil and sauté the mushroom stems, onions, and garlic on medium heat until the onions are translucent, about 5 minutes. Stir in the breadcrumbs, oregano, parsley, and cheese (if desired). Season with salt and pepper.

4 Distribute the filling equally among mushroom caps, pressing lightly to set filling into each cap.

5 Place mushroom caps on an oiled baking sheet. Bake for about 20 minutes, or until the mushrooms are hot. Remove from the baking sheet and place on a serving dish. Garnish with fresh rosemary or basil sprigs.

PER SERVING: Calories 97 (From Fat 47); Fat 5g (Saturated 1g); Cholesterol 0mg; Sodium 179mg; Carbohydrate 11g (Dietary Fiber 1g); Protein 3g.

TIP: This appetizer goes well with Bruschetta with Fresh Basil and Tomatoes (see the recipe earlier in this chapter) and a selection of olives. A mini-chopper or small food processor can make preparation easier and faster.

VARY IT! Experiment with additions to filling mixture. Add a few tablespoons of chopped walnuts or pecans, basil, or sun-dried tomato pesto.

Crispy Kale Chips

PREP TIME: 10 MINUTES | COOK TIME: 20 MINUTES | YIELD: 6 SERVINGS

INGREDIENTS

One large bunch of kale

1 tablespoon olive oil

1 teaspoon coarsely ground salt

DIRECTIONS

1 Preheat the oven to 300 degrees.

2 Thoroughly rinse the whole kale leaves. Cut the kale off the thick stems using a knife or kitchen shears. Cut or tear the leaves into bite-sized pieces. Dry the pieces well by pressing them in paper towels or using a salad spinner.

3 In a large bowl, use a wooden spoon or your clean hands to toss together the kale pieces, olive oil, and salt. Spread the mixture evenly across a large cookie sheet or baking pan.

4 Bake in the oven for about 20 minutes until crispy, taking care not to let the leaves become brown.

PER SERVING: *Calories 42 (From Fat 23); Fat 3g (Saturated 0g); Cholesterol 0mg; Sodium 331mg; Carbohydrate 4g (Dietary Fiber 1g); Protein 1g.*

TIP: These light and crunchy wisps melt in your mouth. They make a great alternative to popcorn as a snack, but you can also serve them as a side with a sandwich or add them to a green salad for texture and flavor. Feel virtuous snacking on them because they are loaded with health-supporting nutrients.

WARNING

Kale chips are super easy to make, but they can also easily flop. The secret to success is three-fold: Be sure the kale pieces are completely dry before baking, and don't add too much oil or the chips will be soggy, not crispy. Finally, don't let them brown; baking them too long will make them bitter.

Rosemary Almonds

PREP TIME: 5 MINUTES	COOK TIME: 25 MINUTES	YIELD: 8 SERVINGS

INGREDIENTS

2 cups whole almonds

1½ tablespoons finely chopped fresh rosemary

1 tablespoon olive oil

1 teaspoon coarsely ground salt

DIRECTIONS

1 Preheat the oven to 325 degrees. Line a large baking pan with aluminum foil or parchment paper.

2 In a small bowl, combine all of the ingredients. Toss to coat the nuts.

3 Spread the nut mixture evenly across the pan. Bake for about 25 minutes or until the nuts are lightly browned. Cool before serving.

PER SERVING: Calories 298 (From Fat 235); Fat 26g (Saturated 2g); Cholesterol 0mg; Sodium 313mg; Carbohydrate 11g (Dietary Fiber 6g); Protein 10g.

TIP: Hard to imagine that something that tastes so good could be so good for you. These are a great party snack, and you can add leftovers to a green salad.

VARY IT! Add a teaspoon of cayenne pepper for a spicy treat, or for a sweet and savory variation, add a couple tablespoons of maple syrup to the nut mixture before baking.

Chapter **11**

Enjoying Easy Soups, Salads, and Sides

Soups, salads, and sides complete a meal by complementing the entrée, adding flavor, texture, and color to the plate. They're versatile, too. Alone, a hearty bowl of soup, generous salad, or side — or any combination of two or more — can make the perfect lunch or dinner. Soup is even on the menu in Chapter 9 — for breakfast!

I love the convenience of soups, salads, and sides, so I keep plenty of the ingredients in my pantry and refrigerator. Use them to add variety to meals and as quick, light meals and snacks by themselves.

Serving Soups for All Seasons

Beans and lentils are the foundations of many filling, nutritious vegetarian soups. High in protein and fiber, they give soups a stick-to-your ribs quality that makes them well suited for the main course at meals. Use canned beans or dried, or try your hand at using a pressure cooker, or a multicooker like an Instant Pot, to soften dried beans more quickly (I include more information about pressure cookers and multicookers in Chapter 8). Recipes in this section include traditional lentil soup; a classic, cold vegetable soup (gazpacho); and chili with a twist, made with raisins and cashews.

Lentil Soup

INGREDIENTS

1¼ cups dried lentils (½ pound)

5 cups water

1 medium onion, chopped

1 teaspoon minced garlic

½ teaspoon salt

½ teaspoon black pepper

2 tablespoons olive oil

1 (16-ounce) can stewed or crushed tomatoes

1 bay leaf

DIRECTIONS

1 Rinse the lentils in a colander or strainer.

2 Combine the lentils, water, onion, garlic, salt, pepper, and olive oil in a large saucepan. Cover and cook on medium–high heat until boiling — about 14 minutes.

3 Stir in the tomatoes and bay leaf.

4 Reduce the heat to low, cover, and let simmer for 45 minutes, or until the lentils are tender.

PER SERVING: *Calories 144 (From Fat 36); Fat 4g (Saturated 1g); Cholesterol 0mg; Sodium 325mg; Carbohydrate 22g (Dietary Fiber 3g); Protein 6g.*

TIP: This soup has a rich, savory flavor, and the lentils cook quickly because of their small size and flat shape. If you have leftover cooked spinach, stir it into this soup to add color and a healthful nutrient boost.

VARY IT! In place of regular crushed tomatoes, try fire-roasted crushed tomatoes. Find them canned or frozen at the grocery store.

Classic Gazpacho

PREP TIME: 15 MINUTES, PLUS TIME FOR BREAD TO MARINATE (AND CHILL) | **YIELD: 5 SERVINGS**

INGREDIENTS

1 slice stale white bread

2 tablespoons red wine vinegar

1 tablespoon olive oil

1 teaspoon minced garlic

1 (28-ounce) can whole peeled tomatoes

½ cup finely chopped onion

1 green bell pepper, finely chopped (see Figure 11-1)

1 medium cucumber, peeled and sliced

¼ teaspoon cayenne pepper

1 teaspoon hot pepper sauce

Juice of 1 medium, fresh lemon (about 2 tablespoons)

Chopped onions, green bell peppers, or croutons, for garnish (optional)

DIRECTIONS

1 Break the bread into small pieces and place it in a small cup or bowl. Pour the vinegar and oil on top and add the garlic. Mash with a fork, and then set aside for at least 30 minutes.

2 Place the bread mixture in a blender and add 1 cup of the liquid from the canned tomatoes, plus the onion, green bell pepper, and cucumber (save a few tablespoons of onion and green bell pepper for garnish). Blend at low speed for 1 minute.

3 Add the remaining tomatoes and juice, cayenne pepper, hot pepper sauce, and lemon juice. Give the mixture a whirl in the blender to break up the whole tomatoes. Chill for at least 2 hours.

4 Garnish (if desired) with a sprinkling of chopped onions, green bell peppers, or croutons and serve.

PER SERVING: *Calories 99 (From Fat 27); Fat 3g (Saturated 0g); Cholesterol 0mg; Sodium 409mg; Carbohydrate 14g (Dietary Fiber 3g); Protein 3g.*

TIP: This spicy Spanish soup is served cold. Many variations exist, from very smooth to chunky. Adjust the heat according to your taste by adding more or less cayenne pepper and hot pepper sauce (this version is relatively mild). The soup's color and taste may vary slightly, depending on the tomatoes you use.

How to Core and Seed a Pepper

FIGURE 11-1: Coring, seeding, and dicing a bell pepper doesn't have to be difficult; just follow these steps.

Illustrations by Elizabeth Kurtzman

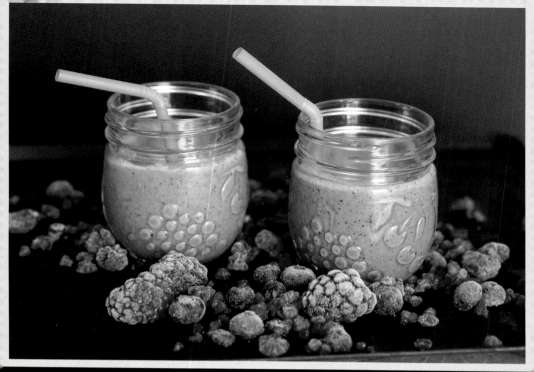

Very Berry Smoothie (Chapter 9)

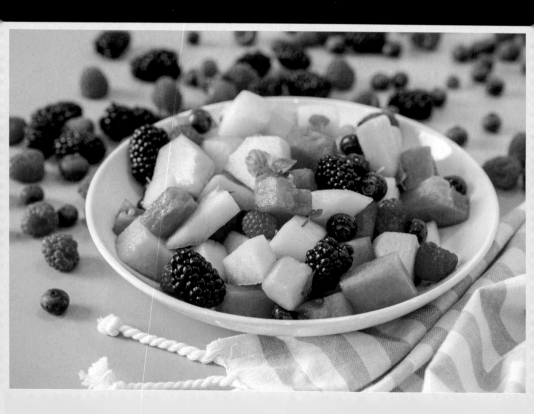

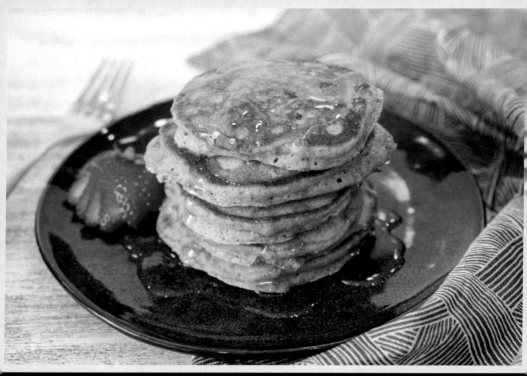

Mom's Healthy Pancakes (Chapter 9)

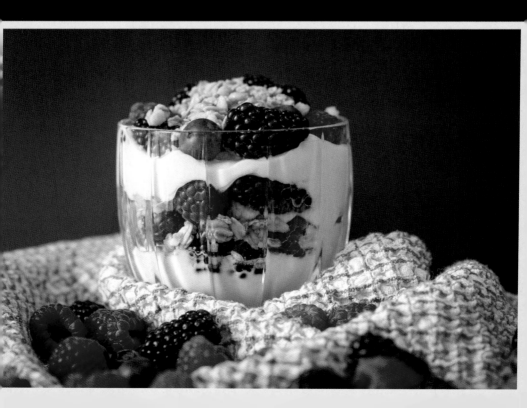

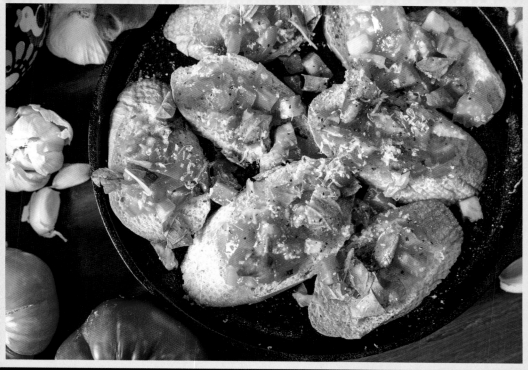

Bruschetta with Fresh Basil and Tomatoes (Chapter 10)

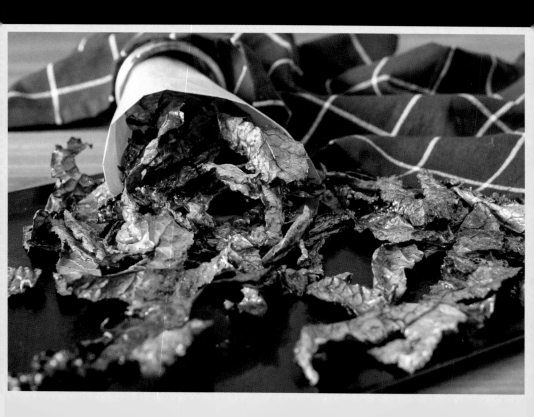

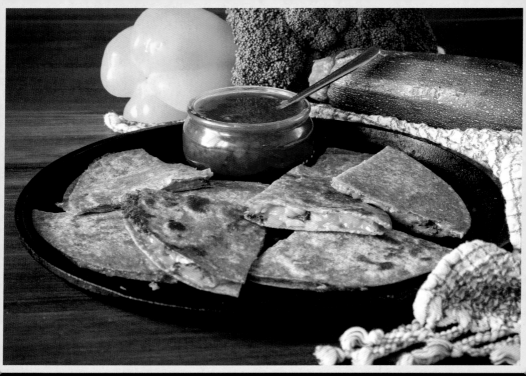

Grilled Vegetable Quesadilla (Chapter 10)

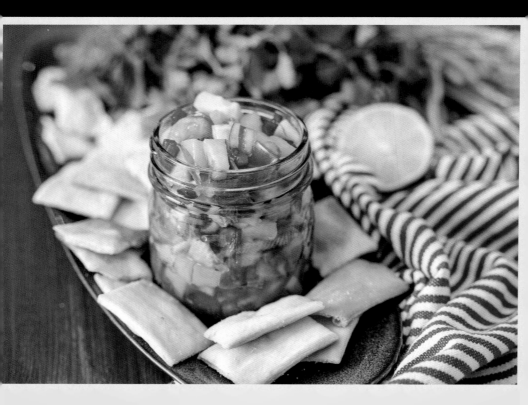

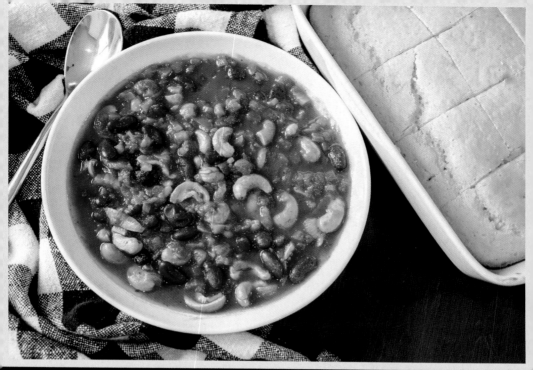

Cashew Chili (Chapter 9) and Easy Cornbread (Chapter 13)

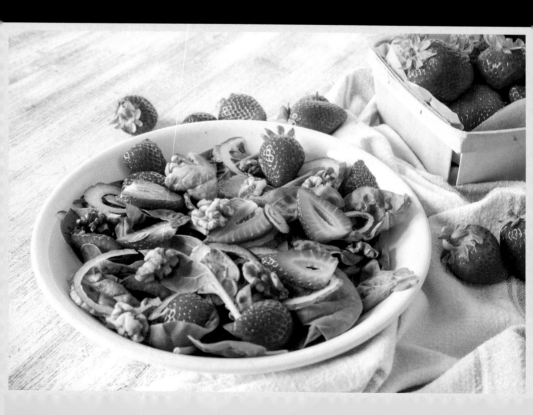

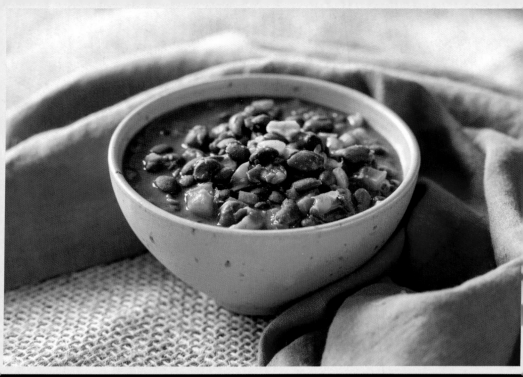

Cuban Black Beans (Chapter 12)

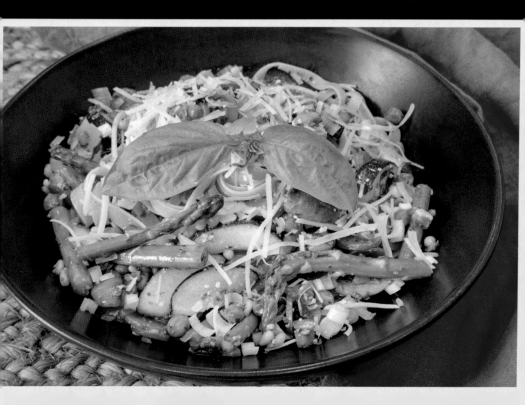

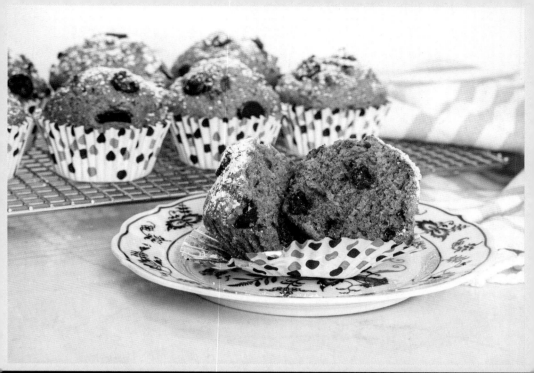

Cocoa Pink Cupcakes (Chapter 14)

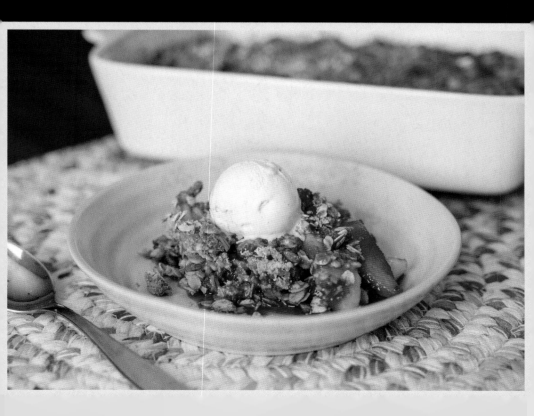

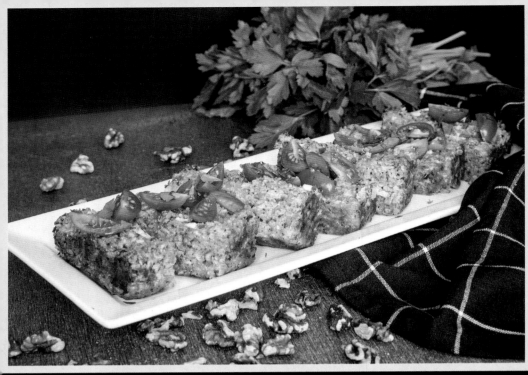

Everybody's Favorite Cheese and Nut Loaf (Chapter 15)

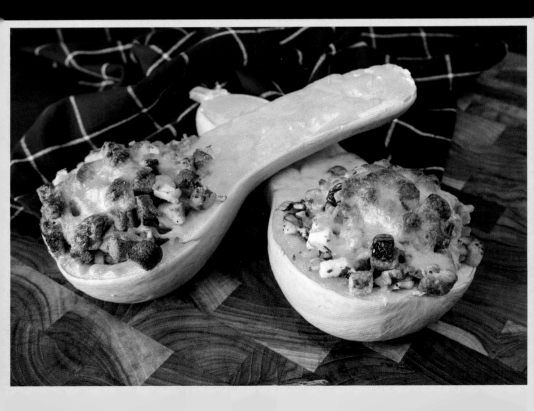

Cashew Chili

PREP TIME: 20 MINUTES	COOK TIME: ABOUT 55 MINUTES	YIELD: 6 LARGE SERVINGS

INGREDIENTS

2 tablespoons olive oil

4 medium onions, chopped

2 large green bell peppers, seeded and chopped

2 stalks celery, minced

4 teaspoons minced garlic

1 teaspoon dried basil

1 teaspoon oregano

½ teaspoon chili powder

1 teaspoon ground cumin

1 teaspoon black pepper

1 (15-ounce) can tomato sauce

1 (16-ounce) can stewed tomatoes or whole peeled tomatoes

2 tablespoons red wine vinegar

1 bay leaf

1 cup cashew pieces

⅓ cup raisins

3 cups cooked dark red kidney beans (two 15-ounce cans)

DIRECTIONS

1   In a large pot, heat the olive oil. Add the onions, bell peppers, and celery and cook over medium heat until the onions are translucent — about 10 minutes.

2   Stir in the garlic, basil, oregano, chili powder, cumin, and pepper.

3   Add the tomato sauce, tomatoes (with their juice), vinegar, and bay leaf. Reduce the heat to low and continue cooking for 2 to 3 minutes.

4   Stir in the cashews and raisins and cook over low heat for another 16 to 17 minutes.

5   Add the beans and cook for an additional 25 minutes, stirring frequently. The chili is done when all the ingredients are well blended and soft and the chili is thick and bubbly.

PER SERVING: *Calories 401 (From Fat 144); Fat 16g (Saturated 3g); Cholesterol 0mg; Sodium 1,067mg; Carbohydrate 57g (Dietary Fiber 11g); Protein 14g.*

NOTE: Raisins add a touch of sweetness to this chili, and cashews add a rich, nutty flavor.

TIP: Serve this Cashew Chili by itself or over steamed rice with cornbread and a green salad on the side. This chili is thick, and it thickens considerably more if left overnight. This is my favorite vegetarian chili of all time. I've been making it to rave reviews for decades.

VARY IT! In place of dark red kidney beans, try using a mixture of garbanzo beans, pinto beans, and red kidney beans for a change of pace. A handful of fresh or frozen corn kernels adds color.

Going Beyond Iceberg Lettuce

Chilled salads made with fresh, seasonal ingredients are palate-pleasing refreshments in summer months and add contrast to the warmth and texture of cooked foods in cold-weather months. These dishes are delicious and very easy to make.

Arugula Salad with Pickled Beets and Candied Pecans

INGREDIENTS

6 ounces goat cheese or chèvre

2 tablespoons freshly ground black pepper for dipping

6 heaping cups arugula, washed, with heavy stems removed

1 cup sliced pickled beets

1 cup candied pecan halves

Vinaigrette dressing

DIRECTIONS

1 Divide the goat cheese or chèvre into 12 portions. Let the cheese sit at room temperature for 10 to 15 minutes, and then roll it into balls.

2 Place the pepper into a small bowl and dip one side of each ball into the pepper.

3 Arrange the arugula on six plates. Cut the beet slices in half, and then distribute the beets and pecans evenly over the arugula. Put two balls of cheese on each plate.

4 Drizzle the salad with your favorite vinaigrette dressing and serve immediately.

PER SERVING: *Calories 351 (From Fat 291); Fat 32g (Saturated 9g); Cholesterol 22mg; Sodium 404mg; Carbohydrate 22g (Dietary Fiber 1g); Protein 9g.*

NOTE: This salad is a delicious and nutritious alternative to mixed green salads. Bottled, pickled beets from your pantry and candied pecans available in many supermarkets make this special salad a snap to assemble.

VARY IT! Vegans omit the goat cheese. Also good: Sprinkle the salad with dried cherries or dried cranberries.

ARUGULA

Arugula, also called *rocket salad* or *roquette,* is a dark, leafy green known for its distinctive sharp, spicy, peppery flavor, similar to that of mustard greens. Arugula is native to the Mediterranean and grows wild throughout southern Europe. You can serve it cooked, but it's most popular as a salad green. Arugula is becoming very popular in the U.S., and you can find it in many supermarkets.

Easy Four-Bean Salad

PREP TIME: 10 MINUTES (PLUS CHILL TIME) | YIELD: 8 TO 10 SERVINGS

INGREDIENTS

1 (15½-ounce) can cut green beans, drained and rinsed

1 (15½-ounce) can cut wax beans, drained and rinsed

1 (15½-ounce) can dark red kidney beans, drained and rinsed

1 (15½-ounce) can garbanzo beans, drained and rinsed

½ cup chopped green bell pepper

½ red onion, chopped

½ cup sugar (or less to taste)

⅔ cup red wine vinegar

⅓ cup vegetable oil (avoid olive oil, as it solidifies in the refrigerator)

½ teaspoon salt

2 teaspoons black pepper

DIRECTIONS

1 Place the green beans, wax beans, kidney beans, garbanzo beans, bell pepper, and onion in a large bowl.

2 Combine the sugar, vinegar, and oil in a small bowl or cup, stir well, and pour over the bean mixture. Add the salt and pepper and toss to coat.

3 Chill overnight. Toss again to coat the beans before serving.

PER SERVING: *Calories 218 (From Fat 88); Fat 10g (Saturated 1g); Cholesterol 0mg; Sodium 399mg; Carbohydrate 29g (Dietary Fiber 5g); Protein 5g.*

TIP: My advice: Double this recipe. It's delicious, and the leftovers taste even better after a day or two in the refrigerator. If you prefer a less sweet salad, reduce the amount of sugar to your taste.

Italian Chopped Salad

INGREDIENTS

1 large head of romaine lettuce, chopped into ½-inch squares

1 cup canned garbanzo beans, rinsed, drained, and chopped

½ medium cucumber, peeled and minced

½ green bell pepper, seeded and finely chopped

½ yellow or orange bell pepper, seeded and finely chopped

2 or 3 radishes, minced

1 stalk celery, finely chopped

½ medium red onion, minced

1 large tomato, seeded and chopped into ¼-inch pieces

2 or 3 tablespoons of finely chopped fresh parsley

⅓ cup chopped black olives

½ cup grated Parmesan cheese or finely chopped, reduced-fat Swiss cheese (optional)

Vinaigrette dressing to taste

Freshly ground black pepper

DIRECTIONS

1 Mix all the vegetables and cheese (if desired) in a salad bowl. Add your favorite Italian or vinaigrette dressing, and toss well.

2 Divide the salad into six bowls and add pepper to taste. Serve immediately.

PER SERVING: *Calories 205 (From Fat 128); Fat 14g (Saturated 3g); Cholesterol 5mg; Sodium 519mg; Carbohydrate 14g (Dietary Fiber 4g); Protein 7g.*

TIP: I love this salad so much that I remember the first time I tried it. It was at a pizza joint in the beach town of Lahaina on the western coast of Maui. Exact proportions or measurements aren't necessary. The key is that you chop everything into tiny pieces. That's what makes this salad so addictive — the texture. You'll eat heaping bowls full of this salad — a good thing, because it's as nutritious as it is delicious.

VARY IT! Use up whatever salad ingredients you have on hand. Finely chopped yellow summer squash or zucchini, banana peppers, grated carrot, and jicama are good in this salad.

Spinach and Strawberry Salad

PREP TIME: 15 MINUTES (PLUS CHILL TIME) | YIELD: 6 LARGESERVINGS

INGREDIENTS

10 ounces (about 9½ cups) of fresh baby spinach leaves, washed and patted or spin-dried

1½ cups fresh, ripe strawberries, sliced

⅓ cup walnut halves

½ small red onion, peeled and sliced into rings

½ cup balsamic vinaigrette dressing or poppyseed dressing, or as desired

DIRECTIONS

1 Place the spinach leaves in a large bowl. Add the strawberries slices, nuts and onion. Toss gently with a wooden spoon or rubber spatula.

2 Chill for at least two hours before serving. Serve with your favorite balsamic vinaigrette dressing or poppyseed dressing.

PER SERVING: *Calories 150 (From Fat 107); Fat 12g (Saturated 2g); Cholesterol 0mg; Sodium 125mg; Carbohydrate 10g (Dietary Fiber 2g); Protein 3g.*

TIP: As a salad favorite that is bright, fresh, and cheerful, it's also full of flavor and nutrition. It keeps in the refrigerator for two to three days.

VARY IT! Leave out the onion if you are not a fan. Add a handful of fresh blueberries if you have them. You can also substitute pecans or sliced almonds for walnuts.

Tofu Salad

PREP TIME: 10 MINUTES (PLUS CHILL TIME) | **YIELD: 6 SERVINGS**

INGREDIENTS

1 pound firm tofu

½ teaspoon salt

½ cup soy mayonnaise

2 teaspoons yellow mustard

½ teaspoon garlic powder

½ teaspoon black pepper

¼ teaspoon turmeric

¼ cup finely chopped celery

2 green onions, finely chopped

DIRECTIONS

1 Mash the tofu with a fork or potato masher until crumbly.

2 Add the salt, mayonnaise, mustard, garlic powder, pepper, and turmeric and mix well.

3 Add the celery and green onions and mix well. Chill before serving.

PER SERVING: *Calories 110 (From Fat 63); Fat 7g (Saturated 1g); Cholesterol 0mg; Sodium 132mg; Carbohydrate 6g (Dietary Fiber 1g); Protein 6g.*

NOTE: If you've never tried tofu salad, you're in for a nice surprise. Many variations exist. This recipe is similar to traditional egg salad, but tofu takes the place of egg whites, and turmeric and mustard provide the color. The result is a mock egg salad that tastes and looks very much like the real thing.

TIP: Serve it as a sandwich filling on bread, crackers, or rolls, or in a pita pocket with grated carrots. This salad also works well served on a bed of salad greens or as stuffing for a fresh, ripe tomato.

On the Side

You can serve any of the soups or salads I include in this chapter as simple side dishes at almost any meal. A small cup of soup on the side of the plate, a scoop of tofu salad, or a handful of green salad serve as nutritious garnishes — a touch of color or cool crunch — at the same time that they round out your meals.

I wrap up this chapter with two popular side dishes that you can serve with a variety of foods.

Tabbouleh

PREP TIME: 30 MINUTES, INCLUDING TIME TO COOK BULGUR WHEAT AND LET IT COOL (PLUS CHILL TIME)

COOK TIME: 10 MINUTES

YIELD: 6 SERVINGS

INGREDIENTS

2 cups water

1 cup bulgur wheat

¼ cup olive oil

Juice of 1 large, fresh lemon (about ¼ cup)

½ teaspoon salt

3 green onions, chopped (white and green parts)

¼ cup chopped fresh mint leaves

½ cup chopped fresh parsley

½ cup canned garbanzo beans, drained and rinsed

2 medium tomatoes, finely chopped

DIRECTIONS

1 Bring the water to a boil in a saucepan. Add the bulgur wheat, reduce the heat to low, cover, and simmer until the bulgur absorbs all the water — about 8 to 10 minutes.

2 Remove the bulgur wheat from the stovetop and set it aside to cool for about 15 minutes.

3 In a medium bowl, combine the cooled bulgur wheat and the remaining ingredients (except the tomatoes) and toss well.

4 Chill the tabbouleh for at least 2 hours before serving. It's best when you chill it overnight. Add tomatoes and toss again just before serving.

PER SERVING: *Calories 238 (From Fat 90); Fat 10g (Saturated 1g); Cholesterol 0mg; Sodium 206mg; Carbohydrate 34g (Dietary Fiber 7g); Protein 5g.*

TIP: Lemon juice gives this Middle Eastern dish its tangy flavor, and mint provides its characteristic fragrance. You can serve tabbouleh as a side dish with sandwiches and burgers, or add it to hummus in a pita pocket.

VARY IT! Reduce the mint (or leave it out entirely) if you're not a fan.

Seasoned Home Fries

| PREP TIME: 10 MINUTES | COOK TIME: 40 MINUTES | YIELD: ABOUT 8 SERVINGS |

INGREDIENTS

Vegetable oil spray or olive oil

6 medium white potatoes (see tip)

Several shakes each of garlic powder, dried oregano, cayenne pepper, and paprika

DIRECTIONS

1 Preheat the oven to 350 degrees.

2 Coat a baking sheet with vegetable oil spray or a thin layer of olive oil.

3 Wash the potatoes. Leaving the peels on, cut the potatoes into wedges and place them in a mixing bowl.

4 Sprinkle the potato wedges with several shakes of each of the spices, more or less to your taste. Toss to coat.

5 Spread the potatoes in a single layer on the baking sheet. Spray the tops with a thin film of vegetable oil spray, or brush with olive oil.

6 Bake for about 40 minutes, or until the potatoes are soft. Serve plain, with ketchup or salsa, or with malt vinegar for dipping.

PER SERVING: Calories 117 (From Fat 9); Fat 1g (Saturated 0g); Cholesterol 0mg; Sodium 6mg; Carbohydrate 26g (Dietary Fiber 2g); Protein 2g.

TIP: Make this recipe with whatever potatoes you have on hand. You can quarter small potatoes. Cut fist-sized potatoes into 6 or 8 wedges each.

NOTE: This is the ultimate easy recipe — you don't have to measure anything, and it comes out great every time. These potatoes are hugely popular with everyone I serve them to, and the leftovers are good reheated. The cayenne pepper and paprika give the potatoes a nice coppery color, but you can leave out or reduce the amount of the cayenne pepper if you like your food less spicy. You can pair this dish with Scrambled Tofu from Chapter 9, or with any sandwich and many entrées.

Chapter **12**

Making Meatless Main Dishes

I f you're new to a vegetarian diet, visualizing meatless meals may be hard at first. Western culture tends to define meals by the meat that's served. Ask some nonvegetarian friends what they're having for dinner tonight, and they're likely to mention the chicken or fish — not the salad or the peas and carrots.

In fact, vegetarian meals often have no main dish or entrée. Instead, vegetarians can make a meal of any number of side dishes. Beans, rice, vegetables, and other foods come together and fill the plate in colorful combinations of healthful, tasty foods.

Who says you need a focal point?

When there is a focal point, vegetarian entrées often resemble meat-based entrées — minus the meat. Lasagna, burritos, and pizza, for example, can all be made meat-free.

Other vegetarian main dishes reflect cuisines from cultures around the world. Delicious stir-fries, bean and rice dishes, and soy foods are some examples I include in this chapter.

Beans: Versatility in a Can

Beans are a staple ingredient that nearly every culture uses. Inexpensive and one of the most nutritious sources of protein, they should be a mainstay on your vegetarian menus. I include two favorite recipes here.

Basic Bean Burrito

INGREDIENTS

2 cups canned vegetarian refried beans, plain mashed pinto beans, or black beans

4 (10-inch) whole-wheat flour tortillas

¼ cup unflavored nonfat yogurt or low-fat sour cream (vegans can use plant-based yogurt or plant-based sour cream alternatives)

1 cup salsa

Chopped tomato, romaine lettuce or spinach, and green onions (any combination, about 1 cup total)

DIRECTIONS

1 In a small saucepan, warm the beans over medium heat until heated through— about 7 minutes.

2 For each burrito, follow these instructions:

3 Lay a tortilla flat on a dinner plate. (Warm it first, if you like, by heating it on each side for a minute or two in a hot skillet). Spoon about ½ cup of the beans onto the center of the tortilla.

4 Fold one end of the tortilla toward the middle, and then fold the sides toward the middle. Leave the burrito on the plate with the end of the fold tucked underneath so that the burrito doesn't unroll (see Figure 12-1).

5 Top with salsa, chopped tomato, greens, and green onion. Add a dollop of yogurt and serve immediately.

PER SERVING: *Calories 275 (From Fat 41); Fat 5g (Saturated 0g); Cholesterol 0mg; Sodium 197mg; Carbohydrate 45g (Dietary Fiber 6g); Protein 14g.*

TIP: You can doctor up this burrito anyway you like, but here's a bare-bones version that virtually everyone loves. If you use whole beans, mash them with a potato masher or fork and mix them until they're smooth in consistency. Cheese eaters can add a couple tablespoons of grated, low-fat cheddar cheese or plant-based cheese alternative to the topping if desired.

VARY IT! Express yourself by adding banana or jalapeño peppers, sliced black olives, sliced avocado, mashed sweet potatoes, strips of cooked tempeh . . . or whatever suits your fancy.

Cuban Black Beans

PREP TIME: 15 MINUTES | COOK TIME: 50 MINUTES | YIELD: 8 SERVINGS

INGREDIENTS

¼ cup olive oil

1 large onion, chopped (see Figure 12-2)

1 green bell pepper, chopped

2 stalks celery, including green leaves, chopped

4 garlic cloves, minced

4 cups (two 20-ounce cans) black beans, drained and rinsed (or 2 cups dried black beans, soaked and cooked in a pressure cooker)

2 teaspoons salt, or to taste

1 bay leaf

2 teaspoons ground cumin

½ teaspoon dried oregano

2 tablespoons fresh lemon juice

DIRECTIONS

1 In a large skillet, heat the olive oil. Add the onions, bell pepper, celery, and garlic and cook over medium heat until the onions are translucent — about 10 minutes.

2 Add the beans, salt, bay leaf, cumin, and oregano, and stir well to combine.

3 Cover and simmer on low heat for another 35 or 40 minutes, stirring occasionally to prevent sticking. Stir in the lemon juice. Remove the bay leaf and serve.

PER SERVING: *Calories 195 (From Fat 63); Fat 7g (Saturated 1g); Cholesterol 0mg; Sodium 593mg; Carbohydrate 25g (Dietary Fiber 9g); Protein 8g.*

TIP: Serve these beans over a plate of your favorite steamed rice, or thin the beans with vegetable broth and serve them as black bean soup. This flavorful, hearty dish goes well with a refreshing green salad and a chunk of crusty bread.

FOLDING A BURRITO

1.

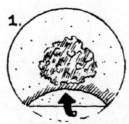

FOLD ONE END OF THE
TORTILLA TOWARD THE
MIDDLE.

2.

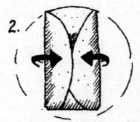

AND THEN FOLD THE SIDES
TOWARD THE MIDDLE.

3.

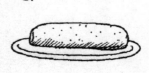

LEAVE THE BURRITO
ON YOUR PLATE WITH
THE ENDS TUCKED
UNDERNEATH SO IT
DOESN'T UNROLL
ON YOUR PLATE.

FIGURE 12-1:
How to fold a
burrito so that it
doesn't unroll
on the plate.

CHOPPING ONION

1. CUT ONION IN HALF, STEM TO
   BOTTOM. SLICE OFF TIP.

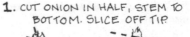

2. PLACE ONE HALF, CUT
   SIDE DOWN, ON A
   CUTTING BOARD.

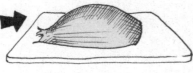

3. SLICE IN 1/8" PARALLEL
   SLICES, STOPPING ABOUT
   A HALF AN INCH FROM THE
   ROOT END.

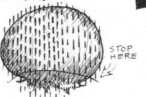

STOP
HERE

4. TURN THE ONION HALF
   AND SLICE ACROSS THE
   PARALLELS SO THAT THE SMALL
   ONION PIECES FALL AWAY.

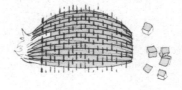

FIGURE 12-2:
Follow these
steps to chop an
onion.

MAKING VEGETARIAN-STYLE BEANS AND FRANKS

If you loved beans and franks as a nonvegetarian, you'll love this vegetarian version. Add two sliced meatless vegetarian hot dogs, a handful of minced onion, and a couple of tablespoons of molasses to a 15-ounce can of vegetarian baked beans. If you like, you can also add a couple of tablespoons of ketchup and dark brown sugar. Stir, pour into a 1½-quart casserole dish, and bake, uncovered, at 350 degrees for 40 minutes, or until hot and bubbly.

Pasta-Mania

Pasta is a fun food. Multi-colored, multi-shaped varieties served with different types of sauce and extras make pasta almost endlessly versatile. There's a variation to suit nearly every palate. Leftover pasta keeps in the refrigerator for several days or in the freezer for several months.

Pesto Pasta Primavera

PREP TIME: 15 MINUTES | COOK TIME: ABOUT 20 MINUTES | YIELD: 6 SERVINGS

INGREDIENTS

Pesto:

3 cups chopped fresh basil leaves, lightly packed

4 cloves garlic, peeled

4 tablespoons pine nuts

6 tablespoons Parmesan cheese or a combination of Parmesan and Romano cheeses

¼ teaspoon black pepper

⅓ cup olive oil

Pasta:

1 pound whole-wheat fettuccine or other pasta

2 tablespoons olive oil, divided

½ cup pine nuts

1 medium onion, minced

1 clove garlic, minced

1 pound asparagus, trimmed and sliced diagonally in ¼-inch pieces

1 medium zucchini, sliced

1 medium carrot, sliced very thin

½ pound fresh mushrooms, sliced

1 cup frozen peas, thawed

2 green onions, chopped

½ teaspoon black pepper

½ cup grated Parmesan cheese

6 cherry tomato halves and several sprigs of parsley, for garnish

DIRECTIONS

1 Place the basil, garlic, pine nuts, cheese, and pepper in a blender or food processor. Process until well blended and smooth, and then dribble in the olive oil. Continue processing until the mixture is the consistency of a smooth paste. Set aside.

2 In a large pot, cook the pasta according to package instructions. Drain and set aside. (Follow Steps 2 through 5 while the pasta is cooking.)

3 In a small skillet, heat 1 tablespoon of olive oil. Add the pine nuts and cook on medium heat, stirring frequently, until the pine nuts begin to sizzle. Continue cooking until they become golden brown (about 3 minutes), taking care not to let them burn. Remove them from the heat and set them aside.

4 In a large skillet, heat the remaining olive oil over medium heat. Add the onion and garlic and cook until the onions are translucent — about 7 minutes.

5 Add the asparagus, zucchini, carrot, and mushrooms, and cook over medium heat for 5 minutes.

6 Stir in the peas and green onions. Heat for 2 minutes.

7 Add the pepper, and then add the cooked pasta, cheese, pine nuts, and about half of the pesto, tossing until the ingredients are well mixed. Serve immediately. Garnish with cherry tomato halves and parsley.

PER SERVING: *Calories 627 (From Fat 271); Fat 30g (Saturated 6g); Cholesterol 9mg; Sodium 264mg; Carbohydrate 73g (Dietary Fiber 15g); Protein 25g.*

(continued)

NOTE: *Primavera* means "spring" in Italian. In culinary circles, primavera dishes are made with a variety of fresh vegetables and herbs.

TIP: *Pesto* is a sauce that's traditionally made with basil, pine nuts, Parmesan cheese, garlic, and olive oil. This dish is best in the summertime, when basil is fresh and you can make a batch of pesto from scratch. Pesto is a snap to make, and it fills your home with the wonderful aroma of fresh basil.

TIP: This recipe makes about double the amount of pesto that you use for a pound of pasta. Store the leftover pesto in an airtight container for one week in the refrigerator, or freeze it in a small jar or airtight plastic bag for several months. When you can't make your own pesto, substitute ready-made pesto from the supermarket and have dinner ready in minutes.

VARY IT! For a vegan version, omit the Parmesan cheese, or substitute nutritional yeast for all or part of it. Alternatively, leave out the pesto sauce and instead toss the pasta with herbs, spices, vegetables, and an additional 2 to 3 tablespoons of olive oil. You can also substitute chopped walnuts for toasted pine nuts.

Rotini with Chopped Tomatoes and Fresh Basil

PREP TIME: 15 MINUTES	COOK TIME: 10 MINUTES OR LESS FOR PASTA	YIELD: 6 SERVINGS

INGREDIENTS

3 cups diced ripe Roma tomatoes (scoop out and discard most of the seeds)

½ cup chopped fresh basil

8 ounces shredded part-skim mozzarella cheese (about 2 cups)

1 cup grated Parmesan cheese

½ cup chopped walnuts

1 pound whole-wheat rotini (spiral-shaped) pasta

4 tablespoons olive oil

Freshly ground black pepper

Black olives and parsley, for garnish

DIRECTIONS

1 In a medium bowl, toss together the tomatoes, basil, mozzarella cheese, Parmesan cheese, and walnuts.

2 In a large pot, cook the rotini according to package instructions and drain.

3 In the pot or in a large bowl, toss the pasta with the olive oil. Next, add the tomato mixture and toss until well combined.

4 Serve on six individual plates and add freshly ground black pepper to taste. Garnish each plate with a black olive and a sprig of parsley.

PER SERVING: *Calories 585 (From Fat 242); Fat 27g (Saturated 9g); Cholesterol 33mg; Sodium 439mg; Carbohydrate 64g (Dietary Fiber 8g); Protein 28g.*

NOTE: You can make this light, simple dish any time of the year, but I like to make it in the summertime, when tomatoes and basil are in season and fresh.

TIP: Vegans can substitute soy cheese for regular cheese, or leave out the cheese entirely. You can also substitute nutritional yeast for all or part of the Parmesan cheese. Leftovers are delicious the next day, after the pasta has absorbed the flavors of the sauce.

etarian Lasagna

INGREDIENTS

1 large head or 2 small heads broccoli

2 medium zucchini and/or yellow (summer) squash

1 tablespoon olive oil

1 large onion, chopped

1 cup carrots, grated

3 cups reduced-fat ricotta cheese

4 egg whites

1 teaspoon dried oregano

1 teaspoon thyme

2 tablespoons dried parsley

½ teaspoon black pepper

¾ cup grated Parmesan cheese, divided

1 jar (about 24 ounces) prepared pasta sauce

8 ounces no-boil whole-wheat lasagna noodles

12 ounces shredded part-skim mozzarella cheese (3 cups), divided

DIRECTIONS

1 Preheat the oven to 350 degrees.

2 Chop the broccoli and zucchini or squash into small pieces. In a medium skillet, heat the olive oil. Cook the onions in the oil over medium heat until they're translucent — about 7 minutes. Add the broccoli, zucchini, and carrots, and steam for 2 to 3 minutes to partially cook. Remove from the heat.

3 In a medium bowl, mix the ricotta cheese, egg whites, oregano, thyme, parsley, pepper, and half the Parmesan cheese.

4 In a lightly oiled, 13-x-17-inch pan, layer the lasagna as follows:

Put a generous layer of pasta sauce on the bottom of the pan.

Lay four uncooked lasagna noodles on the sauce (or the number of noodles needed to fit the pan in a single layer; break the noodles if necessary to fit).

Add a layer of the ricotta cheese mixture, and then half the vegetable mixture, followed by half the mozzarella cheese.

Repeat the layers, and then top it off with another layer of noodles, more pasta sauce, and the remaining Parmesan cheese.

5 Bake for 1 hour, or until brown and bubbly.

PER SERVING: *Calories 354 (From Fat 126); Fat 14g (Saturated 7g); Cholesterol 43mg; Sodium 666mg; Carbohydrate 32g (Dietary Fiber 7g); Protein 25g.*

NOTE: Bottled pasta sauce and no-boil lasagna noodles make the preparation for this dish quick and easy. This dish appeals to vegetarians and nonvegetarians alike. Serve it with a simple green salad and crusty bread.

VARY IT! If you have sun-dried tomato pesto or basil pesto on hand, spread some of that on top of the lasagna along with the pasta sauce (or mixed in with the pasta sauce) in Step 4.

All-Time Favorites

Who says you can't enjoy a slice of pizza or a sloppy Joe on a vegetarian diet? These days, just about any old favorite recipe has a vegetarian counterpart. I include three popular examples in this section.

Roasted Vegetable Pizza

PREP TIME: ABOUT 50 MINUTES (INCLUDING TIME FOR DOUGH TO RISE)	COOK TIME: 70 MINUTES	YIELD: 2 LARGE PIZZAS (4 SERVINGS, OR 8 SLICES PER PIZZA)

INGREDIENTS

Pizza Dough:

1½ teaspoons yeast

1¾ cups warm water (110 degrees)

1 tablespoon honey or sugar

1 teaspoon olive oil

½ teaspoon salt

2 cups whole-wheat flour

2 cups all-purpose flour

Pizza Toppings:

2 cups combined of your choice of washed, chopped vegetables (whatever you have on hand): broccoli, mushrooms, green bell peppers, onions, black olives

2 tablespoons olive oil

2 tablespoons balsamic vinegar

¾ cup bottled pizza sauce (more or less to suit your taste)

8 ounces shredded reduced-fat mozzarella cheese (about 2 cups)

DIRECTIONS

1　Preheat the oven to 375 degrees.

2　In a large mixing bowl, dissolve the yeast in warm water (about 110 degrees) and add the honey or sugar. Add the oil and salt and stir.

3　Gradually add the flour, alternating between whole-wheat and white. Mix well after each addition using a wooden spoon or your hands to make a soft dough.

4　Turn out the dough onto a floured board and knead for 5 minutes, adding more flour if needed. The finished dough should be soft and springy but not sticky.

5　Lightly oil the sides of the mixing bowl. Put the dough in the bowl, turn the dough over once, cover with a towel or waxed paper, and let set in a warm place for about an hour.

6　While the dough rises, wash and chop the vegetables for the pizza toppings.

7　Pour olive oil and balsamic vinegar onto the bottom of a 13-x-9-inch baking dish. Add the vegetables and toss to coat them with oil and vinegar. Spread evenly on the bottom of the baking dish and roast in the oven for 35 to 40 minutes, stirring occasionally, until the vegetables are cooked and browned. Set aside.

8　Divide the dough in half. If you would like to reserve one half for later, store it in the refrigerator or freezer and reduce pizza toppings accordingly.

(continued)

9 Give the dough a quick knead, and then pull and stretch it out onto an oiled, 14-inch pizza pan. You can also roll the dough out first on a floured surface, or simply press the ball of dough onto the pizza pan and distribute it evenly by using your hands. If it springs back too much, let it rest for 5 minutes, and then stretch it again.

10 Spoon on the pizza sauce and spread it to within ½ inch of the edge of the dough.

11 Sprinkle the shredded cheese evenly over the pizza, and then add the vegetable toppings.

12 Place the pizza in the oven and bake for 30 minutes, until the crust and/or cheese begins to brown lightly. Do not overcook.

13 Remove from the oven and let set for 5 minutes.

14 Cut into slices and serve.

PER SERVING: *Calories 362 (From Fat 85); Fat 9g (Saturated 3g); Cholesterol 10mg; Sodium 479mg; Carbohydrate 54g (Dietary Fiber 6g); Protein 17g.*

TIP: Pizza in its simplest form — with fresh tomato sauce and mozzarella cheese — is vegetarian. In this recipe, I show you how to take it one step further, adding roasted vegetables for rich flavor. But don't stop there. With a homemade base of pizza dough, you can be creative and try many different topping combinations. Another option: Leave off the cheese. You'll be surprised how good a vegan, cheeseless pizza tastes. And without all that high-fat dairy cheese, pizza can be a guiltless indulgence.

TIP: This recipe makes two pizzas. Make both pizzas at the same time, or save half the dough for another day. Pizza dough keeps in the freezer for up to three months.

VARY IT! An even easier and quicker option — with a sweet n' spicy edge — is pineapple jalapeño pizza. I'd go so far as to call it a cult favorite. Instead of the roasted vegetables, arrange several canned pineapple rings on top of the pizza. Scatter a handful of jalapeño pepper slices over the pineapple. For extra color and kick, add sliced red onion, too.

Tempeh Sloppy Joes

PREP TIME: 15 MINUTES | COOK TIME: ABOUT 20 MINUTES | YIELD: 4 SERVINGS

INGREDIENTS

1 tablespoon olive oil

1 clove garlic, minced

1 medium onion, chopped

½ green bell pepper, chopped

1 (8-ounce) package tempeh (any variety), crumbled into small pieces

2 tablespoons reduced-sodium soy sauce

½ cup pasta sauce

1 teaspoon brown mustard (or other mustard)

2 tablespoons apple cider vinegar

2 teaspoons sugar

4 whole-grain burger buns

DIRECTIONS

1 In a medium saucepan, heat the olive oil. Add the garlic, onion, and bell pepper, and cook over medium heat until the onions are translucent — about 10 minutes. Add the tempeh and soy sauce and stir well. Cook for an additional 2 minutes.

2 Add the pasta sauce, mustard, vinegar, and sugar. Mix well and simmer for 10 minutes. Serve on whole-grain buns.

PER SERVING: *Calories 301 (From Fat 99); Fat 11g (Saturated 2g); Cholesterol 0mg; Sodium 634mg; Carbohydrate 39g (Dietary Fiber 3g); Protein 17g.*

NOTE: Sloppy Joe filling made with tempeh tastes similar to — but not as greasy as — the kind made with meat.

TIP: This is many people's favorite alternative to burgers and hot dogs. Serve this sandwich filling on whole-grain burger buns. It's also good served on whole-grain toast.

Baked Potato

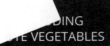

COOK TIME: 1 HOUR	YIELD: 4 SERVINGS

INGREDIENTS

2 medium russet potatoes

3 tablespoons olive oil, divided.

½ cup unflavored yogurt, divided

¼ cup grated Parmesan cheese

Salt and pepper

1 cup chopped broccoli, steamed for one minute on high in a microwave oven

¼ cup sliced, fresh mushrooms

½ medium zucchini or yellow squash, sliced thinly

½ green or red bell pepper, chopped

¼ cup sliced black olives

¼ cup of salsa

DIRECTIONS

1 Preheat the oven to 400 degrees.

2 Rub potatoes with ½ teaspoon olive oil each and pierce each potato several times with the tines of a fork.

3 Place potatoes directly on the oven grates and bake for one hour. Potatoes are cooked well enough when a fork can pierce the potato easily.

4 Remove potatoes from the oven and transfer them to a cutting board or serving platter. Cut the potatoes in half, placing each half with the cut side up. Gently scoop out a little more than half of the potato in each half, transferring the potato from all four halves to a medium-sized bowl.

5 Mash the potato filling with a fork, adding half of the yogurt and the Parmesan cheese. Spoon the filling back into the potato skins, dividing the filling as evenly as possible. Season with salt and pepper to taste.

6 Sauté the steamed broccoli, mushrooms, squash, and bell peppers in 2 tablespoons olive oil over medium heat for several minutes or until softened. Top the potato halves with the sautéed vegetables. Add a dollop of the remaining yogurt and a dollop of salsa to each potato half. Serve hot.

PER SERVING: *Calories 248 (From Fat 126); Fat 14g (Saturated 3g); Cholesterol 9mg; Sodium 296mg; Carbohydrate 26g (Dietary Fiber 3g); Protein 7g.*

NOTE: It's potato-y comfort food, and it's good for you, too. Even better, it's easy to make. This version of the loaded baked potato is packed with health-supporting nutrients and is lower in calories than many traditional varieties filled with fatty cheeses, butter, bacon, or sour cream.

Asian Alternatives

The two recipes in this section are good examples of easy, tasty, Asian-style vegetable dishes that incorporate soy foods as rich, healthful protein sources. Enjoy these often.

ble Stir-Fry

INGREDIENTS

4 tablespoons reduced-sodium soy sauce

1 teaspoon sugar

¼ teaspoon ground ginger

2 cloves garlic, minced

2 tablespoons vegetable oil

1 pound firm or extra-firm tofu, sliced into rectangles (approximately ¼ inch x 1½ inch)

1 large onion, chopped

3 stalks celery, thinly sliced

3 carrots, thinly sliced

1 cup broccoli florets

½ cup sliced canned water chestnuts

1 cup sliced fresh mushrooms

3 cups sliced bok choy (Chinese cabbage)

2 cups mung bean sprouts

1 tablespoon creamy peanut butter

1 tablespoon cornstarch

¼ cup water

DIRECTIONS

1 In a small bowl, combine the soy sauce, sugar, ginger, and garlic. Set aside.

2 In a large skillet, heat the vegetable oil over medium heat. Add the tofu and fry it on both sides for about 5 minutes or until browned. Remove, place on a plate lined with paper towels, and set aside.

3 Add the onion, celery, and carrots to the skillet, and cook over medium heat for 3 to 4 minutes, stirring frequently.

4 Add the remaining vegetables, peanut butter, and the soy sauce mixture, and continue to cook for an additional 2 minutes. Stir.

5 Add the cornstarch and water and continue to cook for about 4 minutes or until the liquid thickens and all the ingredients are steaming hot. Serve immediately over rice.

PER SERVING: *Calories 238 (From Fat 117); Fat 13g (Saturated 1g); Cholesterol 0mg; Sodium 144mg; Carbohydrate 22g (Dietary Fiber 7g); Protein 13g.*

NOTE: Chinese stir-fries traditionally use peanut oil to cook and flavor the vegetables. More convenient and just as effective for flavor is peanut butter, which this recipe uses.

TIP: Feel free to vary the amounts or varieties of vegetables according to your preferences and what you have on hand. This meal is highly nutritious — full of vitamins, minerals, and fiber. Leftovers aren't a problem — this dish tastes great reheated.

Soy–Ginger Kale with Tempeh

INGREDIENTS

1 bunch kale (about 1 pound)

2 tablespoons olive oil

2 cloves garlic, minced

½ cup chopped onion (about half of a medium-sized onion)

⅓ cup plus ¼ cup of your favorite bottled soy-ginger sauce

1 (8-ounce) block tempeh (any variety), chopped into ½-inch cubes

A few tablespoons of water

DIRECTIONS

1 Rinse the kale leaves well, removing and discarding the thick stems. Cut the rinsed leaves into ½-inch-wide strips (do not pat dry). Set aside.

2 In a large skillet, heat the olive oil over low heat. Add the garlic and onions and cook for about 5 minutes, stirring to prevent sticking.

3 Add the kale, and then pour ⅓ cup of the soy-ginger sauce over the mixture. Cover and cook over medium heat for about 10 minutes, or until tender, stirring occasionally to make sure the kale doesn't stick (add a few extra tablespoons of soy-ginger sauce, if necessary).

4 In a small skillet over medium heat, add ¼ cup of soy-ginger sauce, followed by the tempeh cubes. When the sauce and tempeh begin to sizzle (about 5 minutes), turn the tempeh using a spatula. Reduce heat, add a few tablespoons of water, and cook for an additional 5 minutes, or until the tempeh is browned on both sides. Be careful not to let the sauce burn. Remove from heat.

5 Remove the lid from the kale. Lift and stir the mixture with a spatula, and then transfer it to a shallow serving bowl. Top with the tempeh cubes and serve.

PER SERVING: *Calories 167 (From Fat 89); Fat 10g (Saturated 2g); Cholesterol 0mg; Sodium 3839mg; Carbohydrate 13g (Dietary Fiber 4g); Protein 9g.*

NOTE: This is a staple in my home from spring through fall, when the CSA (community- supported agriculture) farm to which I subscribe delivers organic kale nearly every week. (See Chapter 7 for additional information on CSA farms.) The soy-ginger sauce makes this dish slightly sweet and delicious. I serve it with steamed brown rice or seasoned couscous.

VARY IT! Replace kale with other greens, such as Swiss chard or collards.

Chapter **13**

Baking Easy Breads and Rolls

Bread — the "staff of life" — is a dietary staple around the world. It's hard to think of anything more inviting in a home than the fragrance of freshly baked bread.

There's room for bread on the table at breakfast, lunch, or dinner. Muffins, quick breads, and homemade biscuits make good snacks anytime, too. I discuss in more detail in Chapter 6 the different types of cereal grains used to make breads and rolls, and in Chapter 3 I cover the nutritional merits of grains (plenty!). The recipes I include in this chapter are a sampling of the many types of breads you can enjoy on a vegetarian diet.

WARNING

If you eat out, be aware that meats such as bacon and minced ham are sometimes added to biscuits, loaf breads, and rolls. In the American South, cracklin' cornbread is made by stirring small, crunchy pieces of fried pork fat into the batter.

REMEMBER

Breads are easy to bake and enjoy at home. They complement and round out many vegetarian meals. Enjoy a slice or share a batch!

Whole-Wheat Crescent Rolls

PREP TIME: 15 MINUTES (PLUS TIME FOR THE DOUGH TO RISE)	COOK TIME: 20 MINUTES	YIELD: 32 ROLLS

INGREDIENTS

1 package (¼ ounce) active dry yeast

¼ cup warm water

¾ cup warm milk (nonfat cow's milk or unflavored plant milk)

2 tablespoons sugar

2 tablespoons honey

1 teaspoon salt

2 egg whites

¼ cup vegetable oil

1½ cups whole-wheat flour

2 cups unbleached all-purpose flour

Olive oil

DIRECTIONS

1 In a large mixing bowl, dissolve the yeast completely in the warm water.

2 Add the milk, sugar, honey, salt, egg whites, vegetable oil, and whole-wheat flour. Stir until all the ingredients are well combined and the dough is smooth.

3 Add the all-purpose flour and mix until the dough forms a ball. If the dough is too sticky to handle, add several more tablespoons of flour as necessary.

4 Place the dough on a floured surface and knead for several minutes until it's smooth and elastic. (See Figure 13-1 for the proper technique for kneading bread dough.)

5 Oil a large bowl with olive oil. Place the dough ball in the bowl and turn it over once so that you lightly coat the top of the dough ball with oil. Cover with a towel or waxed paper and let the dough rise in a warm place until it doubles in size — about 2 hours.

6 Punch down the dough ball with your fist; then divide the ball into two pieces.

7 Place the dough balls one at a time on a floured surface. Roll each piece of dough into a circle approximately 12 inches in diameter. Lightly brush each circle with olive oil. With a sharp knife, cut the circle in half, and then in quarters, continuing until you have 16 wedges of dough (see Figure 13-2).

8 Preheat the oven to 350 degrees. Beginning at the wide end of each wedge, roll the dough into a crescent shape, ending by pressing the tip onto the roll. Set each roll on a lightly oiled baking sheet and bend the ends slightly to give the roll a crescent shape.

(continued)

9 Cover and let the rolls rise for about 30 minutes before baking. Bake for 20 minutes, or until the rolls are lightly browned. Do not overcook.

PER SERVING: *Calories 74 (From Fat 18); Fat 2g (Saturated 0g); Cholesterol 0mg; Sodium 80mg; Carbohydrate 12g (Dietary Fiber 1g); Protein 2g.*

TIP: These rolls fill the house with the delicious aroma of yeast bread and make any meal special. Their texture is soft and slightly chewy. They stay fresh for two or three days, and they also freeze well.

NOTE: The addition of whole-wheat flour makes these rolls more nutritious and flavorful than rolls made only with refined white flour. It also gives them a nice light brown color.

THE PROPER WAY TO KNEAD DOUGH

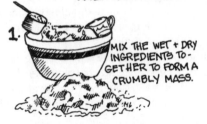

1. MIX THE WET + DRY INGREDIENTS TOGETHER TO FORM A CRUMBLY MASS.

TRANSFER TO A LIGHTLY FLOURED SURFACE.

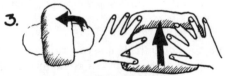

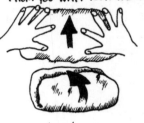

2. PUSH THE DOUGH DOWN AND AWAY FROM YOU WITH YOUR PALMS.

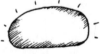

3. LIFT THE DOUGH AND GIVE IT A QUARTER TURN. FOLD OVER, KNEAD AND GIVE IT ANOTHER QUARTER TURN. KEEP REPEATING THE PROCESS.

THE DOUGH WILL APPEAR SMOOTH AND ELASTIC WHEN IT HAS BEEN KNEADED WELL.

FIGURE 13-1: Use these steps to knead bread dough.

Illustration by Elizabeth Kurtzman

MAKING WHOLE-WHEAT CRESCENT ROLLS

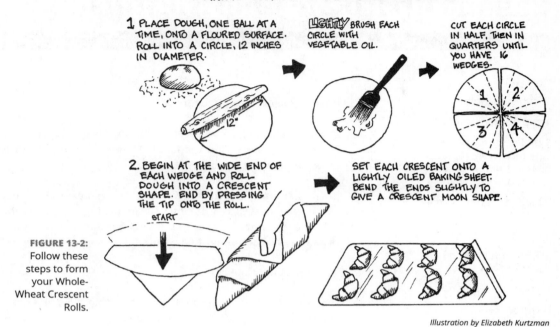

1. PLACE DOUGH, ONE BALL AT A TIME, ONTO A FLOURED SURFACE. ROLL INTO A CIRCLE, 12 INCHES IN DIAMETER.

LIGHTLY BRUSH EACH CIRCLE WITH VEGETABLE OIL.

CUT EACH CIRCLE IN HALF, THEN IN QUARTERS UNTIL YOU HAVE 16 WEDGES.

2. BEGIN AT THE WIDE END OF EACH WEDGE AND ROLL DOUGH INTO A CRESCENT SHAPE. END BY PRESSING THE TIP ONTO THE ROLL.

START

SET EACH CRESCENT ONTO A LIGHTLY OILED BAKING SHEET. BEND THE ENDS SLIGHTLY TO GIVE A CRESCENT MOON SHAPE.

FIGURE 13-2: Follow these steps to form your Whole-Wheat Crescent Rolls.

Illustration by Elizabeth Kurtzman

Banana Chocolate Chip Muffins

PREP TIME: 15 MINUTES | COOK TIME: 20 MINUTES | YIELD: 12 MUFFINS

INGREDIENTS

½ cup vegetable oil

1 cup packed brown sugar

1 tablespoon powdered vegetarian egg replacer blended with 4 tablespoons water, or 4 egg whites

2 teaspoons pure vanilla extract

2 ripe bananas, mashed

1½ cups unbleached all-purpose flour

½ cup whole-wheat flour

¼ cup wheat germ (optional)

1 teaspoon baking powder

1 teaspoon baking soda

½ teaspoon salt

6 ounces chocolate chips (about 1 cup)

DIRECTIONS

1   Preheat the oven to 350 degrees.

2   In a medium bowl, whisk together the oil, sugar, egg replacer/water, and vanilla. Add the bananas and blend well with a whisk or an electric mixer. Set aside.

3   In another bowl, add the all-purpose and whole-wheat flour, wheat germ (if desired), baking powder, baking soda, and salt. Fold the dry ingredients into the wet ingredients with quick strokes — be careful not to overmix.

4   Stir in the chocolate chips.

5   Spoon the batter into 12 lined or oiled muffin cups and bake for 20 minutes, or until muffins are golden brown. When cool enough to handle, remove muffins from cups.

PER SERVING: *Calories 309 (From Fat 120); Fat 13g (Saturated 3g); Cholesterol 0mg; Sodium 200mg; Carbohydrate 47g (Dietary Fiber 3g); Protein 4g.*

TIP: Everyone loves these muffins, and they're a great way to use up bananas that are becoming too ripe. They freeze well, so make a batch whenever you have extra bananas and you'll have muffins on hand when you want them.

VARY IT! Substitute dairy-free chocolate chips or butterscotch chips for the chocolate chips. Add a handful of chopped walnuts or pecans.

Easy Cornbread

PREP TIME: 10 MINUTES | COOK TIME: 30 MINUTES | YIELD: 4 SERVINGS

INGREDIENTS

2 tablespoons olive oil

¾ cup cornmeal

2 egg whites

1½ cups unflavored nonfat yogurt

½ teaspoon baking soda

½ teaspoon salt

½ cup chopped onion

¼ teaspoon black pepper

DIRECTIONS

1 Preheat the oven to 425 degrees. Oil a 1-quart casserole dish or skillet.

2 Combine all the ingredients in a medium-sized bowl and stir until completely mixed.

3 Pour the batter into the oiled casserole dish or skillet and bake for 30 minutes, or until set. Do not overcook.

PER SERVING: *Calories 210 (From Fat 72); Fat 8g (Saturated 1g); Cholesterol 2mg; Sodium 554mg; Carbohydrate 27g (Dietary Fiber 2g); Protein 9g.*

TIP: This cornbread is flavorful and moist. Serve it warm alongside Cashew Chili (see Chapter 11), with vegetable stews and casseroles, or with a bowl of soup.

VARY IT! Add ¼ cup chopped sun-dried tomatoes.

Cinnamon Applesauce Muffins

PREP TIME: 15 MINUTES | COOK TIME: 20 MINUTES | YIELD: 12 MUFFINS

INGREDIENTS

⅓ cup vegetable oil

⅓ cup packed brown sugar

1 tablespoon powdered vegetarian egg replacer blended with 4 tablespoons water, or 4 egg whites

1½ cups unsweetened applesauce

2 cups whole-wheat flour

2 teaspoons baking powder

½ teaspoon baking soda

¼ teaspoon salt

1 teaspoon cinnamon

½ teaspoon nutmeg

DIRECTIONS

1 Preheat the oven to 375 degrees.

2 In a medium bowl, whisk together the oil, sugar, and egg replacer/water. Add the applesauce and blend well with a whisk or an electric mixer. Set aside.

3 In a separate bowl, add the flour, baking powder, baking soda, salt, cinnamon, and nutmeg. Fold the dry ingredients into the wet ingredients with quick strokes — be careful not to overmix.

4 Spoon the batter into lined or oiled muffin cups and bake for 20 minutes, or until muffins are golden brown. When cool enough to handle, remove muffins from cups.

PER SERVING: *Calories 163 (From Fat 60); Fat 7g (Saturated 1g); Cholesterol 5mg; Sodium 175mg; Carbohydrate 24g (Dietary Fiber 3g); Protein 3g.*

NOTE: These simple muffins are good for breakfast and in bag lunches. The whole-wheat flour adds dietary fiber. They taste even better the second day, and they freeze well.

VARY IT! Add a handful of chopped walnuts or pecans, chopped dates, dried cranberries, cherries, currants, or raisins.

Zucchini Bread

PREP TIME: 30 MINUTES	COOK TIME: 1 HOUR	YIELD: 2 LOAVES (24 SLICES)

INGREDIENTS

2 cups sugar

1 cup vegetable oil

4½ teaspoons powdered vegetarian egg replacer blended with 6 tablespoons water, or 6 egg whites

3 teaspoons pure vanilla extract

2 cups coarsely grated, unpeeled zucchini, packed

2 cups unbleached all-purpose flour

¼ teaspoon baking powder

2 teaspoons baking soda

3 teaspoons cinnamon

1 teaspoon salt

1 cup chopped walnuts

DIRECTIONS

1 Preheat the oven to 350 degrees.

2 Combine the sugar, oil, egg replacer/water, and vanilla in a large bowl. Add the zucchini and mix well.

3 In a separate bowl, combine the flour, baking powder, baking soda, cinnamon, and salt. Stir to blend the dry ingredients well.

4 Add the dry ingredients to the zucchini mixture, mix well, and then stir in the nuts.

5 Pour into two greased and floured 9-x-5-x-3-inch loaf pans (make sure that the pans are well greased!). Bake for 1 hour, or until the tops of the loaves are golden brown.

PER SERVING: *Calories 215 (From Fat 108); Fat 12g (Saturated 1g); Cholesterol 0mg; Sodium 207mg; Carbohydrate 25g (Dietary Fiber 1g); Protein 2g.*

NOTE: This is another good breakfast or snack bread in the summer, when zucchini is in season and abundant. The recipe makes two loaves — serve one and freeze the other or give it to a friend.

VARY IT! If you prefer a lighter, less oily bread, reduce the amount of vegetable oil to ¾ cup.

Pumpkin Biscuits

PREP TIME: 15 MINUTES | COOK TIME: 20 MINUTES | YIELD: 12 BISCUITS

INGREDIENTS

1 cup unbleached all-purpose flour

½ cup whole-wheat flour

3 teaspoons baking powder

1 teaspoon salt

¼ cup sugar

1 teaspoon cinnamon

¼ teaspoon nutmeg

¼ teaspoon allspice

⅓ cup margarine (make sure margarine is cold and hard)

¾ cup canned pumpkin or mashed sweet potatoes

¾ cup unflavored plant milk or nonfat cow's milk

DIRECTIONS

1 Preheat the oven to 450 degrees.

2 In a medium bowl, sift together the all-purpose flour, whole-wheat flour, baking powder, and salt. Stir in the sugar, cinnamon, nutmeg, and allspice.

3 Using a pastry blender, cut the margarine into the dry ingredients until crumbly.

4 Fold in the pumpkin, and then gradually add milk, stirring to make dough. Use your clean hands if necessary to shape the dough into a ball.

5 Roll the dough out onto a cool, floured surface to about ½ inch thick. Using a juice glass or a small, round cookie cutter, cut the dough into rounds and place them onto an oiled baking sheet. Push together and roll the dough scraps to cut out the remaining biscuits.

6 Bake for about 20 minutes, or until lightly browned. Be careful not to overcook the biscuits.

PER SERVING: *182 Calories (From Fat 104); Fat 12g (Saturated 5g); Cholesterol 0mg; Sodium 412mg; Carbohydrate 17g (Dietary Fiber 2g); Protein 2g.*

TIP: Serve these with honey for breakfast in the fall, or with the Cashew Chili in Chapter 11 in lieu of cornbread for a change of pace.

VARY IT! Add a handful of chopped pecans or dried cranberries.

Chapter **14**

Dishing Out Delicious Desserts

Most people think of dessert as a guilt-inducing indulgence that's not very nutritious and is loaded with calories. Where most commercial cakes, cookies, and pies are concerned, this is usually true!

Though most desserts contain no meat, many do contain oodles of artery-clogging saturated fat and calories from rich dairy ingredients and eggs. Desserts made with gelatin — a vegetarian no-no — are usually junky, with lots of added sugar and artificial colors and flavors, too.

That's where the vegetarian alternative can help. Make no mistake — just because a dessert is vegetarian doesn't mean it's guaranteed to be better for your health. In general, though, desserts made from scratch at home using wholesome ingredients and fewer animal products tend to be better for you.

The recipes in this chapter will convince you to extend the vegetarian way to the desserts you bake every day. Many of these recipes incorporate fruit to boost the nutritional value and lower the calorie content, and, where possible, whole-wheat flour replaces white.

Chocolate Desserts

Sometimes, nothing but chocolate will do. The desserts in this section will satisfy the chocolate lovers in your life and add a delicious finishing touch to any meal.

The first two recipes are kid-pleasers and lunchbox staples — cupcakes and cookies. They freeze and travel well. The remaining two recipes include a decadent — but much more healthful — tofu version of a classic cheesecake and a foolproof, make-it-in-minutes chocolate cake that I guarantee everyone will love.

Cocoa Pink Cupcakes

INGREDIENTS

½ cup whole-wheat flour

2½ cups unbleached all-purpose flour

1 tablespoon cocoa

1 teaspoon salt

¾ cup vegetable oil

1¼ cup sugar

1 tablespoon powdered vegetarian egg replacer blended with 4 tablespoons water, or 4 egg whites

1 teaspoon pure vanilla extract

1 teaspoon baking soda

1 cup cold water

6 ounces (1 cup) semi-sweet chocolate chips, divided

½ cup chopped walnuts, divided

Confectioners' sugar

DIRECTIONS

1 Preheat the oven to 375 degrees.

2 In a small bowl, combine both types of flour with the cocoa and salt, stir to blend, and then set aside.

3 In a large mixing bowl, cream the oil and sugar together, and then add the egg replacer/water and vanilla.

4 In a cup, combine the baking soda and cold water and stir to dissolve.

5 Add the baking soda mixture alternately with the dry ingredients to the creamed mixture, beginning and ending with the dry ingredients and blending well on low speed after each addition.

6 Stir half the chocolate chips and nuts into the batter.

7 Line muffin cups with paper liners and fill each a little more than half full with batter.

8 Sprinkle the remaining chocolate chips and nuts over the tops of the cupcakes.

9 Bake for about 25 minutes. The cupcakes should appear done but no more than very lightly browned. Be careful not to overcook them, or they'll become dry.

10 After the cupcakes cool, sift confectioners' sugar over the tops.

PER CUPCAKE: *Calories 234 (From Fat 108); Fat 12g (Saturated 3g); Cholesterol 0mg; Sodium 165mg; Carbohydrate 29g (Dietary Fiber 1g); Protein 3g.*

NOTE: I adapted this recipe from one that has been a favorite in my family since I was a little girl. These cupcakes have a not-too-sweet, mild cocoa flavor. The cocoa gives them a rosy brown color on the inside.

TIP: Using egg replacer and dairy-free chocolate chips would make these cupcakes vegan.

Vegan Chocolate Chip Cookies

PREP TIME: 30 MINUTES	COOK TIME: 12 MINUTES PER BATCH	YIELD: ABOUT 6 DOZEN COOKIES

INGREDIENTS

¾ cup margarine, softened

½ cup packed brown sugar

½ cup granulated sugar

1 tablespoon powdered vegetarian egg replacer blended with 4 tablespoons water, or 4 egg whites

1 teaspoon pure vanilla extract

1¼ cups unbleached all-purpose flour

¾ cup whole-wheat flour

¼ teaspoon salt

1 teaspoon baking soda

½ teaspoon baking powder

½ teaspoon cinnamon

2 cups rolled oats

1½ cups (12 ounces) dairy-free chocolate chips

DIRECTIONS

1 Preheat the oven to 350 degrees.

2 In a mixing bowl, cream the margarine, sugars, egg replacer/water, and vanilla until smooth.

3 In a separate bowl, mix all-purpose and whole-wheat flour with the salt, baking soda, baking powder, and cinnamon. Add to the creamed mixture and mix well.

4 Stir in the oats. The batter will be very stiff.

5 Add the dairy-free chocolate chips and mix thoroughly using clean hands.

6 Drop the dough by rounded teaspoonfuls about 3 inches apart on an ungreased cookie sheet. Bake each batch for 10 to 12 minutes, or until the cookies are lightly browned.

PER SERVING: *Calories 71 (From Fat 26); Fat 3g (Saturated 2g); Cholesterol 0mg; Sodium 52mg; Carbohydrate 10g (Dietary Fiber 1g); Protein 1g.*

NOTE: A slightly healthier version of the classic chocolate cookie, these drop cookies are chewy and moist.

Rich Chocolate Tofu Cheesecake

PREP TIME: 30 MINUTES	COOK TIME: 48 MINUTES (PLUS CHILL TIME)	YIELD: 8 SERVINGS

INGREDIENTS

Filling:

1¼ pounds firm tofu

1½ cups sugar, divided

3 ounces (3 squares) semi-sweet baking chocolate

1 teaspoon pure vanilla extract

½ teaspoon pure almond extract

⅛ teaspoon salt

Crust:

1¼ cups graham cracker crumbs

1 tablespoon sugar

⅓ cup margarine

DIRECTIONS

1 Remove the tofu from packaging and place between two paper towels. Place the paper towel–covered tofu in a clean sink, then put a heavy weight, such as a cast-iron skillet, on top. Let the tofu drain for 20 minutes. While it drains, make the crust.

2 For the crust, combine the graham cracker crumbs and sugar in a medium bowl. Melt the margarine in a saucepan over low heat, and then add it to the crumb mixture. Stir until blended, and then press the crumbs into the bottom and sides of an 8-inch, nonstick springform pan. Set aside.

3 In a blender or food processor, blend the drained tofu, ¼ pound at a time, with 1 cup of the sugar, adding ¼ cup sugar with each addition of tofu (set aside the remaining ½ cup sugar for later). Process until the ingredients are well blended.

4 Pour the tofu-sugar mixture into a bowl. Preheat the oven to 350 degrees.

5 In a double boiler or saucepan, melt the chocolate. While the chocolate is melting, place the graham cracker crust in the oven and bake for about 8 minutes; then remove, set aside, and let cool.

6 After the chocolate has melted, add it to the tofu-sugar mixture. Mix in the vanilla, almond extract, salt, and remaining ½ cup sugar. Blend well.

7 Pour the mixture into the graham cracker crust and bake for about 40 minutes. When the cheesecake is done, the edges will rise slightly, with small cracks on the surface. The middle won't rise, but it will be springy to the touch and have a dry, firm appearance. Chill the cheesecake for at least 2 hours after baking.

(continued)

PER SERVING: *Calories 380 (From Fat 144); Fat 16g (Saturated 6g); Cholesterol 0mg; Sodium 201mg; Carbohydrate 56g (Dietary Fiber 1g); Protein 7g.*

NOTE: Tofu makes a fabulous replacement for cream cheese in cheesecake recipes. This cheesecake has a rich chocolate flavor and a smooth, creamy texture. I adapted it from a recipe in *Tofu Cookery* (25th Anniversary Edition) by Louise Hagler (Book Publishing Company).

TIP: You can also use a ready-made 9-inch graham cracker crust (which holds the same volume as the 8-inch springform pan used in this recipe).

VARY IT! Top the cheesecake with fresh raspberries or a thawed bag of frozen raspberries mixed with a few tablespoons of sugar. You can also top the cheesecake with canned cherries.

Easy Vegan Chocolate Cake

PREP TIME: 6 MINUTES	COOK TIME: 30 MINUTES	YIELD: 8 SQUARES

INGREDIENTS

1½ cups unbleached all-purpose white flour

⅓ cup unsweetened cocoa powder

1 teaspoon baking soda

½ teaspoon salt

1 cup sugar

½ cup vegetable oil

1 cup cold water or cold coffee

2 teaspoons pure vanilla extract

2 tablespoons apple cider vinegar

Confectioners' sugar

DIRECTIONS

1 Preheat the oven to 375 degrees.

2 Oil an 8-inch square cake pan. Sift together the flour, cocoa, baking soda, salt, and sugar directly into the cake pan.

3 In a 2-cup measuring cup, mix the oil, cold water or coffee, and vanilla.

4 Pour the liquid ingredients into the cake pan and mix the batter with a fork or a small whisk. When the batter is smooth, add the vinegar and stir quickly. The batter will have pale swirls as the baking soda and vinegar react. Stir just until the vinegar is evenly distributed throughout the batter.

5 Bake for about 30 minutes and set aside to cool. Using a mesh strainer, shake confectioners' sugar on top of the cake immediately before serving. (If the sugar stands on the cake too long before serving, it will melt into the cake.)

PER SERVING: *Calories 317 (From Fat 132); Fat 15g (Saturated 1g); Cholesterol 0mg; Sodium 304mg; Carbohydrate 45g (Dietary Fiber 2g); Protein 3g.*

NOTE: This is the recipe I turn to when there's nothing in the house for dessert, and I want to make something delicious — fast. This family favorite is a no-fail, quick-and-easy recipe using common ingredients you probably have in your pantry. Add your own frosting if you'd like, but I just dust with confectioners' sugar before serving. I adapted this recipe from the Moosewood Collective's *Moosewood Restaurant Book of Desserts* (Three Rivers Press).

VARY IT! Serve with nonfat or nondairy ice cream or sliced fruit.

Fruit Desserts

Fruit desserts are a good choice because they add fiber and other health-supporting nutrients while still satisfying a sweet tooth. They also tend to be lower in calories than desserts made with lots of refined flour, sugar, and fat.

The desserts that follow are wholesome enough that you can even enjoy them for breakfast or as a snack.

Baked Apples

PREP TIME: 10 MINUTES (PLUS CHILL TIME, IF DESIRED)	COOK TIME: 1 HOUR	YIELD: 4 SERVINGS

INGREDIENTS

4 large, tart apples

½ cup packed brown sugar

1 teaspoon cinnamon

1 tablespoon margarine

½ cup apple juice (optional)

DIRECTIONS

1 Preheat the oven to 350 degrees.

2 Wash and core the apples, stopping the coring just before the bottom of the apple (so that the hole doesn't go all the way through). Using a paring knife, cut away the peel from the top to about one-third of the way down each apple (see Figure 14-1).

3 In a small dish or cup, combine the brown sugar and cinnamon. Spoon one-quarter of the mixture into the center of each apple.

4 Divide the margarine into quarters and put one chunk in the center of each apple.

5 Set the apples in an 8-inch square baking dish or a 1-quart casserole dish and add water or apple juice (if desired) to a depth of about ½ inch.

6 Bake uncovered for 1 hour, or until the apples are soft. Serve warm or chilled.

PER SERVING: *Calories 255 (From Fat 32); Fat 4g (Saturated 1g); Cholesterol 0mg; Sodium 41mg; Carbohydrate 60g (Dietary Fiber 6g); Protein 0g.*

TIP: Baked apples are quick and convenient to make when you already have the oven heated to bake a casserole or loaf of bread. They keep in the refrigerator for up to three days, and they're good any time of the day or night — warm with ice cream, cold for breakfast, or as a snack.

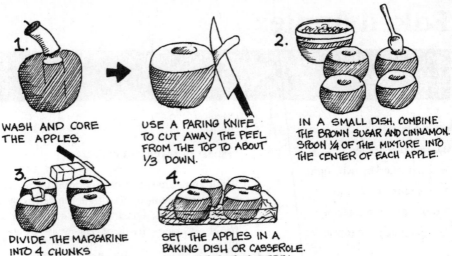

1. WASH AND CORE THE APPLES.

USE A PARING KNIFE TO CUT AWAY THE PEEL FROM THE TOP TO ABOUT 1/3 DOWN.

2. IN A SMALL DISH, COMBINE THE BROWN SUGAR AND CINNAMON. SPOON 1/4 OF THE MIXTURE INTO THE CENTER OF EACH APPLE.

3. DIVIDE THE MARGARINE INTO 4 CHUNKS AND PUT 1 INTO THE CENTER OF EACH APPLE.

4. SET THE APPLES IN A BAKING DISH OR CASSEROLE. ADD WATER TO A DEPTH OF ABOUT 1/2 INCH.

FIGURE 14-1: Filling Baked Apples.

Illustration by Elizabeth Kurtzman

Pear Cranberry Crisp

PREP TIME: 20 MINUTES (PLUS CHILL TIME, IF DESIRED)	COOK TIME: 40 MINUTES	YIELD: 12 SERVINGS

INGREDIENTS

Filling:

6 large, soft, ripe pears, peeled, cored, and sliced

1½ cups fresh or frozen cranberries

¾ cup sugar

2 tablespoons unbleached all-purpose flour

Topping:

1 cup rolled oats

½ cup packed brown sugar

⅓ cup unbleached all-purpose flour (or mix half and half with whole-wheat flour)

¼ cup margarine

½ cup chopped pecans

DIRECTIONS

1 Preheat the oven to 375 degrees. Oil a 9-x-13-inch baking dish.

2 In a large bowl, combine the pears, cranberries, sugar, and flour. Toss to coat the fruit. Spread the fruit over the bottom of the oiled baking dish.

3 In a small bowl, combine the oats, brown sugar, flour, and margarine. Using a fork or pastry blender, combine the ingredients until the mixture is crumbly and the margarine is well incorporated. Stir in the pecans.

4 Sprinkle the topping evenly over the fruit and pat it down with your fingers.

5 Bake for 40 minutes, or until the fruit is bubbly and the topping is browned. Serve warm or chilled.

PER SERVING: *Calories 222 (From Fat 70); Fat 8g (Saturated 2g); Cholesterol 0mg; Sodium 46mg; Carbohydrate 38g (Dietary Fiber 3g); Protein 2g.*

NOTE: This beautiful dish is sweet, tart, and totally satisfying. The cranberries add a festive color and flavor, so this dish works well as a simple but lovely dessert for holidays and other gatherings.

VARY IT! Use tart apples in place of the pears and walnuts in place of the pecans.

Mixed Berry Cobbler

PREP TIME: 15 MINUTES	COOK TIME: 25 MINUTES	YIELD: 9 SERVINGS

INGREDIENTS

5 to 6 cups fresh or frozen berries (boysenberries, blackberries, blueberries, strawberries, raspberries, or a mixture)

1 cup plus 3 tablespoons, divided, unbleached all-purpose flour (or mix half and half with whole-wheat flour)

½ cup plus 2 tablespoons sugar, divided

1½ teaspoons baking powder

¼ teaspoon salt

2 tablespoons vegetable oil

½ cup unflavored plant milk, or nonfat cow's milk

DIRECTIONS

1 Preheat the oven to 400 degrees.

2 Spread the berries in a 9-inch square baking dish. Mix in 3 tablespoons of flour and ½ cup of the sugar.

3 In a separate bowl, mix the remaining cup of flour and the remaining 2 tablespoons of sugar with the baking powder and salt.

4 Add the oil to the flour mixture and mix it with a fork or your fingers until the mixture resembles coarse cornmeal.

5 Add the milk and stir to combine.

6 Spread this mixture over the berries (don't worry if they're not completely covered) and bake for about 25 minutes, or until golden brown.

PER SERVING: *Calories 304 (From Fat 36); Fat 4g (Saturated 0g); Cholesterol 0mg; Sodium 141mg; Carbohydrate 68g (Dietary Fiber 5g); Protein 3g.*

NOTE: I adapted this recipe from one of my favorite vegetarian cookbooks, *The Peaceful Palate* by Jennifer Raymond (Heart & Soul Publications). It's delicious, easy to make, and much lower in fat than a berry pie. It's one of the staple desserts at my house.

VARY IT! For a real treat, top the hot cobbler with a spoonful of nondairy or reduced-fat ice cream.

Other Classic Comforts

Rice pudding and oatmeal cookies are two of my favorite comfort foods. The recipes in this section are variations of two traditional recipes. These versions are healthful enough to eat every day.

TIP

Notice that the rice pudding recipe that follows calls for soymilk in place of the cow's milk traditionally used in puddings and custards. Any plant milk alternative, including rice milk, coconut milk and almond milk — unflavored or vanilla — would work, though. Use whatever you have on hand. I like vanilla soymilk in this recipe because of its creaminess and the extra vanilla flavor it adds.

Rice Pudding

PREP TIME: 5 MINUTES (PLUS CHILL TIME, IF DESIRED)	COOK TIME: 50 MINUTES	YIELD: 6 SERVINGS

INGREDIENTS

3 cups vanilla soymilk or other plant milk, or nonfat cow's milk

½ cup long-grain white rice

¼ teaspoon salt

1 tablespoon margarine

¼ teaspoon ground cinnamon

¼ teaspoon ground nutmeg

¼ cup sugar

DIRECTIONS

1 In a medium saucepan over high heat, bring the soymilk to a boil, stirring constantly — about 5 minutes.

2 Add the rice, salt, margarine, cinnamon, nutmeg, and sugar, and stir to combine. Reduce the heat to low and cover.

3 Cook, covered, for about 45 minutes, or until all the liquid has been absorbed. Lift the lid and stir every 15 minutes, covering again tightly each time you remove the lid.

4 After all the liquid has been absorbed, remove the pudding from the heat. Cool to warm, and then serve or place in the refrigerator to chill for at least 2 hours before serving.

PER SERVING: *Calories 186 (From Fat 32); Fat 4g (Saturated 1g); Cholesterol 0mg; Sodium 163mg; Carbohydrate 33g (Dietary Fiber 0g); Protein 4g.*

NOTE: This rice pudding requires no eggs because it thickens in the pan as the rice absorbs the liquid in the recipe. The result is a rich, creamy rice pudding that's simple to make and requires minimal time supervising the stovetop.

Cherry Oatmeal Cookies

PREP TIME: 20 MINUTES	COOK TIME: 12 MINUTES PER BATCH	YIELD: 36 LARGE COOKIES

INGREDIENTS

1 cup margarine

1 cup packed dark brown sugar

½ cup sugar

2 large eggs

1 teaspoon pure vanilla extract

¾ cup whole-wheat flour

¾ cup unbleached all-purpose flour

½ teaspoon salt

½ teaspoon baking soda

½ teaspoon baking powder

1 teaspoon cinnamon

2 cups rolled oats

1 cup dried cherries

½ cup chopped walnuts or pecans

DIRECTIONS

1 Preheat the oven to 350 degrees.

2 In a large mixing bowl, cream the margarine and sugars. Add the eggs and vanilla and beat until light and fluffy.

3 In a separate bowl, combine whole-wheat flour and the all-purpose flour with the salt, baking soda, baking powder, and cinnamon. Add the dry ingredients to the wet mixture and beat until combined.

4 Stir in the oats, cherries, and nuts and blend well.

5 Drop the cookie dough by the tablespoonful onto lightly greased cookie sheets. Bake for 12 minutes, or until lightly browned.

PER SERVING: *Calories 142 (From Fat 60); Fat 7g (Saturated 2g); Cholesterol 12mg; Sodium 110mg; Carbohydrate 19g (Dietary Fiber 1g); Protein 2g.*

NOTE: The cherries in these thick, chewy cookies are a nice surprise. The cookies freeze well and are a healthful and delicious treat to bring to family and friends when you visit.

Chapter **15**

Celebrating the Holidays, Vegetarian-Style

Holidays are made special by the family and friends we share them with and by the traditions that accompany those special days. Chief among those traditions is the food, of course!

We associate certain foods with specific holidays. What's the centerpiece of most Thanksgiving tables? The turkey, of course. That is, unless you're a vegetarian, in which case you can make use of a variety of plants to round out your holiday meals.

The selection of recipes I include in this chapter underscores the diversity of the vegetable world. Meatless holiday meals are characterized by an abundance of colorful, flavorful, and festive foods.

Adopting New Traditions and Adapting the Old

Food traditions vary, and some even change over time. Christmas dinner may mean antipasto and ravioli to one family and a tofu turkey with all the trimmings to another. It's all a matter of what has become familiar to you and your family or friends over the years.

Many of the recipes in this book are well suited to special-occasion meals. They're colorful and will fill your home with delicious aromas. Some make use of seasonal foods that evoke a particular mood or time of year. Pear Cranberry Crisp, for instance (see Chapter 14), may bring late autumn and the winter holidays to mind.

TIP

If you're new to a vegetarian diet and your traditions still center on foods of animal origin, don't worry. Choose the aspects of special-occasion meals that still fit and find replacements for those that don't.

For example, most of a traditional Thanksgiving dinner is already vegetarian. Mashed potatoes, candied sweet potatoes, green peas, cranberry sauce . . . these foods can stay on the menu. You can easily swap the turkey for Everybody's Favorite Cheese and Nut Loaf, or Stuffed Squash (recipes for both are in this chapter), or any of a number of other main dishes.

REMEMBER

To supplement your menu, add Whole-Wheat Crescent Rolls (Chapter 13), Arugula Salad with Pickled Beets and Candied Pecans (Chapter 11), and Stuffed Mushrooms or Roasted Garlic Spread (Chapter 10). Use your imagination and think about the foods that you enjoy most. Over time, these will become your new traditions, as dear to you as the old ones once were.

Tips for Entertaining for Special Occasions

When you peruse the recipes that follow, think about what makes holiday meals special for you. Do you eat in the dining room rather than the kitchen? Do you place candles or a centerpiece on the table? Do you cover the table with your best linen tablecloth and fine china? Maybe you play soft music in the background.

The atmosphere you create in the room where you eat and the manner with which you present the food set the tone for the meal and can set a meal apart from the everyday routine. You can serve the recipes in this chapter anytime, but if you reserve them for special occasions and serve them with flair, they say, "This meal is special!"

REMEMBER

Be mindful that friends or family members who prepare holiday foods may think their dishes are safe for vegetarians/vegans to eat but contain animal products such as butter, gelatin, bacon grease, lard (in pie dough, for example), and so on. Apply your diplomacy skills, but consider inquiring if you'd like to be sure that what you're eating meets your expectations.

Holiday Recipes to Savor

Many vegetarians have traditions of their own that are linked with specific holidays. In my family of longtime vegetarians, we make Everybody's Favorite Cheese and Nut Loaf at Thanksgiving, for Christmas Eve, and for some special events. The dish is so good that it's become legendary among my extended circle of family and friends. Some of the nonvegetarians who sometimes join us for holiday meals have adopted the tradition for themselves.

Everybody's Favorite Cheese and Nut Loaf

| PREP TIME: 20 MINUTES | COOK TIME: 30 MINUTES | YIELD: 8 SERVINGS |

INGREDIENTS

2 tablespoons olive oil

1 large onion, chopped fine

½ cup water

1½ cups whole-wheat breadcrumbs, plus extra for topping

2 cups grated, reduced-fat cheddar cheese

1 cup chopped walnuts

Juice of 1 large, fresh lemon (about ¼ cup)

6 egg whites (or about 1½ tablespoons powdered vegetarian egg replace blended with 6 tablespoons of water)

Parsley sprigs, bell pepper rings, and cherry tomato halves, for garnish

DIRECTIONS

1 Preheat the oven to 400 degrees.

2 In a large skillet, heat the olive oil over medium heat. Add the onions and cook until they're translucent.

3 Add the water and breadcrumbs and mix well. Remove from the heat.

4 Add the cheese, walnuts, lemon juice, and egg whites and mix well.

5 Scoop the mixture into a greased, 9-x-5-x-3-inch loaf pan or casserole dish. Top with a sprinkling of breadcrumbs.

6 Bake for about 30 minutes, or until golden brown.

7 Turn out onto a platter and garnish with parsley sprigs and cherry tomatoes, or slices of red and yellow bell peppers.

PER SERVING: *Calories 260 (From Fat 180); Fat 20g (Saturated 3g); Cholesterol 0mg; Sodium 509mg; Carbohydrate 11g (Dietary Fiber 1g); Protein 11g.*

NOTE: This savory dish is reminiscent of meatloaf in texture and has a nutty flavor. It's festive if it's presented on a platter garnished with parsley and cherry tomatoes.

TIP: My family makes two loaves to ensure we have enough for second helpings — leftovers are wonderful reheated or eaten cold in a sandwich. You can also serve this dish with ½ cup ketchup mixed with ½ cup salsa.

VARY IT! Experiment with this recipe by replacing part of the walnuts with an equal amount of chopped water chestnuts, or a portion of the cheese with an equal portion of grated carrots.

Stuffed Squash

PREP TIME: 30 MINUTES	COOK TIME: 50 MINUTES (INCLUDING 30 MINUTES TO PREBAKE)	YIELD: 4 SERVINGS (¼ SQUASH PER SERVING)

INGREDIENTS

1 large butternut squash, cut in half, seeds and strings removed (or use 2 small acorn squashes for 4 individual servings — see Figure 15-1 for an illustration of both types of squash)

2 tablespoons olive oil

1 medium onion, chopped

½ cup sliced fresh mushrooms

1 clove garlic, minced

¼ cup finely minced celery (leaves and stem)

¼ teaspoon black pepper

2 tablespoons minced fresh parsley

½ teaspoon sage

½ teaspoon thyme

Juice of 1 large, fresh lemon (about ¼ cup)

¼ cup diced, peeled Granny Smith apple

¼ cup chopped walnuts

¼ cup golden raisins

3 slices whole-wheat bread, coarsely crumbled

¾ cup grated, reduced-fat cheddar cheese (use nonfat cheese or a mix to lower the saturated fat content further)

DIRECTIONS

1 Preheat the oven to 350 degrees.

2 Cut the squash in half. Scoop out and discard the seeds and strings.

3 Place the squash halves in a small, baking dish and fill the dish ½ inch high with water. Place the dish in the oven and bake, covered loosely with foil, for 30 minutes, or until the squash is tender but still firm. (Don't let it overcook because the squash might fall apart when you move it later.)

4 While the squash is baking, heat the olive oil in a small skillet over medium heat. Add the onions, mushrooms, garlic, and celery and cook until the onions are translucent. Stir in the pepper, parsley, sage, thyme, and lemon juice and remove from the heat.

5 Transfer the onion mixture to a mixing bowl. Add the apples, walnuts, raisins, bread, and cheese. Mix until well combined.

6 Remove the squash from the oven and transfer it, cut side up, to a decorative baking or casserole dish. Fill each squash half with half the stuffing mixture and press down lightly.

7 Cover tightly with foil and bake the squash for another 20 minutes, or until the cheese is melted and the stuffing is browned.

PER SERVING: *Calories 412 (From Fat 162); Fat 18g (Saturated 5g); Cholesterol 15mg; Sodium 320mg; Carbohydrate 56g (Dietary Fiber 11g); Protein 12g.*

(continued)

NOTE: Stuffed squash makes a festive main course for holiday meals and is a convenient and colorful centerpiece for the table. Any kind of squash will do, but acorn and butternut squash are the easiest to find in supermarkets.

TIP: Double or triple the recipe as needed to make enough servings to feed the number of guests you expect. You can also use the filling to make several small (3 to 4 inch), individual stuffed pumpkins if you prefer.

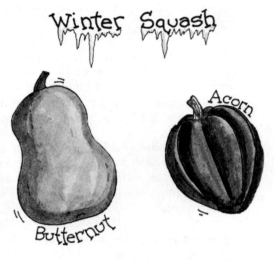

FIGURE 15-1:
These two common types of squash are great for stuffing.

Illustration by Elizabeth Kurtzman

Fluffy Mashed Potatoes
with Mushroom Gravy

INGREDIENTS

Potatoes:

5 pounds Yukon Gold potatoes, peeled and cut into 2-inch chunks (or halved if they're small)

¼ cup melted margarine

1 cup unflavored plant milk or nonfat cow's milk

¼ teaspoon salt

¼ teaspoon black pepper

Mushroom Gravy:

1 tablespoon olive oil

1 pound mushrooms, thinly sliced

1 medium onion, chopped

2 tablespoons unbleached all-purpose flour

1 vegetable bouillon cube

¼ teaspoon salt (if using a sodium-free bouillon cube; otherwise omit)

¼ teaspoon black pepper

1 cup unflavored plant milk or nonfat cow's milk

DIRECTIONS

1 Place the potatoes in a pot and fill with cold water to cover them. Cover and cook over medium-high heat until boiling; then reduce the heat, tilt the cover to allow steam to escape, and simmer for 30 minutes, or until the potatoes are tender.

2 While the potatoes are cooking, prepare the Mushroom Gravy. Heat the olive oil in a medium-sized skillet over medium heat. Add the mushrooms and onions and cook until the onions are translucent — about 5 minutes.

3 Add the flour, and crumble the bouillon cube into the skillet. Stir in the salt (if needed) and pepper.

4 Add the soymilk. Cook and stir for 2 to 3 minutes, until the gravy thickens and the ingredients are well blended. Pour into a small pitcher or serving dish and set aside until the potatoes are ready. If you don't serve it immediately, the gravy may need to be reheated in a microwave oven, or you can hold it on the stovetop, warming, until ready to eat.

5 When the potatoes are done, drain them. In a large bowl, combine the potatoes, margarine, milk, salt, and pepper. Mash with a potato masher until smooth and well blended. Use a wooden spoon to help blend the ingredients if necessary. Transfer to a serving dish and serve with the Mushroom Gravy.

PER SERVING: *Calories 346 (From Fat 77); Fat 9g (Saturated 3g); Cholesterol 0mg; Sodium 282mg; Carbohydrate 56g (Dietary Fiber 5g); Protein 10g.*

TIP: Yukon Gold potatoes lend a rich color to this dish. The gravy goes well on the potatoes, as well as over Everybody's Favorite Cheese and Nut Loaf (see the recipe earlier in this chapter).

VARY IT! Add 1 tablespoon chopped parsley or chives in Step 5.

Roasted Roots

INGREDIENTS

2 medium carrots, peeled and sliced into 1-inch pieces

1 medium turnip, peeled and sliced into 1-inch wedges

3 to 4 beets, peeled and quartered

1 parsnip, peeled, cut lengthwise, and then sliced

1 medium onion, quartered

2 small leeks, split and washed

1 medium white potato, peeled and cut into eighths

1 medium sweet potato, peeled and cut into eighths

1 bulb fennel, quartered

⅓ cup olive oil

4 cloves garlic (chopped or whole cloves)

3 (2-inch) sprigs fresh rosemary, chopped

½ teaspoon salt

½ teaspoon black pepper

5 tablespoons balsamic vinegar

DIRECTIONS

1 Preheat the oven to 350 degrees.

2 Place the vegetables and olive oil in a bowl and toss. Add garlic, rosemary, salt, and pepper. Set the fennel and leeks aside and arrange the remaining vegetables in one layer in an oiled roasting pan or on a greased cookie sheet. Do not cover.

3 Roast the vegetables for 15 minutes, and then add the fennel and leeks. Roast all the vegetables for an additional 50 minutes, or until tender. Pay particular attention to the beets and make sure that they're soft before removing them from the oven.

4 Toss the vegetables with the balsamic vinegar and serve.

PER SERVING: *Calories 198 (From Fat 81); Fat 9g (Saturated 1g); Cholesterol 0mg; Sodium 216mg; Carbohydrate 27g (Dietary Fiber 5g); Protein 3g.*

NOTE: Herbs and the roasting process bring out the delicious flavors of the root vegetables in this dish. The beets stain the other vegetables a rich red color.

Candied Sweet Potatoes

PREP TIME: 5 MINUTES | COOK TIME: 14 MINUTES | YIELD: 6 SERVINGS

INGREDIENTS

8 medium sweet potatoes
(about 3 pounds)

¾ cup packed brown sugar

2 tablespoons margarine

Juice of a fresh lemon
(optional)

DIRECTIONS

1   Cut the potatoes into ½-inch segments. Place the segments in a medium saucepan, cover with water, and bring the water to a boil. Let the potatoes simmer until tender — about 12 to 14 minutes. Cook longer if necessary, but don't let the potatoes get mushy.

2   Remove the potatoes from the heat and drain. Add the sugar and margarine, and stir gently with a large wooden spoon to coat the potatoes.

3   Spoon the potatoes into a serving bowl. Squeeze the juice of one lemon over the tops of the potatoes before serving (if desired).

PER SERVING: *Calories 349 (From Fat 40); Fat 5g (Saturated 1g); Cholesterol 0mg; Sodium 81mg; Carbohydrate 76g (Dietary Fiber 4g); Protein 3g.*

VARY IT! Substitute 1⁄3 cup maple syrup for the brown sugar. Add ¼ teaspoon ground ginger in Step 2. Another option: Add a handful of chopped pecans and/or 1⁄3 cup crushed pineapple in Step 2.

Maple Pecan Pumpkin Pie

PREP TIME: 15 MINUTES | **COOK TIME: 40 MINUTES** | **YIELD: 8 SERVING**

INGREDIENTS

1 (15-ounce) can pumpkin (about 2 cups)

8 ounces silken firm tofu

½ cup pure maple syrup

½ teaspoon ground ginger

1 teaspoon cinnamon

¼ teaspoon nutmeg

1 tablespoon unbleached all-purpose flour

1 (9-inch) pie shell

¼ cup chopped pecans

DIRECTIONS

1 Preheat the oven to 350 degrees.

2 Place the pumpkin, tofu, maple syrup, ginger, cinnamon, nutmeg, and flour in a blender or food processor and process until smooth.

3 Pour the pumpkin mixture into the pie shell.

4 Sprinkle the chopped nuts evenly over the top of the pie.

5 Bake for about 40 minutes, or until set. Cool and then serve.

PER SERVING: *Calories 236 (From Fat 99); Fat 11g (Saturated 2g); Cholesterol 0mg; Sodium 137mg; Carbohydrate 31g (Dietary Fiber 3g); Protein 5g.*

NOTE: Tofu replaces the eggs and milk in this pumpkin pie recipe. The filling is thick, rich, and smooth. If you use a ready-made pie shell, read the product label to ensure it does not contain lard.

4

Living — and Loving — the Vegetarian Lifestyle

Understand more deeply how best to make the transition to a vegetarian lifestyle complete.

Identify strategies for keeping the peace in households where you may be the only vegetarian at the table.

Discuss how to deal with the nonvegetarians you encounter every day outside your home.

Apply knowledge and skills to support your vegetarian diet when you're a guest at someone else's home or when you eat out.

Chapter **16**

Getting Along When You're the Only Vegetarian in the House

S ome food fights are easy to settle. He likes chunky and she likes creamy? Keep two jars of peanut butter in the cupboard. Butter versus margarine, or mayo against Miracle Whip? Not a problem — just keep both on hand.

If only all differences in food preferences were so easy to handle.

If you're a vegetarian, chances are good that you're the only vegetarian in your household. Like May–December romances, partnerships between a steak-and-potatoes type and a veggie lover can present challenges. If you're going vegetarian alone at home, you, your partner, and other immediate family members have to address several issues. Some will be unique to your living situation, but other problems are common in many people's experiences. An awareness of the issues and the manner in which you approach them can have a significant effect on your relationships.

Managing Family Meals

Should you make a standard meat-two-vegetables-a-starch-and-a-salad meal, dodge the meat, and fill up on the rest? Or do you make a separate vegetarian entrée for yourself?

Some families feel burdened by this problem. Nobody wants to get stuck cooking two meals for the same table every night. Should all meals be vegetarian, so that everyone can eat them? After all, most nonvegetarians enjoy many meatless dishes.

I don't have all the answers. The situation requires discussion and negotiation among all parties concerned. Unless you face it head on, though, it will bite you from behind.

Thinking through some of the options may help.

Making both meat and vegetarian foods

Serving both a meat entrée and a vegetarian alternative is the most obvious solution to the problem of preparing meals that everyone can eat. It's also the most work. For vegetarians who happen to be the family cook, it may also be out of the question if they don't want to handle and cook meat.

Deciding who prepares what

If you're the head cook in your household and you're a vegetarian, should you be expected to prepare meat for the nonvegetarians? Maybe it's time for a nonvegetarian family member to learn how to cook their own food. Another option: Prepare meals together. You can be in charge of everything but the meat.

On the other hand, maybe you don't want to subject yourself to the smell of cooking meat, or you don't want meat to touch your kitchen counter or pots and pans. I can relate to that point of view, but you'll have to hash this one out with your family. It may help to know that you're not alone — lots of people like you are out there.

If your household has meat-eaters, sit down and try to work out compromises that everyone can live with. Some options include the following:

>> You may agree that any meat brought into the house is prepared on waxed paper so that it doesn't touch the countertops, and that it's cooked in a pan dedicated solely to meat.

» You may decide to cook meats outdoors on a grill to keep offending odors and drippings out of the house.

» You may choose to buy only precooked meats such as deli or luncheon meats, which can be kept wrapped in the refrigerator and need no cooking or further preparation in the house.

TIP

If you're having difficulty negotiating meal issues with family members, it may help to talk to other vegetarians who've dealt with the same challenge. Consider joining an online vegetarian chat group, participating in a blog, or joining a local vegetarian society. The Vegetarian Resource Group maintains a list of these and other resources online at www.vrg.org/links/.

Respecting others' food preferences

What you eat is a highly personal decision. I've found over the years that it's best to let friends and family members make their own food choices without pressure from me — a strategy you may want to consider as well.

For a while, you may have to live with two variations at every meal. However, preparing both vegetarian and nonvegetarian options for family meals has its advantages. As any experienced vegetarian knows, the vegetarian option tends to look really tasty. Try setting a vegetarian pizza on the table with other pizzas at a party or any gathering. If you're a vegetarian, claim a slice quickly, because the nonvegetarians often want the vegetarian choice. If you're not quick enough, you may find your vegetarian option is gone.

Likewise, put a bowl of pasta topped with marinara sauce on the table side by side with pasta and meat sauce. Conduct a bit of research, and see which bowl empties fastest. I'll put my money on the marinara — I've seen it happen too many times.

So the idea is that if you set out vegetarian entrées, nonvegetarians are going to want them, too. Eventually, you may be making nothing but vegetarian meals, and the other people in your household may not even notice the transition. And all that arguing and teeth gnashing will have been for nothing.

Making do when you need to

Instead of making two meals, another option is for the vegetarian to eat large servings of whatever meatless foods are on the table. Mashed potatoes, steamed broccoli, salad, and a dinner roll make a great meal. You don't have to have a hole on your plate where the meat should be — you can cover up that bare spot with extra servings of the foods you like.

Many vegetarians use this same approach when they eat out at the homes of friends or others who don't serve vegetarian meals. They eat what they can of the available meatless foods. They don't draw attention to themselves (some vegetarians prefer it that way), and they don't give others the impression that it's hard to be a vegetarian by whining about not having an entrée.

This approach is passive and fairly nonconfrontational. Problems are most likely to arise if another family member is bothered by the fact that you're behaving outside the norm of the family. For some, it may appear that you're rejecting family values and traditions. You're not, of course — you're just changing them.

Finding the vegetarian least common denominator

Another sensible strategy is to consider vegetarian foods to be the least common denominator. In other words, everyone — vegetarians and nonvegetarians alike — can eat vegetarian foods, so when you plan meals, start with vegetarian choices. Choose foods that are vegetarian as prepared but to which a nonvegetarian can add meat as desired.

For example, make a stir-fry using assorted vegetables, and serve it on steamed rice. A nonvegetarian can cook chicken, shrimp, pork, or beef separately and add it to the dish. Rather than actually making two different entrées, you're modifying an entrée for a meat-eater. That should be considerably easier than making two distinct dishes.

The following foods are vegetarian, and meat-eaters can add small bits of meat if they so desire:

>> Bean burritos, nachos, or tacos

>> Italian stuffed shells, manicotti, cannelloni, or spaghetti with marinara sauce

>> Mixed green salad (large dinner-style)

>> Pasta primavera

>> Pesto pasta

>> Vegetable jambalaya

>> Vegetable lasagna with marinara sauce

>> Vegetable soup or stew

>> Vegetable stir-fry

>> Vegetarian chili

>> Vegetarian pizza

Gaining Support from Nonvegetarians

When it comes to handling family meals, several options that have worked for others may work for you, too. Because every family is different, though, you may have to adapt these ideas to fit your own circumstances.

For starters, take some simple steps (which I outline in this section) to make the other members of your household more receptive to vegetarian meals. Remember that you're asking them to trade in some of their favorite foods.

What would it take for you to give up something that you like and are comfortable with? You'd probably want a substitute that tastes as good as or better than the food you gave up. You wouldn't want to be inconvenienced. And you wouldn't want the change to leave you feeling dissatisfied.

Keep these points in mind when you ask for your family's support.

Employing strategies for compromise

If your family is agreeable, you may be able to get away with serving nothing but vegetarian meals, provided that everyone likes the choices. Whether you go vegetarian all the time or part of the time, it's a good idea to go out of your way to make foods that everyone likes.

Begin by making a list of family members' favorite foods that just happen to be vegetarian. For instance, your list may include vegetable-topped pizza, bean soup, chili, stuffed baked potatoes, macaroni and cheese, and pasta primavera.

To that list, add some transition foods — foods that look and taste like familiar meat-based foods — that appeal to most people. These alternatives taste good, and you can use them in the same ways as their meat counterparts. Let them serve as crutches or training wheels until people become more comfortable planning meals without meat. Here are some foods you might try:

>> Vegetarian burger patties and hot dogs

>> Vegetarian cold cuts for sandwiches

>> Vegetarian bacon, sausage links, and patties

>> Frozen, crumbled, textured vegetable protein to replace ground beef

REMEMBER

Let family members have input into planning, and incorporate their preferences into the menu. People who are involved in any aspect of meal planning are more likely to be interested in eating the food. Before long, you'll have a list of family favorites a mile long.

Setting a positive example

Don't push. It's that simple. When you preach to people and push them to do something they aren't ready to do — like change the way they eat — you're likely to get the opposite of the result you want.

REMEMBER

Instead, teach by your own example. If your family or partner isn't ready to make a switch to a vegetarian diet, quietly go about it by yourself. Your actions will make an impression, and chances are good that, given time, the others will notice, get interested, and make some dietary changes of their own.

I know this from experience. I grew up in Michigan in the 1960s and 1970s in a typical, traditional, meat-and-potatoes household. One day, just as my family was sitting down to dinner, my mother briefly announced that from that day forward she would be a vegetarian. She didn't say another word about it. No explanation except, "This is what I've decided is right for me." She sat down, and we ate our dinner.

My mother didn't discuss her vegetarianism with anyone. With the exception of her family and close friends, most people didn't even realize that she didn't eat meat. At family meals, she continued to prepare meat for my father and siblings, but she would make a cheese omelet or toasted cheese sandwich for herself (a Wisconsin native, she was stuck in the cheese-and-eggs rut!) and eat the same salad and vegetables that the rest of us ate.

Time went by. Then, one by one, my sisters and brother and I quietly went vegetarian ourselves. Nobody offered more of an explanation than to say to our mother, "You don't have to fix meat for me anymore." Eventually, the only person my mother was preparing meat for was my father. Many years later, meat faded out of his diet, too. Decades later, my parents are in their 90s and the rest of us are a whole lot older. And . . . we're still vegetarians.

This process has repeated itself with others I have known throughout my life. People notice what you eat, even if you never point it out. As the saying goes, "Actions speak louder than words." Those actions make an impression. Many times, they inspire others to reflect, and maybe even to make a change. In their own time. At their own pace.

The only reasonable alternative if you want others to change is to let them decide for themselves.

Negotiating the Menu When Guests Come

In addition to working out a family meal plan that promotes harmony, you may want to discuss how to handle such events as guests staying at your house and friends dropping in for dinner.

For some people, this kind of situation can cause friction, particularly when the lifestyle of the vegetarian in the household is seen as an intrusion or unwelcome deviation from the norm. Having outsiders come in can cause built-up tensions to flare. The meat-eater's point of view may be that if eating meat is the norm of the guests, the preferences of the majority should rule.

In other circles, vegetarianism may be no big deal. In fact, some of your guests may well be vegetarians themselves.

REMEMBER

If you live with someone who doesn't support your diet choice, it's a good idea to get the issue on the table and resolved before your guests arrive. You may decide to eat out, or you may opt to bring takeout food home. However you solve the dilemma, the important thing is to anticipate the problem and try to find a solution ahead of time.

Then enjoy the visit.

Giving your guests options

Many people are comfortable having some vegetarian dishes and some meat dishes available, with everyone free to choose what they please. This works well when the household already has a custom of serving two entrées — one meat-based and one meatless.

But nonvegetarians will often have a serving of the meatless choice. You want the nonvegetarians to have the option of tasting that delicious-looking vegetarian entrée if they care to, but you also want to ensure that enough is left for the vegetarians. So when you invite guests to come to your home, ask ahead of time whether anyone has special dietary needs. Do your best to estimate the number of people who may be interested in the vegetarian option — and then double that amount.

I once spent several days on a small boat on the Great Barrier Reef on a scuba diving trip. I was one of two vegetarians in a group of about 15 divers and crew. For our first meal — spaghetti — the cook set aside a small amount of pasta with meatless sauce for me and the other vegetarian on board. She labeled it as meatless and set it out on the serving table alongside the larger bowl of pasta with meat sauce.

I made the mistake of being near the end of the serving line. By the time I got to the head of the line, the vegetarian spaghetti was gone. From that day forward, the two vegetarians were permitted to go through the serving line first.

And I made an important realization — the vegetarian option often appeals to everyone, vegetarian or not.

Serving meals with mainstream appeal

One easy way to handle meals for guests is to rely on old standbys — such as vegetable lasagna or pasta primavera — that are familiar to both vegetarians and nonvegetarians alike. Serve either with a loaf of good bread and a fresh, colorful mixed green salad or bowl of minestrone soup, and finish the meal with coffee and a delectable dessert.

Nobody will notice the meat was missing.

Minimizing the focus on meat-free

Another strategy to redirect guests' attentions away from the fact that they're eating a meatless meal is to knock their socks off with a delicious, sophisticated, gourmet vegetarian meal, or an ethnic entrée such as an Indian curry dish or a Middle Eastern spinach pie. Many guests would be impressed and also enjoy the change of pace.

Don't forget about the importance of setting the mood, too. Dim the lights and put on some soft music. Set an attractive table. Use a tablecloth or placemats. Place a vase with a sprig of foliage or flowers from the yard on the table. Arrange foods in serving bowls or plates using sprigs of fresh herbs and sliced fruit as garnishes.

REMEMBER

Emphasize the experience of enjoying good food with good company. The fact that there's no meat on the table will be irrelevant.

Chapter **17**

Vegetarian Etiquette in a Nonvegetarian World

Maintaining a vegetarian lifestyle at home is one thing. Doing it away from home with style and grace is quite another thing.

You owe no one an explanation of your eating preferences. Keep in mind, though, that despite the fact that vegetarianism has become more mainstream in recent years, the vast majority of people still eat meat. You'll likely stand out, especially if you eat a vegan diet. For that reason, you're the one who has to do most of the adapting in social situations.

This chapter focuses on common situations for which you need to develop skills to relate with nonvegetarians. You'll become more comfortable managing these situations as you gain experience.

Mastering the Art of Diplomacy

You may be quite content to live a vegetarian lifestyle without explaining your choice to people or attempting to convert them. If so, you're probably the type who doesn't rub people the wrong way. You're an undercover vegetarian, not a walking-and-talking advocate, and that's fine. Even in your relative silence, you're making a statement.

On the other hand, if you frequently find yourself engaged in debates or earnest discussions about the merits of a vegetarian diet — whether you initiate the conversations or not — you should give some thought to your approach in handling these interactions.

Diplomacy is key, whether you prefer to do your own thing quietly or hope to inspire others to go vegetarian. You're going to need skills in dealing with social situations in which your vegetarian lifestyle converges with the nonvegetarian world. That takes time and experience. To help you get started, consider some of the ideas I share in this section.

Considering how you present yourself

Think about how people today may be perceived positively or negatively based on their social media posts, such as on Instagram or Facebook. Your physical appearance can give people the impression that you have it all together or that you're a frazzled wreck.

Similarly, the manner in which you conduct yourself in the presence of others affects the way they perceive you. If you're belligerent, bossy, or brash, you come off as being uncouth. Even if your point of view is valid, others are likely to discount your message at best, or be totally repulsed and reject it outright at worst.

Bumper stickers, buttons, and shirts with vegetarian slogans can express your politics loudly and clearly. One makes a statement. Two emphasize the point. But when your car and body are blanketed with these items, you're shouting. Some people may perceive you to be hysterical, depending on the degree of coverage of your car and clothing. Consider that you may reach a point of diminishing returns in terms of the extent to which people will listen to you when you express your views this way.

ACTIVISM DONE RIGHT

Some people feel that the in-your-face approach has a place. Opinions are neither right nor wrong, of course. The bra burners of the 1960s drew attention to women's rights issues with their very visible demonstrations of activism, and other women advocated for change in subtler ways. Likewise, a peace activist may wage a hunger strike to draw attention to the cause, while others promote peace behind the scenes. Ultimately, it's up to you whether — and how — you advocate for vegetarianism. Attacking others, however, is a negative approach that's likely to alienate people and make them less receptive to your message.

Responding to questions about your vegetarianism

"Why did you become a vegetarian?"

Most vegetarians have heard that question at least 25 times.

"If you don't eat meat, how do you get enough protein?"

They've heard that one just as many times.

"What do you eat for dinner?"

"Don't you just want a good steak once in a while?"

"If you're a vegetarian, why do you wear leather shoes?"

When someone inquires about your vegetarianism, the best response is a simple, straightforward answer. You don't have to expound on the basics — just the facts will do. This is generally also not the time for the hard sell, nor is it the time to push someone else's buttons by criticizing their lifestyle.

You need to use your own judgment, but most of the time when people ask questions such as these, they're just curious. They may not know much about vegetarianism, but you've piqued their interest. They may also be testing to determine what you're all about. Answer their questions concisely, but leave 'em wanting more. They'll ask when they want to know — and they may start asking you how they can become vegetarians themselves.

Being an effective role model

The world would be a better place if more people were vegetarians. Those of us who've already made the switch know how nice it can be to live a vegetarian lifestyle. A vegetarian lifestyle is good for you, good for the animals, and good for the environment and planet.

REMEMBER

As much as possible, try to be positive in the way you interact with others where food is concerned. Your attitude affects how people feel about you, and people will associate that feeling with how they feel about the concept of vegetarianism.

The truth is, being a vegetarian isn't particularly difficult, and vegetarianism has many benefits. Why not advertise that fact? Some vegetarians present themselves in a way that makes it appear that living a vegetarian lifestyle is difficult and problematic. Instead, aim to show people how easy and pleasurable a vegetarian lifestyle can be. Take the positive tack if you want other people to give vegetarianism serious consideration.

Filling your plate to showcase vegetarian variety

Show people that eating a vegetarian diet doesn't mean you have to go hungry when you eat meals away from home. Fill your plate with food. Let people see how colorful and appealing a meal without meat can be. Don't leave a hole on your plate or allow it to look empty, as if you're deprived.

Demonstrating flexibility in difficult situations

All vegetarians get stuck at a truck stop or a fast food restaurant occasionally, where the menu has nothing for them to eat. Those are the times when you kick into survival mode and take a can of juice, a side order of slaw, and a bag of chips and just hang on until the next opportunity to eat some real food.

Most of the time, though, vegetarians have plenty of food choices, or they can make do with what there is. Whether you're a guest at someone's home, eating out on business, traveling, or out with friends, try to be flexible when it comes to your meals. By being flexible, you show others that you can be a vegetarian in a nonvegetarian society without your lifestyle creating too much conflict. Send a positive message.

REMEMBER

Flexibility and planning are especially important for vegans. Vegans may find it more difficult than other types of vegetarians to eat away from home, especially in small or rural communities or when they're in the company of nonvegetarians or nonvegans and don't have total control over where a group goes to eat.

I was once with a group of people, including two vegans, at a conference in Kansas City. When it came time to find a place to have dinner the first night, we literally roamed the streets for over an hour, wearily walking into one restaurant after another, reading the menus, finding few vegan options, and walking out again. Eventually, after everyone was frustrated and overly hungry, we settled on a Chinese restaurant. We ended up eating there every night thereafter for the rest of that week. The impression I was left with was that it was no fun at all to be a vegan, and that it was tiresome and difficult to find something to eat away from home.

TIP

In a mixed group of vegetarians and nonvegetarians, or vegans and nonvegans, try to anticipate the limitations and preempt them. Steer your party to a restaurant at which you'll be most likely to have numerous choices. If you can't do that, do your best to make do wherever you land.

Some vegetarians eat a vegan diet at home but occasionally make exceptions and eat foods containing dairy and/or eggs when they're away and have limited choices. The reason? They prefer not to isolate themselves socially from nonvegans. They feel that by being 90 percent of the way there, they're achieving most of the benefits of a vegan lifestyle without sending others a negative message. (Does this make them a lacto-ovo vegetarian rather than a vegan? Technically, yes, but one that is closer to the vegan end of the vegetarian spectrum!)

REMEMBER

When you're setting an example for others, inspiring lots of people to drastically reduce their intake of animal products may be more important than inspiring one or two to go vegan.

Reconciling your approach and withholding judgment

Just as your decision to live a vegetarian lifestyle is a personal one, the manner in which you interact with people is also your call. You can be tolerant or intolerant, compassionate or confrontational.

Your approach may be different from someone else's. A concession on the part of one near-vegan to eat a food containing dairy or eggs when away from home may be completely unacceptable to another vegan, just as a flexitarian's decision to eat a piece of turkey on Thanksgiving may be an abhorrent choice to other vegetarians.

REMEMBER

In understanding others' choices, remember how complicated and deeply personal the subject of vegetarianism can be for everyone. Reconcile your approach as you see fit. Then work at projecting a positive image. Show others that you're confident, content, and at ease with your lifestyle.

Handling Dinner Invitations

Being invited to a nonvegetarian's home for dinner is one of the most common and most stressful events that many vegetarians encounter. How you approach the situation depends on the degree of formality of the occasion and how well you know your host.

WARNING

If you're a dinner guest at a nonvegetarian's home, carrying on about the evils of meat is a major faux pas. Even if another guest eggs you on and attempts to engage you in an earnest discussion or debate about the merits of vegetarianism, resist the temptation to participate. To do otherwise is just plain uncouth.

Informing your host about your diet

You're a vegetarian. Out with it.

You need to find the right moment to tell your host that you're a vegetarian, but do say something right away. If the invitation comes by phone or in person, the best time to say something is when you get the invitation.

Say something as simple as, "Oh, thanks, I'd love to come. By the way, I'd better tell you that I'm a vegetarian. You don't have to do anything special for me — I'm sure I'll find plenty to eat — but I just didn't want you to go to the trouble of fixing meat or fish for me."

The chances are good that your host will ask whether you eat spaghetti, lasagna, or some other dish that they're familiar with serving and thinks will suit your preferences. If your host suggests a shrimp stir-fry, you can also nip that one in the bud by letting them know that you don't eat seafood (if you don't). In that case, you may want to toss out a few more suggestions of foods you do eat, or you could reassure your host that you'll be fine with extra servings of whatever vegetables, rice, potatoes, salad, and other side dishes they plan to serve.

If you get an invitation to dinner by email, through a spouse or partner, or in some other indirect way, you have two choices:

>> Show up for dinner and eat what you can.

>> Call your host, thank them for the invitation, and mention that you're a vegetarian.

If you're invited as the guest of the invitee (your spouse, partner, date, and so on), you may want that person to call the host on your behalf. Examine the situation and do what feels most appropriate and comfortable.

REMEMBER

Initiating a conversation about your vegetarianism may feel a bit awkward, but telling your host upfront that you're a vegetarian may be less uncomfortable than showing up for dinner and finding nothing you can eat, or discovering that the host made something special for you that you have to decline. In either of these situations, not only do you run the risk of not getting enough to eat, but you also risk disappointing your host, or causing them to puzzle over why you aren't eating what they served.

Some people may get a little anxious when you say that you're a vegetarian. Most people who invite guests to dinner want them to enjoy the food and have a good time, and they may not be very familiar with what a vegetarian will and won't eat.

Reassure your host that you'll be fine. Most people appreciate knowing ahead of time that you won't be eating the meat or fish, as it saves them from preparing something that won't be eaten. It also saves everyone the disappointment or embarrassment of scurrying to find something for you to eat.

You don't want to be in a situation where the rice is cooked with chicken stock, the salad is sprinkled with bacon, the appetizer is shrimp cocktail, and steak is the main course. You can be a bit conspicuous if all you have on your plate is a dinner roll.

TIP

If you think you may have trouble finding something you can eat at your host's house, have a snack before you leave home. That way, you won't be starving if you discover that there isn't much to eat.

Offering to bring a dish

Another way to handle dinner invitations is to offer to bring a dish that you and everyone else can share. This works best in casual situations when you know your host well or the setting is relatively informal. You may not feel as comfortable suggesting this, for instance, if you're invited to a formal company function at the home of someone with whom you don't interact regularly. In that case, bringing your own food could look tacky.

Offer, but don't push. If you tell your host that you're a vegetarian and he sounds worried or unsure about how to handle it, you might say something like this:

> "If you'd like, I'd be happy to make my famous vegetable paella and saffron rice for everyone to try. It often complements other entrées, and a salad and bread would go well with it."

If your host bites, great. If they brush the suggestion aside, just consider your job done and leave it at that. Reassure them that you think you'll be fine eating the salad and side dishes that don't contain meat or seafood and that you're looking forward to coming.

Graciously declining nonvegetarian foods

Sometimes you tell your host you're a vegetarian, and they try to fix a special vegetarian meal for you but "miss." For example, they may prepare a gelatin mold salad, use eggs in the baked goods, put bacon on the salad, or serve the salad with Caesar dressing (it contains anchovies). What should you do?

Be the best actor that you can be and just eat whatever you can of the other parts of the meal. Make your plate look as full as you can so your host doesn't feel as though you don't have enough to eat. Assure them that you're fine. Enjoy the company, and eat when you get home.

If you can't finesse a refusal without your host detecting it, go ahead and fess up. Explain as gently and simply as possible that you prefer to pass up the dish and why. You might acknowledge that many people are surprised to discover that vegetarians don't eat gelatin (or lard, or beef broth, for example). Be sure to thank your host for their efforts and reassure them that you have plenty to eat.

Being a stealth vegetarian: What to do if your host doesn't know

If you decide for whatever reason not to tell your host in advance that you're a vegetarian, downplay the fact during the meal or stay undercover. Pointing out that you can't eat the food will make everyone uncomfortable and may put a damper on the gathering. Your host may feel badly and may even ask why you didn't say something sooner.

Eat what you can. If you have to ask about ingredients in the food or can't eat something because it's not vegetarian, be sure to play down any inconvenience. Reassure your host that you'll be just fine with what there is.

Managing Invitations to Parties and Other Special Events

It's fairly easy to manage invitations to weddings, banquets, and other functions with lots of people where the food is served from a buffet line. Even if a sit-down meal is served, a hotel or restaurant usually caters the food. You may find it much easier to speak to hotel or restaurant staff about getting a vegetarian meal than to ask the host directly.

Handling parties at private homes

If the function happens to be held at a private residence, follow the advice I give earlier in this chapter for dinner invitations. If the occasion involves a large number of guests, lots of food will likely be served and your host won't have to do anything special for you.

Making your way through public venues

If the event is at a hotel, club, community center, or restaurant, call ahead and ask to speak with the person in charge of food service. You don't have to say anything to your host. It's perfectly fine to speak to the chef or caterer and request a vegetarian or vegan entrée as a substitute for whatever the other guests are served. Most places will provide an alternate dish at no extra charge, but if you're worried, you can ask to be sure.

Be clear about what you can and can't eat. For example, if you eat no meat, fish, or poultry, say so. Otherwise, you may end up with fish or chicken, because vegetarian only means "no red meat" to some people. You might also ask about how the chef will prepare other items. For instance, if Caesar salad is on the menu, see whether a different type of dressing or salad can be set aside for you (and remind the kitchen that you don't eat bacon on your salad).

REMEMBER

When talking with a member of the food service staff, be sure to mention whether you eat dairy products or eggs. If you aren't explicit and you're vegan, you may end up with egg pasta, an omelet or a quiche, grated cheese on your salad, or cheese lasagna.

TIP

If you call the restaurant or hotel kitchen to request a vegetarian meal for an event, feel free to suggest a dish that you know you can eat and that the kitchen is likely to be able to make. For example, most kitchens have the ingredients on hand to make pasta primavera or a large baked potato topped with steamed vegetables. Those foods are simple to fix, and they can be preferable to that ubiquitous steamed vegetable plate.

As service begins and the waiter arrives at your table, quietly mention that you've ordered a vegetarian meal. If a plate containing meat lands at your place before you can say a word, let the food sit there until you can flag the waiter down to request your vegetarian meal.

If the meal is a buffet, you may not even need to mention to your host that you're a vegetarian, unless you think the menu may be limited. If the buffet is at a restaurant or hotel, it will likely include a wide variety of dishes and plenty of foods you can eat.

TIP

If you're vegan, however, it may still be wise to phone ahead and ask about the menu, just to be certain that it will have dairy- and egg-free choices. You may have to request that some rice, pasta, or vegetables are set aside for you if everything on the buffet line is doused with butter or cream sauce. The chef may even be able to make you a separate, suitable dish.

Dating Nonvegetarians

If your date is also a vegetarian, you're off to a good start. All you have to worry about (food-wise, anyway) is whether you're in the mood for Mexican or Thai or Ethiopian food. Even if you're a lacto ovo vegetarian and they're vegan, at least you're simpatico — you'll work it out.

On the other hand, if your date isn't a vegetarian, broach the subject early on. You don't have to make a big deal of the fact that you don't eat meat, but it's probably best to mention that fact sooner rather than later, and probably before you get together for a meal.

TIP

If you think the relationship has the potential to become serious, ask yourself the following:

>> Do I expect this person to stop eating meat eventually?

>> What would the ground rules be if we decided to live together?

>> Would I be willing to have meat in the house?

>> Would we cook two different meals or fend for ourselves?

>> What would we do if nonvegetarian guests came over for dinner — serve them meat or not? How would we resolve the conflict if we had different views about what to do?

>> Can I live and let live, or would I want my partner to see things as I do and maintain a vegetarian lifestyle?

This last question is especially important if your vegetarianism is rooted in ethical beliefs or attitudes. Compromising is difficult to do when your personal philosophy is on the line. You have to decide whether your life has room for someone who lives differently.

Some vegetarians find it harder to connect with a partner who doesn't share the same sensitivities. If it doesn't matter now, it may later. You don't have to arrive at any hard-and-fast conclusions about these issues today, but if you've never faced them before, it's a good idea to begin thinking about them.

If you do decide to get serious with a nonvegetarian, be sure to think about how to make the relationship work over the long run. If you want children, talk about whether you'd raise them as vegetarians.

Some vegetarians won't even date a nonvegetarian. (Kiss someone with greasy cheeseburger lips? No way!) Would you? If you restrict yourself to dating only fellow vegetarians, you may spend many a Saturday night alone in front of a screen. After all, vegetarians make up only a single digit percentage of the population, and only a fraction of that number is in the market for a date.

TIP

Vegetarian singles groups are active in some cities. Check with your local vegetarian society to see whether such a group exists in your area. These groups plan restaurant outings, outdoor activities, and other events with the needs and interests of singles in mind.

Working It Out: Vegetarianism on the Job

In many professions, your success at the office is partly dependent on how well you blend into the organization's culture. If your job involves entertaining clients or meeting with colleagues over lunches and dinners, your eating habits will be on display for all to observe.

If you're a vegetarian, the manner in which you conduct yourself can lead others to mark you as either sensible and health-conscious or eccentric and difficult to get along with. Your vegetarianism may be an asset or a liability, depending on how you play it.

To tell or not to tell?

Your dietary preferences may matter more in some work settings than in others. An advertising agency or a marketing department within a company, for instance, is likely to be comfortable with creative people who do things differently.

On the other hand, if you're in a more conservative line of work such as law or banking — especially in rural areas and parts of the country where vegetarianism may be less prevalent — it may be more important for you to appear compatible with your peers. Attitudes about vegetarianism have changed considerably in recent years, but some people are still likely to be less receptive to your lifestyle than others.

Why should you care about what your co-workers think of your eating habits?

In general, it's helpful in any work setting to be collegial and share a sense of camaraderie with your coworkers. Make people comfortable when they're with you. Enjoying a meal together is often part of that. If you play your cards right, you can turn the difference in your lifestyle into an asset that will reflect positively on you and enhance others' impressions of you.

TIP

To increase your likelihood of success, don't preach about the benefits of being a vegetarian. With your actions as a model, you can communicate an understated message to your co-workers that they'll get loud and clear. Show them that you care about your health, that you're socially and environmentally conscious, and that you have the self-discipline and determination to persevere with healthy lifestyle habits.

Handling meals during job interviews

Job interviews often involve lunching with your prospective employer and colleagues. If that happens, you don't need to hide the fact that you're a vegetarian. At the same time, you don't need to make a big deal of it. Just approach the subject in a confident, matter-of-fact way. Remember the following:

>> First impressions count. In job interviews, you want your prospective employer and colleagues to focus on your skills and ideas, not on the fact that you don't eat meat. When they reflect back on their meeting with you, you want them to think about how well you'll fit into their environment and how your unique set of abilities will be an asset to their organization.

>> When you're on a job interview, the people interviewing you often choose the restaurant where you'll eat. As a result, you may not have an opportunity to steer them to a restaurant with lots of vegetarian choices. If that happens, size up your menu options as quickly as possible, and downplay inconveniences due to your diet.

TIP

If you have plans to go to a restaurant that's unfamiliar to you, try to look at the menu ahead of time. Most restaurants post their menus online. If you don't see an obvious vegetarian option, call the restaurant and ask for recommendations about what may be possible for you to order. Given enough notice, finer restaurants are usually happy to prepare a special meal for you.

It's fine to ask the waiter whether the soup is made with chicken stock or a beef base, or if the beans contain lard. But if you do, make it as low-key as you can. If the answer is affirmative, have an alternative choice in mind so that you don't hold up the table's order while you struggle to find another dish.

>> Have an off-menu choice in mind, in case you have trouble finding something on the menu. In a restaurant that serves pasta, for example, it's usually easy for the kitchen to whip up pasta tossed with olive oil, garlic, and vegetables, or pasta served with a marinara sauce. If you find yourself at a steakhouse, go for a baked potato, salad, and vegetable side dishes.

You may find yourself at a job interview being served a catered luncheon in a conference room. If you're served a preplated ham sandwich, eat what you can from your plate and leave the rest. No explanation is necessary unless someone asks why you've left the food. In that case, all you have to say is, "I don't eat ham." Reassure your host that you're okay. The key is not to make a big deal out of the fact that they served you meat and you aren't eating it.

Leaving a positive impression

The best way to handle your dietary difference is to present yourself with confidence and in a matter-of-fact way. Let your co-workers view you as being sensible and health conscious, virtues that would reflect upon you positively in most business settings.

Just keep it low-key. After all, if one of your co-workers had values that didn't suit you, would you want to hear about it every day?

WARNING

Whatever you do, don't allow yourself to be sucked into silly conversations or debates about the political or ethical issues relating to vegetarianism. These subjects have great merit, but you'll be a loser if you bring them up in a business setting.

IN THIS CHAPTER

» **Taking a positive approach**

» **Considering restaurant options**

» **Combining vegetarian menu items**

» **Advocating for yourself at restaurants**

» **Staying on course when you travel**

Chapter **18**

Eating in Restaurants and Other Venues

Despite the 16-ounce steaks and entire chicken halves that you may find on the menu, ordering vegetarian entrées when you go out to eat is much easier now than it was in the past. Even so, keep a few tricks up your sleeve to ensure that you get what you want when you order meals away from home.

This chapter covers some of the strategies and know-how that seasoned vegetarians rely on when they go out to eat in the nonvegetarian world, whether at a neighborhood restaurant or farther away from home.

Adopting the Right Attitude

Eating out is one of life's great pleasures. Your vegetarian diet shouldn't get in the way of enjoying good food in the company of other people.

In fact, you may find just the opposite is true: Living vegetarian can open up a wide range of new food options at restaurants that serve foods you don't make or can't easily make at home.

Eating out on a vegetarian diet can be fun. It's all a matter of your perspective and of understanding some ways to expand your choices wherever you go.

Staying flexible

One key to enjoying vegetarian meals away from home is your ability to adapt to the environment you find yourself in. At certain times and in certain circumstances, you may find that you don't have much control over where you eat out.

Keep an open mind-set. If you find yourself at a restaurant where the closest thing to a vegetarian entrée is the macaroni and cheese side dish, get creative. Order a few side dishes and piece together your own meal. Eat less for dinner but enjoy a favorite dessert. Be ready to adapt to your setting as needed.

Savoring the atmosphere and the companionship

Enjoy your surroundings and the people you're with when you eat out. The setting and company are as much a part of the experience as the food.

Let's face it: Most of us aren't at risk of withering away from lack of food. If you find yourself in a situation where you have few good meatless menu options, order what you can. Then turn your attention to the beautiful view, the soothing music, and the stimulating conversation. Have a snack later if you get hungry before your next meal.

Choosing the Restaurant

The good news for vegetarians is that the restaurant industry has gotten the word that a sizable proportion of the population wants meatless foods when they eat out. Not all these people are full-fledged vegetarians, but they see vegetarian meals as being healthful and tasty alternatives.

Even some of the most traditional restaurants have responded by adding at least one or two vegetarian options to their menus. Many have added veggie burgers because burgers are so familiar and popular.

Wherever you go, you have options now. Look for vegetarian restaurants, and try cafes nestled into natural foods supermarkets, where high-quality, delicious, meatless entrées are nearly always available. Mix it up by eating at ethnic restaurants serving Middle Eastern, Chinese, Indian, and other cultural cuisines known for their many good meatless dishes. (For more on different cultural cuisines, see the "Ethnic options" section later in the chapter.)

Chains versus fine dining

Finer restaurants and family-run venues are often in a good position to accommodate special requests. They tend to prepare their menu items at the time you order, so you usually have an opportunity to make substitutions or other modifications, such as ordering a salad without bacon bits or a plate of pasta without the meat sauce.

In contrast, chain restaurants are less likely to be able to help you out, because many of their menu items are premade. They may not be able, for instance, to cook the rice without chicken stock — the rice may have been made in a large batch the day before — or to make the pasta without meat in the sauce.

REMEMBER

Ask questions about how the food is prepared *before* you order. If you prefer to avoid cream, butter, grated cheese, anchovies, and other animal products, check to be sure that the restaurant doesn't add these ingredients to the food, rather than sending the food back after it comes to the table with the offending ingredient.

TIP

Be aware of cooking terms that can be clues that a menu item contains an animal product. For example, *au gratin* usually means that the food contains cheese, *scalloped* means that the dish contains cream, *sautéed* can mean that the food is cooked in butter, and *creamy* usually means that the item is made with cream or eggs.

REMEMBER

Be reasonable about special requests, especially if you can see that the restaurant is very busy. If it's a Friday or Saturday night and the place is packed, make your requests as simple as possible.

VEGETARIAN CHOICES ON THE RUN

Fast-food restaurants usually have only limited vegetarian options, but some have several. Examples include pancakes with syrup, muffins, mixed green salads, bean burritos (you can order them without the cheese), bean soft tacos or regular tacos, bean tostadas, beans-and-cheese, veggie burgers, baked potatoes with toppings from the salad bar, and veggie wrap sandwiches. Note that yogurt served at some fast-food restaurants may contain gelatin.

Vegetarian restaurants and natural foods cafes

Many natural foods stores have a cafe tucked away in a corner where you can get a quick bite to eat. Some carry cold salads and ready-made sandwiches, and others have a more extensive menu, including a salad bar, hot foods, and baked goods. These cafes are popular places for many people to pick up a takeout meal for lunch during the workweek or for dinner on the way home from work.

Vegetarian restaurants, on the other hand, can run the gamut from homey little vegetarian hideaways to large metropolitan restaurants that stay packed for lunch and dinner. Some are raw foods specialists or macrobiotic eateries, others concentrate on vegan cuisine, and many serve foods with an ethnic bent, such as Indian or Middle Eastern, or a blend of various ethnic cuisines.

Some vegetarian restaurants have an atmosphere that harks back to the counterculture feel of the 1960s and 1970s, with an earthy environment that's usually quite casual. You're likely to find brown rice rather than white rice on the menu, and whole-grain breads rather than white, refined dinner rolls. Even desserts such as cookies and pie crusts may be made from whole grains.

Many vegetarian restaurants flag menu items that are vegan. You'll find packets of raw sugar on the table, and the menu will offer natural soft drinks, herbal teas, dishes made with tempeh and tofu, and foods made with minimally processed ingredients. You may find soymilk or other plant milks on the menu, too. All of these features — as well as a rustic, homey atmosphere — give many vegetarian restaurants a distinctive personality that sets them apart from other restaurants.

TIP

Many "old-school" cafeteria-style restaurants have a vegetable plate option that lets you assemble your own "veggie plate" comprised of three or four of the meatless side dish choices. To be the on safe side, especially in rural areas, you may want to confirm with the wait staff that vegetables such as green beans or cooked greens aren't cooked with bacon or other meats.

Ethnic options

Many countries, such as India and China, have vegetarian traditions. Not everyone in these countries is vegetarian, but many are, and everyone — vegetarian or not — is familiar with the concept of vegetarianism and vegetarian foods.

Other countries — including those along the Mediterranean Sea, in the Middle East, and in parts of Latin America — have some traditional foods that happen to be vegetarian, despite the fact that the diets in these cultures often rely heavily on meats and other animal products. For example, people in the Middle East eat lamb in large amounts, but falafel, spanakopita (you know it as "spinach pie"), and hummus are also traditional favorites that happen to be vegetarian.

What you order when you eat at an ethnic restaurant depends on what type of vegetarian diet you follow and how that restaurant prepares specific foods.

In one Italian restaurant, for example, the pasta with marinara sauce may be topped with cheese, and in another restaurant, it may not. If you're vegan, you probably won't eat the spanakopita at a Greek restaurant, because it's usually made with cheese. On the other hand, you may be perfectly happy with a Greek salad (minus the feta cheese), some pita bread, and an order of boiled potatoes with Greek seasonings.

REMEMBER

Wherever you eat, ask the wait staff for specifics about how the restaurant prepares the food, especially if you're vegan. One restaurant's baked ziti in marinara sauce may be free of all dairy products, while another's may come to the table smothered in melted mozzarella. Some restaurants prepare marinara sauce using beef broth, or use pasta made with eggs.

The following are common vegetarian foods served in a variety of ethnic restaurants:

At Italian restaurants, try:

>> Fresh vegetable appetizers (sometimes called antipasto) with or without mozzarella cheese

>> Mixed green salads

>> Minestrone soup, lentil soup, or pasta e fagioli (pasta with beans)

>> Focaccia and Italian bread with olive oil or flavored oil for dipping

>> Vegetable-topped pizzas (with or without cheese)

>> Pasta primavera

>> Spaghetti with marinara sauce

>> Pasta with olive oil and garlic

>> Italian green beans with potatoes

>> Cappuccino or espresso

>> Italian ices and fresh fruit desserts

At Mexican restaurants, try:

>> Tortilla chips with salsa and guacamole

>> Bean nachos

>> Mixed green salads

>> Gazpacho

>> Bean soft tacos, tostadas, and burritos

>> Spinach burritos or enchiladas

>> Cheese enchiladas

>> Bean chalupas (fried tortillas layered with beans, lettuce, tomato, and guacamole)

>> Chiles rellenos (cheese-stuffed green pepper, usually batter-dipped and fried, topped with tomato sauce)

>> Flan (custard dessert made with milk and eggs)

WARNING

Vegetarians should make it a habit to ask whether beans are cooked with lard, a common practice at Mexican restaurants. Restaurant menus don't always note whether the beans are prepared vegetarian–style.

At Chinese restaurants, try:

>> Vegetable soup or hot and sour soup

>> Vegetarian spring rolls or egg rolls

>> Sweet and sour cabbage (cold salad)

>> Vegetable dumplings (fried or steamed)

>> Minced vegetables in lettuce wrap

>> Sesame noodles (cold noodle appetizer)

>> Sautéed greens

>> Chinese mixed vegetables with steamed rice

>> Broccoli with garlic sauce

>> Vegetable lo mein

>> Vegetable fried rice

>> Szechwan-style green beans or eggplant (spicy)

>> Family-style tofu or Buddha's Delight

>> Other tofu and seitan (gluten) dishes

At Indian restaurants, try:

>> Dal (lentil soup)

>> Cucumber and yogurt salad

>> Chapati, pappadam, naan, and roti (Indian breads)

>> Samosas and pakoras (vegetable-filled appetizers)

>> Mutter paneer (tomato-based dish made with cubes of cheese and peas)

>> Vegetable curry with steamed rice

>> Palak paneer (spinach-based dish with soy cheese)

>> Lentil, chickpea, and vegetable entrées

>> Rice pudding

At Ethiopian restaurants, try:

>> Fresh vegetable salads

>> Injera (large, round, flat, spongy bread — tear off small pieces and use them to pinch bites of food from a communal tray)

>> Bean, lentil, and vegetable-based dishes served directly on a sheet of injera on a tray or platter

At Middle Eastern restaurants, try:

>> Hummus

>> Spinach salad

>> Dolmades (stuffed grape leaves)

>> Baba ghanoush (a blended eggplant dip or appetizer)

>> Fatoush (minced fresh green salad)

>> Tabbouleh salad (wheat salad)

>> Spanakopita (spinach pie)

>> Lentil soup

- » Falafel plate or sandwich (chickpea patties)

- » Vegetarian stuffed cabbage rolls (filled with rice, chickpeas, and raisins)

- » Halvah (sesame dessert)

- » Muhallabia (ground rice pudding; contains milk but no egg)

- » Ramadan (cooked, dried fruit with nuts, often served with cream and nutmeg)

Working with Menu Choices

You may occasionally encounter a menu with virtually nothing for a vegetarian. Some fast-food restaurants, "Southern-style" restaurants and truck stops are good examples — the baked beans contain pork, the biscuits are made with lard, the vegetables are cooked with bacon, and the staff just chuckles and looks incredulous when you ask whether the menu has any meatless items.

You're stuck.

In most cases, though, choices abound — you just have to get creative. With a little practice, getting a vegetarian meal at a nonvegetarian restaurant is a relatively simple matter.

Asking about appetizers

Combine several appetizers to create a vegetarian plate. For example, you might order a mixed green salad, a bowl of gazpacho, an order of stuffed mushrooms, and an appetizer portion of grilled spinach quesadilla.

This approach is a great way to taste a sampling of several foods. It's also a good way to control the amount of food you eat. Restaurant portions — especially for entrées — are often excessively large. By ordering a few appetizers, you can help hold your meal to a reasonable amount of food.

Surveying the sides

Just as you may create a meal from the appetizer menu, you can also piece together a full plate from a sampling of sides.

Pay attention to the descriptions of entrées on the menu, including the sides listed with meat dishes. Choose three or four and check with your server to find out how they're prepared. With a salad and some good bread, your meal may be the envy of the others at your table.

Coming up with creative combinations

When a restaurant isn't vegetarian-friendly, scan the menu to get an idea of the ingredients the restaurant has on hand. In many cases, you can ask for a special order using ingredients that the restaurant uses to make other menu items.

For example, if the restaurant serves spaghetti with meat sauce, you know it has pasta. The tomato sauce may be already mixed with meat, but the restaurant may have vegetables on hand for side dishes. Ask for pasta primavera made with olive oil and garlic and whatever vegetables the chef can add.

If all else fails, ask for a baked potato and a salad, or a salad and a tomato sandwich on whole-wheat toast. Be creative. If the restaurant serves baked potatoes, ask for one as your entrée. You can top it with items from a salad bar, if the restaurant has one. Try adding broccoli florets, salsa, black olives, sunflower seeds, or whatever looks good to you.

Making sensible substitutions

Take a good look at meat-containing entrées and determine whether the restaurant can prepare them as vegetarian dishes instead. For instance, a pasta dish mixed with vegetables and shrimp could easily be made without the shrimp. A club sandwich could be fixed with grilled portobello mushrooms, avocado, cheese, or tomato slices instead of the meat. This is most likely to work at restaurants where the food is made to order and not premade.

Working with Restaurant Staff

Your attitude and level of confidence can make a difference in how well you do when you order a vegetarian meal at nonvegetarian restaurants. Your relationship with the wait staff is key.

Try these tips to make the most of your dining experience:

>> **Be assertive:** When you speak with restaurant staff about your order, be clear about what you want. For instance, instead of just saying, "I'm a

vegetarian," explain specifically what you do and don't eat. Let the wait staff know whether dairy and eggs are okay, or if you don't want your foods flavored with chicken broth or beef broth.

Don't be afraid to press to get the information you need to order effectively. Ask your server whether your special request will increase or decrease the cost of the meal, too.

>> **Smile and say thank you:** As your mother taught you, "please" and "thank you" go a long way. If you need special attention from restaurant staff to get a meal you can eat, ask for it. But be as pleasant as possible. Ask the wait staff for suggestions if you can't figure out what to order.

Traveling Vegetarian

When you travel, you have less control over meals, you may be in unfamiliar surroundings, and you have to contend with the challenges that a change in your normal routine can bring. That can put you at risk of eating poorly, particularly if you can't find the meatless options you need.

For vegetarians, avoiding meat and possibly other animal products away from home requires a set of skills acquired with time and experience. In this section, I help you get started by explaining ways you can improve your chances of getting what you need when you're on the road, in the air, or on the sea.

Tips for trippin' by car, bus, or train

If you get hungry when you're traveling by car or bus, you're usually limited to whatever is near the exit off the highway. Your choices are likely to be a fast-food restaurant, a family chain eatery, or a truck stop with limited choices for vegetarians.

Traveling by train, your food choices may vary, depending on the type of train you're riding. Commuter trains may offer no food service whatsoever. Trains with longer routes may have meal cars serving pre-packaged snacks and drinks, or table service with limited menus.

In all these cases, consider carrying your own food. Pack a cooler or bag of food to take along. On car trips, it'll save you time not having to stop for meals. You'll save money and eat more healthfully, too.

If you do pack your own food, portable, nutritious choices include:

>> Bagels

>> Bottles of mineral water or flavored seltzer water

>> Deli salads

>> Fresh fruit

>> Homemade, whole-grain quick breads, muffins, and cookies

>> Hummus sandwiches

>> Individual aseptic (shelf-stable) packages of soymilk or other plant milk

>> Individual boxes of dry breakfast cereal

>> Instant soup cups or instant hot cereal cups that you can mix with hot water from the coffee maker at a gas station food mart

>> Peanut butter or almond butter sandwiches on coarse, whole-grain bread

>> Peeled baby carrots

>> Small cans or aseptic packages of fruit juice

>> Snack-sized cans of fruit or applesauce

>> Tofu salad sandwiches

TIP

If you like to take trips by bicycle, or if you hike, you need to pack foods that are light and portable and don't require refrigeration. Dried fruit and nut mixtures, small containers of plant or fruit juice, crackers and peanut butter, and fresh fruit are good choices.

Food for fliers

Airlines have cut back on meal service, especially on shorter flights. So don't be surprised if the next time you fly, you aren't served anything more than peanuts or snack mix and a beverage. Be prepared. Many travelers now routinely carry on their own food from home.

WARNING

If you bring food from home for a flight, be prepared for airport security personnel to pull your carry-on aside for an additional search. To avoid delays, consider taking foods out of your carry-on bag and setting them in the bin separately before you go through screening. For more information about what you are allowed to carry onboard, check out the government's TSA website: www.tsa.gov/travel/security-screening/whatcanibring/food.

Most airlines still offer full meal service on most longer and overseas flights, and they'll usually accommodate requests for vegetarian meals if you give them enough notice. Call the airline's reservation desk or, better yet, go online and place an online order with the airline at least 24 hours before your flight. Ideally, you should make the request when you initially book your reservations.

Meal service options are in a state of flux because of continuing cutbacks in service at most airlines. In the past, most airlines offered several options for vegetarians, including lacto ovo, lacto vegetarian meals, and vegan meals. Some even offered fruit plates, Asian vegetarian meals, or Indian vegetarian meals. Check with your airline to find out which options are available.

On most flights, the crew has a list of passengers who've ordered special meals. They may identify you as you're taking your seat, or they may ask you to ring your flight attendant call button just before meal service begins. On other flights, you get served a regular meal unless you speak up and tell the flight attendant that you've ordered a vegetarian meal.

TIP

If you're seated near the back of the plane, you may want to ring your call button early during meal service to let attendants know that you're expecting a vegetarian meal. That ensures that they don't give it away before they get to you, which can happen when someone seated in front of you asks for a vegetarian meal despite not having ordered one, or when the airline hasn't loaded enough of a particular special request onto the aircraft.

Meatless at sea

Many cruise ships are like spas or small communities on the water, with a wide selection of restaurants and foods, including healthful, vegetarian options. Some have separate menus for health-conscious people, or they flag specific entrées and menu items as being "healthy." In many cases, that means meatless.

If meat is included in the dish, it can often be left out of meals that are cooked to order. For example, a large salad topped with chicken strips can be made without the chicken, and a stir-fried vegetable and meat dish can be made with all the same ingredients, minus the meat.

If you find that the menu choices on a particular day don't include enough meatless options, handle the situation the way you would at a fine restaurant. Explain your needs to your server or the chef and ask for a special order. If possible, let the kitchen know what you want the day before, especially if the ship is going to seat a large number of people (for the captain's dinner, for instance).

TIP

If you have concerns about whether a cruise line can accommodate your food preferences, check online, email or call the customer service department, or have your travel agent request information about meals and get sample menus to examine.

In addition to elaborate, sit-down meals, cruise ships are known for their expansive buffets. The sheer volume and variety of foods at these buffets makes it easy for most vegetarians to find enough to eat. You'll have to sidestep the gelatin salads, and vegans may have to bypass items made with cream and cheese. Fill up on good-for-you fresh tropical fruit salads, rice, pasta, vegetables, and breads.

Coming up with alternatives: When plans go awry

Be prepared to improvise when you travel. You may not be able to anticipate every complication that affects your meals, but if you're flexible and creative, you can deal effectively with most of them.

Most travel snafus involving meals happen when you travel by plane. As any frequent flyer will tell you, ordering a vegetarian meal doesn't ensure you'll get it. This isn't always the airline's fault — sometimes a last-minute change of aircraft means that the meals meant for your flight aren't on that plane.

If you miss a flight and have to take an alternate flight, you won't get the meal that you specially ordered. If you upgrade your ticket to first class just before you board your flight, your vegetarian meal may be back in coach, and you may have another (maybe better) menu from which to choose. Your flight attendant can usually retrieve your meal from coach, though, if you still want it.

TIP

If you have a particularly long travel day and want to be extra sure that your vegetarian meal has been ordered, phone the airline or check online a day or two before you leave, just to confirm that the request has been noted. This is especially important if you've made a schedule change, because the agent may not have carried your meal request over to your new reservation.

If you do find yourself stuck with a ham sandwich instead of your vegetarian meal, here are a few things you can do:

>> Eat what you can of the meal you've been served. Picking the meat off a sandwich and eating the rest isn't an option for many vegetarians, nor is pushing the sausage away from the stack of pancakes that it's been leaning against. But your only other option may be peanuts and tomato juice, so if you're really hungry, eat the salad and dessert.

>> Ask your flight attendant for cookies, crackers, nuts, pretzels, or juice. A flight attendant who knows you haven't received your special order will often help you out with some extra snacks or beverages.

>> Pull out the reserves (fresh fruit, nuts, a bagel, or a sandwich) that you took along in your carry-on bag, just in case.

TIP

Whatever your mode of travel, packing your own provisions is good insurance for times when best-laid meal plans fall through. Some good ideas include small containers of aseptically packaged plant milk or fruit juice, packaged crackers, pretzels, nuts, dried fruit, or trail mix. You can sprinkle trail mix over a green salad during in-flight meals or at airport food courts to turn a salad into a substantial meal or snack.

TIP

Take opportunities to restock while you're traveling. Many hotels have bowls of fruit at the checkout desk. Before you leave your hotel, pick up a piece and stow it in your carry-on bag or luggage. If you don't find fruit at your hotel, buy a piece or two in the airport terminal or at a supermarket or cafeteria. Fruit is good to have on hand in case you get hungry while you're traveling, and it's a good source of dietary fiber and other nutrients that people tend to neglect when they travel.

REMEMBER

Also keep in mind that if you stay in hotels that have rooms with a refrigerator, you can pick up a few breakfast or lunch items from a local grocery store. You may save enough money to splurge on a nice dinner, and you may also have something leftover to carry on for your next flight!

5

Living Vegetarian for a Lifetime

Understand what you need to know when you're pregnant and the urge for pickles and nondairy ice cream strikes.

Know how to handle first foods, food fights, and other potential challenges in raising young children on a vegetarian diet.

Explore issues relating to older vegetarian children and teens, including understanding growth rates, balancing nutrition and treats, and getting kids interested in good foods whether they're at home or away.

Discuss the changing needs of adult vegetarians and special health advantages of eating green as you age.

Examine ways to stay active the vegetarian way for as long as you want to, including athletes of all skill levels.

Chapter **19**

When You're Expecting: Managing Your Vegetarian Pregnancy

There's no better time to be a vegetarian than when you're expecting. A healthful vegetarian — and even vegan — diet can provide a woman and her baby with all the nutrients needed for a healthy start in life.

But don't be surprised if your family and friends don't know it.

Tell people you're pregnant and that you're a vegetarian, and all sorts of alarms go off. Your family and friends may not have personal experience with a vegetarian diet, and they may not have a current understanding of the science. They're anxious, and anxieties heighten when a baby's involved.

Of course, vegetarians all over the world have been having healthy babies for centuries. In North America, though, the idea of meat-free diets for babies and children still sounds to some like a radical idea.

That's slowly changing. But until more people have a better understanding of vegetarian diets, concern over your vegetarian pregnancy may seem like an irritating intrusion.

Take comfort in knowing that people care. The information in this chapter will help put to rest some of the most common worries.

Before Baby: Ensuring a Healthy Start

Not every pregnancy is planned, but if you think you may get pregnant soon, it's a perfect time to be proactive and get yourself into great nutritional shape. The longer you have to eat well before you become pregnant, the better for you and your baby.

Prepregnancy advice for vegetarians is similar to advice for nonvegetarians:

TECHNICAL STUFF

>> Follow your health-care provider's advice about taking a regular-dose, daily multivitamin and mineral supplement for several months before you get pregnant. In particular, it's important to have adequate folic acid before pregnancy.

Folic acid may help prevent a *neural tube defect* such as *spina bifida* in your baby. Spinal bifida is a type of birth defect that involves an incomplete closure of the spinal cord.

>> Limit sweets and junk foods. They displace more nutritious foods from your diet.

>> If you drink coffee, limit it to two cups a day. Avoid alcohol and tobacco.

>> Get regular physical activity and drink plenty of water.

REMEMBER

Vegetarians often go into pregnancy with an edge over nonvegetarians, because vegetarians are more likely than other people to have close-to-ideal body weights.

Paying careful attention to your diet and fitness level can go a long way toward ensuring a healthy pregnancy and baby. Drinking plenty of fluids, especially water, and getting plenty of rest round out a healthful prepregnancy lifestyle. In this section, I tell you what you need to know about nutrition and exercise when you're thinking about becoming pregnant.

Maximizing nutrition before you get pregnant

The longer you can eat well before you become pregnant, the better off you and your baby will be. People who are well nourished have strong immune systems, and they're less likely to succumb to common illnesses such as colds and the flu.

By limiting your intake of junk foods and stocking up on plenty of nutritious vegetables, whole grains, and fresh fruits, you can help to ensure that you enter pregnancy as well-nourished as possible. Being in good health *before* pregnancy increases the chances of healthy outcomes for both you and your baby.

WARNING

Ensuring that your iron stores are high before you get pregnant is also important. Many North Americans go into pregnancy with low iron stores and put themselves at risk for iron deficiency while they're pregnant. Maternal blood volume increases by about 50 percent during pregnancy, and those who go into pregnancy with low iron stores risk becoming anemic. See Chapter 3 for more about iron.

If you follow a strict vegetarian or vegan diet, you need to have a reliable source of vitamin B12 before, during, and after pregnancy. See Chapter 3 for details on getting vitamin B12.

Staying physically fit

The beginning of a pregnancy isn't the best time to start a new or vigorous exercise program. If you establish an exercise routine prior to pregnancy, though, it's likely you can continue that level of activity throughout your pregnancy. Get individualized advice from your health-care provider about exercising while you're pregnant.

REMEMBER

Staying physically active helps you maintain muscle tone and strength and promotes normal stools during a time when many people experience problems with constipation and hemorrhoids. The fiber in your vegetarian diet also helps where that's concerned!

Eating Well for Two

Okay, the test strip line indicates that you're on your way to becoming a parent. The questions are beginning to trickle in:

>> Now that you're eating for two, how are you going to get enough protein?

>> Are you getting enough calcium, iron, and other nutrients?

The questions you're being asked now that you're pregnant are probably the same ones you fielded when you first became a vegetarian. Understanding the ways that pregnancy changes your nutritional needs and how you can meet those needs on a vegetarian diet gives you the confidence to enjoy your vegetarian pregnancy with fewer worries. Figure 19-1 shows some vegetarian foods that are especially good for you during pregnancy.

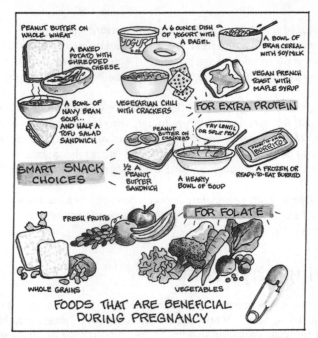

FIGURE 19-1:
Vegetarian foods
to eat during
pregnancy.

Illustration by Elizabeth Kurtzman

In this section, I explain how to maximize the nutritional value of your diet to help ensure a healthy pregnancy for you and your baby.

Watching your weight gain

Vegetarians are more likely than nonvegetarians to go into pregnancy at body weights that are close to ideal. People who become pregnant when they're close to their ideal weight are expected to gain from 25 to 35 pounds. If you're overweight when you become pregnant, you may hear recommendations to gain less — between 15 and 25 pounds. If you're thin when you become pregnant, it's healthy to gain more weight — between 28 and 40 pounds. Weight gain varies with individuals, however, so it's important to get prenatal guidance from a health-care provider, whether that's your medical doctor, nurse practitioner, or midwife.

In the first three months of pregnancy, it's common to gain very little weight — a few pounds at most. Weight gain picks up in the second and third trimesters, and a weight gain of about one pound a week is typical.

When you begin gaining weight after the third month of pregnancy, you need about 300 more calories per day than what you needed before you became pregnant. In the last three months of pregnancy, that figure rises to 450 more calories per day compared to what you needed before pregnancy. Those who need to gain more weight need slightly more calories, and those who need to gain less weight need fewer calories to maintain a healthy pregnancy weight.

Most pregnant vegetarians have weight gains that follow patterns similar to those of pregnant nonvegetarians. However, vegans are more likely to be slender going into pregnancy. They may be more likely than others to have low calorie intakes because their diets tend to be bulky — high in fiber from lots of fruits and vegetables.

If you're having trouble gaining weight, consult your health-care provider for individualized advice. The following tips may also be helpful:

TIP

>> Snack between meals. Foods that are light and easy to prepare are good choices. Examples include a bowl of cereal with fortified plant milk, half a peanut butter sandwich or peanut butter on crackers, a bowl of hearty soup such as lentil or split pea soup, or a frozen, ready-to-heat bean burrito.

>> Substitute starchy, calorie-dense foods for bulkier, low-calorie foods. For example, instead of filling up on a lettuce and tomato salad, try a thick soup made with vegetables and barley. Choose starchy vegetables such as potatoes, sweet potatoes, peas, and corn more often than low-calorie choices such as green beans and cucumbers. (Don't give up the folate- and calcium-rich greens, though!)

>> Drink extra calories. Shakes and smoothies are an easy way to get the calories you need. If you use dairy products, make shakes or smoothies using ice milk or frozen yogurt mixed with fresh fruit. Vegans can use tofu, fortified plant milks, and plant-based ice cream substitutes.

WARNING

If you have the opposite problem and are beginning your pregnancy overweight, now is not the time to actively reduce. At most, you want to control your weight gain by limiting sweets and fatty or greasy foods that are calorie-rich but nutrient-poor. Plan to lose weight gradually with diet and exercise after the baby is born.

Putting nutritional concerns in perspective

Friends and family mean well, but constant badgering about your vegetarian diet can make even the most confident person worry that their diet and pregnancy don't mix. Not true. In this section, I give you some information you can use to reassure others that you're just fine.

During pregnancy, it's important to keep the junk foods in your diet to a minimum to ensure that your diet has enough room for the good stuff.

Protein

Protein is the first thing people ask vegetarians about, but it's the nutrient about which most vegetarians have the least need to be concerned. Even if you're pregnant, protein still should be the least of your concerns, as long as you are eating a variety of wholesome foods and getting enough calories to meet your energy needs.

The recommended level of protein intake during pregnancy is 71 grams per day for most women. That's about 50 percent more protein than a woman needs when she's not pregnant. Most women, including vegans, already meet that level of protein intake before they become pregnant. They typically get even more during pregnancy because their calorie intakes increase by 300 or more calories a day, and protein makes up part of those 300 calories. So you can see that getting enough protein during pregnancy is nothing to worry about.

Each of these food choices adds an extra 10 grams of protein or more to your diet:

>> A peanut butter sandwich on whole-wheat toast

>> A baked potato topped with a scoop of hummus

>> A 6-ounce dish of flavored yogurt (regular or soy-based; both are higher in protein than other plant-based forms of yogurt) with a bagel

>> A bowl of vegetarian chili and a couple of crackers

>> A bowl of bran cereal with fortified soymilk (soymilk is higher in protein than other forms of plant milk)

>> Two pieces of vegan French toast with maple syrup, topped with a generous scoop of soy yogurt

>> A bowl of navy bean soup with half a tofu salad sandwich

Calcium

Counting the milligrams of calcium in your diet wouldn't be much fun, and fortunately, it's not necessary. Getting enough calcium isn't a problem, even if you're a vegetarian.

In general, pregnant people need about the same amount of calcium as people who aren't pregnant. Current recommendations call for 1,000 milligrams of calcium per day during pregnancy and while breastfeeding your baby. Because vegans typically get less calcium than other vegetarians and nonvegetarians, it may be more challenging for them to meet the recommended level of calcium intake.

The RDA for calcium doesn't change in pregnancy because the body becomes more efficient at absorbing and retaining calcium when you are pregnant. All vegetarians should aim for the 1,000-milligram target for calcium intake during pregnancy. The best way to do this is to try hard to get six to eight servings of calcium-rich foods each day. See Chapter 3 for a list of good calcium sources.

If you need help getting enough calcium in your diet when you're pregnant, try these ideas:

>> Go for big portion sizes of calcium-rich foods. Instead of a wimpy half-cup serving of cooked kale, go for the gusto and take a 1-cup helping.

>> It may be easier to drink your calcium than to chew it. Have some calcium-fortified orange juice, or make smoothies with calcium-fortified plant milk, fresh or frozen fruit, and tofu processed with calcium.

Vitamin D

Vitamin D goes hand in hand with calcium to ensure that your baby's bones and teeth develop normally, so be sure that your vitamin D intake is adequate. Vegetarians and nonvegetarians alike need a reliable source of vitamin D, but it's easy to come by. You can get vitamin D from exposure to sunlight, or from fortified foods or a supplement. Just make sure you get it. For more on vitamin D, see Chapter 3.

Iron

If you pumped up your iron stores before you got pregnant (see the earlier section "Maximizing nutrition before you get pregnant" for details), it's more likely you began your pregnancy with adequate iron stores. This is important, because going into pregnancy with low iron stores is associated with iron deficiency anemia in the later stages of pregnancy.

All pregnant people need additional iron during the second and third trimesters of pregnancy when maternal blood volume skyrockets and iron levels plummet. It's common for health-care professionals to recommend taking an iron supplement of 30 milligrams per day during pregnancy.

Iodine

Iodine requirements increase during pregnancy, and even mild to moderate deficiencies have been associated with adverse effects on babies' cognitive functions. Some research suggests that both vegetarians and nonvegetarians alike in the U.S. may have a tendency for mild iodine deficiencies. Therefore, it's best to err on the side of caution and ensure that you are including enough iodine in your diet. That's especially true if you don't use iodized salt, since plant foods typically have low iodine levels.

Pregnant vegetarians should aim for getting a supplement of 150 micrograms of iodine each day, and use iodized salt in cooking and at the table.

WARNING

Be aware that many prenatal supplements do not contain iodine. Check to be sure your prenatal vitamin and mineral supplement contains iodine. If it doesn't, you may need to take an individual iodine supplement.

Vitamin B12

WARNING

A pregnant vegetarian needs no more vitamin B12 than any other pregnant person. However, if you're a vegan, you have to make a special effort to get it. I can't stress this point enough. Vitamin B12 is found in eggs and dairy products, which vegans don't eat. In fact, some evidence indicates that even some lacto ovo vegetarians may have inadequate vitamin B12 status.

Not only does your baby need vitamin B12 from you while they are developing, your baby also needs it while breastfeeding. So, all vegetarians should have a daily reliable source of vitamin B12 before, during, and after pregnancy. See Chapter 3 for more information about vitamin B12.

Omega-3 fatty acids

Getting enough omega-3 fatty acids, including *docosahexaenoic acid (DHA)* or DHA and *eicosapentaenoic acid (EPA)*, may be important for brain and eye development for developing fetuses and babies. Most pregnant people in the U.S., whether vegetarian or not, fall short of recommended levels of intakes of DHA, or DHA and EPA, from foods or supplements. In fact, research suggests that vegetarians and vegans are likely to get substantially less than nonvegetarians.

To be on the safe side, vegetarians should make sure they get a regular dietary supply of *alpha-linolenic acid (ALA)*, a fatty acid that gets converted into DHA in the body. In addition, because conversion of ALA to DHA, even in pregnancy, does not seem to substitute for direct sources of DHA in terms of improving DHA status, it's best for vegetarians to include some direct sources of DHA in their diets.

Eggs are a direct source of DHA, but vegetarians who don't regularly eat eggs can get take a vegetarian DHA supplement or get alpha–linolenic acid from the following sources:

>> Canola, flaxseed, soybean, and walnut oils

>> Cooked soybeans

>> Ground flaxseeds

>> Tofu

>> Walnuts

WARNING

Pregnant vegetarians should limit foods containing *linoleic acid*, another type of fatty acid found in corn, safflower, and sunflower oils. Excess linoleic acid can interfere with your body's ability to convert linolenic acid into DHA.

Keeping mealtime simple

What most pregnant people need is someone to make their meals for them. Now *that's* meal planning made easy! Okay, so you don't see that happening within the next nine months. Here's what you do: Take some shortcuts for a while. Here's how:

TIP

>> Embrace convenience foods. Frozen vegetarian entrées and snacks such as burritos, ready-to-heat sandwiches, and veggie burger patties can reduce meal prep to minutes.

>> Order out when you're too tired to cook. Chinese vegetable stir-fry with steamed rice, a falafel sandwich and a side of tabbouleh, or a vegetarian pizza may be just what you need.

>> Open a can or carton. Eat a can of lentil soup with whole-wheat toast, or have a bowl of cereal with fortified plant milk for dinner. Canned beans, canned soups, breakfast cereals, frozen waffles, burritos, and microwave popcorn are nutritious and quick.

>> Become a weekend cook. Make a big batch of vegetarian chili or lasagna and freeze part of it. You can take it out and reheat it when you don't feel like cooking. Muffins and quick breads freeze well, too. You can also fix a big, fresh fruit salad or mixed green salad one day, and eat it over the next three days.

REMEMBER

When you're pregnant, you don't really have to eat different foods than when you're not pregnant — you just need about 300 *more* calories per day. Give yourself permission to take the easy way out. Forget about fancy meals until a time when you have more energy. For now, eat according to your appetite, and pay attention to the overall quality of your food choices.

Handling Queasies and Cravings

Pregnancy is a time for strange food aversions and even stranger cravings. They're usually harmless and pass by the end of the first three months of pregnancy. Not always, but usually. The same is true of nausea — better known as morning sickness, and known by some as morning, noon, and nighttime sickness!

These aspects of pregnancy are no different for vegetarians than they are for non-vegetarians. In this section, I help you understand how to cope with these issues.

Dealing with morning sickness any time of day

Morning sickness can be one of the most uncomfortable symptoms of pregnancy, whether you're a vegetarian or not. For many people, overcoming nausea is a matter of waiting it out. In the meantime, here are some things you can do to minimize its effects:

TIP

>> Eat small, frequent meals or snacks. Don't give yourself a chance to get hungry between meals, because hunger can sometimes accentuate feelings of nausea.

>> Eat foods that are easy to digest, such as fruits, toast, cereal, bagels, and other starchy foods. Foods high in carbohydrates such as these take less time to digest. In contrast, fatty or greasy foods such as chips, pastries, cheese, heavy entrées, and rich desserts take longer to digest and are more likely to give you trouble.

>> If nausea or vomiting keep you from eating or drinking for more than one day and night, check with your health-care provider for guidance. It's important to get help to ensure you don't become dehydrated.

>> If vitamin or mineral supplements make you nauseous, try varying the time of day you take them, or try taking them with a substantial meal. If the smell of the supplement is offensive, try coating it with peanut butter before swallowing.

Managing the munchies

If you're having cravings for something outlandish — like, say, tofu cheesecake with chocolate sauce, or a hummus and green tomato sandwich — the best thing to do is . . . go for it! This phase isn't going to last forever, and, let's face it, pregnancy is a time when all sorts of hormonal changes are taking place and things can be topsy-turvy for a while. You can't do much about it, it's not necessary to control it, and it's probably not going to hurt you. As long as you aren't chewing on radial tires or the clay in your backyard, you should be just fine.

TIP

What should you do if you crave meat or another animal product that you've banned from your diet? It's your call. But if you want to stay meat-free and you find yourself daydreaming about bacon, try a look-alike. Soy- and vegetable-based substitutes for cold cuts, hot dogs, burgers, and bacon are available in supermarkets. I talk about these in more detail in Chapter 6.

Chapter **20**
Raising Your Vegetarian Baby

Enter a world in which the little people wear mashed potatoes in their hair and toss more of their food onto the floor than into their mouths. Hey, when was the last time you smeared smashed peas up and down your arms and hid cracker bits behind your ears? You were probably 2 feet tall and had three chins. Me, too.

This scenario is pretty much the same whether your child is a vegetarian or not. In this chapter, I help guide you in the progression from breast or bottle to baby food and beyond, and I address special considerations for vegetarians.

REMEMBER

Many health-care providers are neither familiar with nor comfortable with the idea of vegetarian diets for children. Be assured that vegetarian diets are perfectly safe and adequate for children and that they hold numerous advantages over non-vegetarian diets. Although attitudes are changing, vegetarian diets are still largely outside the Western cultural mainstream, and that's the primary reason you may meet with resistance from health-care providers. You may also find unnecessary cautions and a lack of support for vegetarian diets in baby and childcare books. Be assured that these opinions aren't consistent with scientific knowledge. The Academy of Nutrition and Dietetics and the American Academy of Pediatrics (AAP) support the use of well-planned vegetarian diets for children.

Taking Vegetarian Baby Steps

We all begin our lives as vegetarians. Think about it: How many newborns eat hamburgers or chicken nuggets? Milk is our first food. Humans make milk for human babies. The alternative, infant formula, is as close a replica as can be made in a laboratory. Babies should be breastfed or bottle-fed exclusively for the first four to six months of life. They need no other food during this time.

WARNING

In fact, if you start solid foods too soon, your child is more likely to become overweight and to develop allergies. Resist the temptation to start solids too early.

In this section, I walk you through the basics of a vegetarian diet during the first year of life.

First foods: Breast and bottle basics

Breast milk is the ideal first food for babies, because it's tailor-made for them. At no other time in our lives do most of us have a diet so well-suited to our needs. From birth through at least the first six months — and longer, if possible — breastfeeding your baby is the best choice, bar none, for several reasons:

>> The composition of breast milk makes it the perfect food for human babies. Even baby formulas may not compare. It's quite possible that breast milk contains substances necessary for good health that haven't yet been identified and, therefore, aren't available in synthetic formulas. Just as researchers are discovering new phytochemicals and other substances in whole foods that aren't found in synthetic vitamin and mineral supplements, our knowledge about the nutritional value of breast milk continues to evolve.

>> Breast milk contains protective substances that give your baby added immunity, or protection against certain illnesses. Breastfed babies are also less likely than others to have problems with allergies later in life.

>> Breastfed babies are more likely than others to maintain an ideal weight throughout life.

>> Breast milk is convenient and sterile.

>> Breastfeeding is good for Mom because it helps the uterus return to its former size more quickly and aids in taking off excess pregnancy weight gain.

REMEMBER

Babies of vegetarians are at an advantage over babies of nonvegetarians, because vegetarians have fewer environmental contaminants in their breast milk. The diets of vegetarians contain only a fraction of the amount of pesticide residues and other contaminants that nonvegetarians unknowingly consume. These contaminants are concentrated in animal tissues and fat, and people who eat the animal products store the contaminants in their own tissues and fat. Consequently, when they produce breast milk, they pass the contaminants on to their babies through their milk.

Those who breastfeed their babies get lots of applause, but those who can't breastfeed shouldn't be chastised. Some people can't or don't want to breastfeed, for a variety of reasons. They need to feed their babies a synthetic baby formula instead. Just as with breastfed babies who need breast milk, formula-fed babies need their formula — and nothing but their formula — for at least the first four to six months. Once solid foods are added, breastfeeding or formula feeding should continue until at least the first birthday.

Several brands of baby formula are on the market, and your health-care provider may recommend a few to you. Most are based on cow's milk, altered for easy digestibility and to more closely resemble human milk. Vegans don't use these formulas.

However, all commercial baby formulas contain vitamin D derived from lanolin, a waxy substance that comes from sheep wool. These baby formulas are the only choice for infants in vegan families who are not breastfed. These formulas are acceptable for use by vegans. Some vegans will choose to use them, and others will choose to breastfeed.

GETTING THE CALORIES AND NUTRIENTS YOU NEED

You may be surprised to discover that you need even more calories when you're breastfeeding — about 200 more calories per day — than you do when you're pregnant. Therefore, most breastfeeding people need a total of 500 more calories a day than they needed before they were pregnant. No wonder many people find that during the time they're breastfeeding, they begin losing some of the extra weight they gained while they were pregnant.

You also need a few more nutrients when you're breastfeeding compared to when you're pregnant. For instance, you need about 5 grams more protein daily. You can easily get the extra nutrients in the additional calories that you eat. Be sure to include plenty of fluids, too; water is always the best choice. And remember that vegetarians need to be sure to get a reliable source of vitamin B12. (See Chapter 3 for more about getting enough B12.)

These formulas, including such brands as Isomil, Prosobee, Gerber Good Start Soy, and Earth's Best Soy, are acceptable for use by vegans.

WARNING

Plant milk is not the same thing as infant soy-based formula, and it is not appropriate for infants. If you don't breastfeed your baby, be sure that you feed your baby a commercial infant formula, not ordinary plant milks that are meant for general use. When your child is older, these are fine, but not in infancy and toddlerhood. Likewise, cow's milk should not be used to replace commercial infant formula in the first year.

REMEMBER

If you bottle-feed your baby, don't put anything in the bottle except breast milk, formula, or water for the first six months. Sugar water drinks, soft drinks, and iced tea are inappropriate for babies and small children. Nothing is more nutritious or beneficial to your baby for the first six months than breast milk or infant formula.

Solids second

When your baby is about six months old, begin gradually introducing solid foods when any of the following occur:

>> Your baby reaches about 13 pounds in weight, or doubles his birth weight.

>> Your baby wants to breastfeed eight times or more during a 24-hour period.

>> Your baby takes a quart of formula or more in a 24-hour period and acts as if she's still hungry and wants more.

You can also gauge your baby's readiness for solids based on the developmental signs described here: www.healthychildren.org/English/ages-stages/baby/feeding-nutrition/Pages/Bite-Sized-Milestones-Signs-of-Solid-Food-Readiness-.aspx.

You won't find any hard-and-fast rules about how to introduce solid foods to babies — just some general guidelines. For instance, all babies — whether their families are vegetarians or not — start out eating foods that are the easiest to digest and least likely to cause problems, such as allergic reactions or choking. These foods are cooked cereals and mashed or pureed fruits and vegetables.

TIP

Rather than abruptly discontinuing breastfeeding or bottle-feedings, just supplement them by gradually introducing small amounts of solid foods. Begin by mixing baby cereal with breast milk or infant formula and offering a few tablespoons. Work up to two feedings a day, totaling about a half cup. From there, gradually add other foods, one at a time, a little at a time, and your baby will increase the amounts at a self-pace. Introducing foods one at a time helps you pinpoint the culprit if your baby has a sensitivity to a particular food.

REMEMBER

You should wait until a bit later to introduce protein-rich foods and foods that are high in fat. After your baby becomes accustomed to cooked cereals and mashed and pureed fruits and vegetables, moving on to table foods with texture can be adjusted to meet your baby's eating ability.

WARNING

Don't give cow's milk to infants under the age of one year. Cow's milk can cause bleeding in the gastrointestinal tract of human babies and lead to anemia. Studies have also linked cow's milk given to infants with an increased risk for insulin-dependent diabetes.

Adding foods throughout the first year

Table 20-1 suggests schedules for feeding vegan babies from 6 through 12 months of age. Notice that the guide excludes all animal products. If you prefer a lacto ovo vegetarian approach, you can substitute milk-based baby formula for soy formula, eggs for tofu, and low-fat cheese and yogurt for soy varieties.

TABLE 20-1   **Feeding Vegan Babies from 6 to 12 Months of Age**

Food Category	6–8 Months	9–10 Months	11–12 Months
Milk	Breast milk or soy formula	Breast milk or soy formula	Breast milk or soy formula
Cereal and Bread	Begin iron-fortified baby cereal mixed with breast milk, soy formula	Continue baby cereal and add other breads and cereals	Baby cereal, toast, crackers, unsweetened breakfast cereal, rice, pasta, soft bread
Fruits and Vegetables	Introduce strained fruits and vegetables	Pieces of soft/cooked fruits and vegetables	Soft canned or cooked fruit, peeled soft fresh fruit, soft cooked vegetables
Legumes and Butters	Introduce mashed tofu, pureed legumes, yogurt, cooked egg yolks	Tofu, pureed legumes, cheese, soy or dairy yogurt, cooked egg yolks	Tofu, mashed legumes, soy or dairy yogurt, cheese, cooked egg yolks, tempeh, bite-sized pieces of *meat analogs* (soy-based substitutes such as veggie hot dogs, burger patties, and cold cuts; note that hot dogs must be cut up to prevent choking risk.)

Adapted from The Dietitian's Guide to Vegetarian Diets: Issues and Applications, 4th Edition by Reed Mangels, PhD, RD; Virginia Messina, MPH, RD; and Mark Messina, PhD, MS, 2021. (Jones & Bartlett Learning).

WARNING

Rice may contain high levels of arsenic, a natural element found in the environment and linked to some forms of cancer and neurodevelopmental problems in babies. Though manufacturers have lowered the arsenic levels in rice, babies are especially vulnerable to concentrated amounts in their diets. For that reason, it's best to vary the types of grains they eat. Variety in the diet helps to dilute the impact of any single foods or ingredients that may pose risks to health.

Tracking Your Toddler

Vegetarian diets are associated with numerous health advantages, so children who start their lives as vegetarians are more likely to develop good eating habits that will follow them into adulthood. Even so, after young vegetarian children from 1 to 3 years of age begin eating table foods, you need to be aware of a few issues.

Planning meals

No real trick exists for feeding most children a healthful vegetarian diet. The key is to offer a variety of foods and encourage children to explore new tastes. Table 20-2 presents a daily feeding guide for vegetarian toddlers and preschoolers ages 1 through 3 years.

TABLE 20-2   **Meal Planning Guide for Vegetarian Toddlers and Preschoolers from 1 to 3 Years of Age**

Food Category	Number of Servings	Example of One Serving
Grains	6 or more	½–1 slice bread; ¼–½ cup cooked cereal, grain, or pasta; or ½–¾ cup ready-to-eat cereal
Legumes, nuts, and seeds	2 or more	¼–½ cup cooked beans, tofu, tempeh, or textured vegetable protein; 1½–3 ounces meat analog; or 1–2 tablespoons nuts, seeds, or nut or seed butter
Fortified soymilk or the like	3	1 cup fortified soymilk, pea protein-based milk, infant formula, breast milk, cow's milk (whole milk for 1 to 2-year-olds; low-fat or skim milk can be used after 2 years if the child is growing appropriately)
Vegetables	2 or more	¼–½ cup cooked or ½–1 cup raw vegetables
Fruits	3 or more	¼–½ cup canned fruit; ½ cup juice; or 1 medium fruit
Fats	3–4	1 teaspoon margarine or oil; use ¼ teaspoon flaxseed oil or 1 teaspoon canola oil daily to supply omega-3 fatty acids

Adapted from Simply Vegan Fifth Edition, by Debra Wasserman and Reed Mangels, PhD, RD, 2013. Reprinted with permission from The Vegetarian Resource Group, P.O. Box 1463, Baltimore, MD 21203; phone 410-366-8343; website www.vrg.org.

TIP

If you need assistance adapting the food guide for your individual child, or you need more help with menu planning, contact a registered dietitian nutritionist who's familiar with vegetarian diets and accustomed to working with families.

Adjusting to food jags

Young children are notorious for wanting to eat nothing but mashed potatoes one week and shunning them the next. Fixations on certain foods — and aversions to others — are typical at this age, and they sometimes last as long as weeks, or even months.

Toddlers grow out of food jags, and these fickle food preferences seldom do any nutritional harm. Your best strategy is not to overreact. I cover ways to encourage your child to eat vegetables and other healthful foods in Chapter 21.

Getting enough calories

Vegetarian diets — especially low-fat or vegan diets — can be bulky. Many plant foods are high in fiber and relatively low in calories. Because young children have small stomachs, they may become full before they've had a chance to take in enough calories to meet their energy needs. For this reason, it's important to include plenty of calorie-dense foods in the diets of young vegetarian children.

WARNING

Some adults try to keep their fat intakes to a minimum, especially to control their weight, but this very aspect of plant-based diets that helps adults control their weight can backfire for young children. If fat intakes are overly restricted in young vegetarian children, those children may have trouble getting enough calories to meet their energy needs.

Liberally using plant sources of fat can help provide young children with the extra calories they need during a period of their lives in which they're growing and developing rapidly. So, for instance, adding a slice of avocado (nearly all fat) to a sandwich is fine, or using nut and seed butters on sandwiches and vegetable sticks is also a good idea.

Vegan or vegetarian? Determining what's appropriate for young children

After your baby makes the transition to a toddler diet and solid foods, you have to decide the extent to which you'll include animal products in their diet.

Young children can thrive on vegetarian diets that include some animal products or none at all. Table 20-2 shows you what to expect toddlers and preschoolers to eat.

The protein needs of vegan children are a bit higher than those of nonvegan children because of differences in the digestibility and composition of plant and animal proteins. Assuming vegan children get enough calories to meet their energy needs, though, and get a reasonable variety of plant foods, they should get plenty of protein in their diet.

WARNING

An added caution is that vegan children need a reliable source of vitamin B12 in their diet. I list examples in Chapter 3. If a vegan child has limited exposure to sunshine, consult your health-care provider to determine whether you should add a vitamin D supplement or fortified foods to their diet.

Serving sensible snacks

Another way to ensure that vegetarian kids get enough calories is to offer them between-meals snacks.

WARNING

Be sure you don't give toddlers foods they can choke on. For instance, grapes and whole tofu hot dogs are dangerous because they can easily get stuck in the esophagus. If you want to offer these foods to a small child, be sure to slice them in half or into quarters. Also be careful with chips, nuts, and other small snacks that can lodge in a small child's throat. Be sure to supervise young children while they're eating.

A few nutritious snack ideas for vegetarian toddlers include

>> Cooked or dry cereal with fortified plant milk

>> A dab of smooth peanut or almond butter on a cracker

>> Graham crackers

>> Single-serving, shelf-stable boxes of fortified plant milk

>> Small pieces of fresh fruit

>> Plant-based yogurt

>> Tofu processed with calcium, served as cubes or made into smoothies or pudding

>> Unsweetened applesauce

>> Whole grain cereal O's

Chapter **21**

Meatless Meals for Children and Teens

A 2021 poll conducted for the nonprofit Vegetarian Resource Group found that 5 percent of U.S. children ages 8 to 17 consistently report never eating meat, poultry, fish, or seafood. One percent of females and 3 percent of males are vegan. That's a substantial number of young vegetarians and vegans!

Many of these kids are the only vegetarians in their household. You've got to admire their conviction, but when Mom and Dad aren't vegetarians as well, the situation may cause parents to worry about the nutritional adequacy of the diet and how best to manage family meals without meat. Even in homes where vegetarianism is the norm, people have questions about vegetarian nutrition for kids.

REMEMBER

Feeding any child — vegetarian or not — takes time, patience, and care. A haphazard diet that's heavy on chips and soft drinks and light on fruits and vegetables — or otherwise poorly planned — isn't likely to meet the needs of any growing child. On the other hand, a well-planned vegetarian diet offers health advantages over nonvegetarian diets for kids, and it helps put into motion healthful eating habits that can become a pattern for a lifetime.

In this chapter, I discuss the most common questions and concerns about vegetarian diets for children and teenagers.

Watching Your Kids Grow

Some people worry that children who don't eat meat won't grow as well as they should. Reports in the scientific literature over the years have addressed poor growth rates in vegetarian children, but a closer look at those studies should help you put concerns into perspective.

According to these studies, growth problems in vegetarian children occurred when:

>> The children lived in poverty in developing countries and didn't have enough to eat.

>> The children did not live in poverty but had bizarre, inadequate diets that were severely limited in variety and calories.

Malnutrition, not vegetarianism, causes growth retardation. Any child, vegetarian or not, who doesn't have enough to eat will suffer from nutritional deficiencies and may have difficulties developing properly.

I advocate vegetarian diets that contain adequate calories and a range of foods to ensure that children meet their nutritional needs. Reasonable vegetarian diets not only meet nutritional needs but are associated with health advantages as well.

Understanding issues about growth rates

Talking about growth rates in vegetarian children raises the question of what a normal rate of growth is for a child.

Your pediatrician has growth charts that are used to plot your child's height and weight at regular intervals, comparing them to population norms. You may even be doing this yourself at home. Growth rates are usually reported in percentiles. For instance, one child may be growing at the 50th percentile for height and weight, while another child of the same age may be growing at the 90th percentile. Still another same-aged child may be growing at the 25th percentile. Is one child healthier than the others? Not necessarily.

Within any group of people, you should expect to see 50 percent growing at the 50th percentile, 25 percent growing at the 25th percentile, and so on. That's called *normal distribution.* In other words, variation is normal within population groups. A child growing at the 25th percentile isn't necessarily healthier or less healthy than a child growing at the 90th percentile. What's important is for a child growing at a particular rate to continue to grow at that same rate.

However, you want to investigate a decline in your child's growth rate. So a child growing at the 35th percentile who continues to grow at the 35th percentile is probably fine, but if that child's rate of growth falls to the 25th percentile, the parent or health-care provider should look into possible causes.

Putting size into perspective

Parents expect kids who eat a meat-and-potatoes diet to go through growth spurts at certain ages. Most people think of that as a good thing. It's important for your child to grow up to be big and strong, right? Many people hope for football player–sized kids and worry that the playground bully is going to pick on their child if he's too small.

The good news is that the growth rates of lacto and lacto ovo vegetarian children are similar to the growth rates of nonvegetarian children. (I give details about what different kinds of vegetarians eat in Chapter 1.) However, you find very little information about growth rates of vegan children in the U.S., although a peek at the growth rates of children in China eating a near-vegan diet has given scientists some idea of what you may expect to see.

In a population study called the China Project, which began in 1983, scientists found that children eating a near-vegan diet grew more slowly than U.S. children eating a standard, Western-style diet containing meat and milk. The Chinese children attained full adult stature eventually, but they took longer to get there. They grew over a period of about 21 years, as compared to American children, who stopped growing at about the age of 18.

Chinese girls reached *menarche* (had their first menstrual cycle) at an average age of 17, compared to 12 for U.S. girls. This later age of menarche was associated with lower rates of breast cancer in Chinese women, theoretically because they were exposed to high levels of circulating estrogen hormones for a shorter period.

So it's possible that U.S. vegan children may grow more slowly than other children. Nobody knows, though, if that's good, bad, or indifferent.

Two more recent German studies, one from 2019 and another from 2021, lend more clarity to the idea that vegan and vegetarian diets enable children to grow normally.

One study compared groups of vegan, vegetarian, and nonvegetarian children ages 1 to 3 years. The study found no significant differences among the groups in their scores for weight-for-age, height-for-age, and weight-for-height.

The other study examined older children and teens ages 6 to 18 years, comparing vegans, vegetarians, and nonvegetarians. Again, there were no significant differences among the children and teens in terms of their heights, weights, or body mass indexes (BMI), a measure of body fat that is based on one's height and weight.

REMEMBER

The most important thing for you to know if you have a vegetarian child is that your child's growth rate should be constant or increase. If growth takes a nose dive, that's the time to investigate and intervene. In the meantime, if your child is growing and is otherwise healthy, you have no need to worry.

Feeding Fundamentals

People generally associate vegetarian diets with health advantages for everyone, but a few of the characteristics that make vegetarian diets good for you can be pitfalls for children if you aren't aware of them and don't take precautions. The primary issue is the bulkiness of a vegetarian diet and the fact that some children can fill up before they've taken in enough calories.

In this section, I discuss this issue and a few others to be aware of.

Making sure kids get enough calories

It's important to be aware of the potential bulkiness of a vegetarian diet and to give your child plenty of calorie-dense foods. A child whose diet is mostly low-calorie, filling foods such as large lettuce salads and raw vegetables could run into problems getting enough calories. It's okay to include those foods in your child's diet, but don't let them displace too many higher-calorie foods.

Feel free to use vegetable sources of fat in your child's diet, such as seed and nut butters, olive oil, and avocado slices. These fats are a concentrated source of calories. Though some adults may want to limit fatty foods in their own diet to control their weight, kids need the extra calories for growth.

If you and your family have recently switched to a vegan diet and your child loses weight or doesn't seem to be growing as quickly, include more sources of concentrated calories. Add vegetable fats, and serve more starchy foods — whole-grain breads, cereals, peas, potatoes, and corn — and fewer low-calorie, bulky foods such as lettuce and raw vegetables. Smoothies made with higher calorie ingredients mixed with plant milks and plant-based yogurt are another kid-friendly idea. Like other vegetarian diets, vegan diets can be healthful for children.

Reviewing the ABCs of nutrition for kids

When it comes to designing a vegetarian diet for older children and teens, a few key nutrients — protein, calcium, iron, and vitamins B12 and D — deserve special attention. (If you need more information about any of these nutrients, I cover them in detail in Chapter 3.)

I could list numerous other nutrients and discuss their roles in the growth and development of children, as well as the importance of including good food sources in the diet. When it comes right down to it, though, the major points you need to remember are to make sure kids get enough calories, a reasonable variety of foods, a reliable source of vitamin B12 for vegan and near-vegan children, and adequate vitamin D. Kids should limit junk foods, too, so they don't displace more nutritious foods.

Protein power

Protein and calorie malnutrition go hand in hand. When a child's diet is too low in calories, their body will burn protein for energy. When the diet contains sufficient calories, the body can use protein for building new tissues instead of burning it for energy. So, the primary determinant of adequate protein intake is simply ensuring that a child is getting enough calories to meet their energy needs.

Typically, though, getting enough protein on a vegetarian diet is not a problem for children. The average protein intakes of vegetarian children, including vegans, meet or exceed recommendations.

The exact amount of protein your child needs each day depends on several factors, including their size, activity level, and the number of calories they need each day. The Food and Nutrition Board of the National Academy of Medicine estimates that 10 to 30 percent of calories should come from protein for children and teens ages 4 through 18.

SUPPLEMENT WITH SNACKS

Give your kids nutritious snacks between meals. In Chapter 20, I include a list of good snacks for younger children. For older children and teens, you can expand that list to include

- Bagels

- Bean burritos and tacos

- Cereal with soymilk or other plant milks or skim cow's milk

- Dried fruit

- Fresh fruit

- Fresh vegetable sticks with hummus or black bean dip

- Frozen fruit bars

- Frozen waffles with maple syrup or jam or jelly

- Individual frozen vegetarian pizzas

- Muffins

- Popcorn

- Sandwiches

- Smoothies made with soymilk or other plant milks and fresh fruit, ice cream substitute, or nonfat dairy products

- Veggie burgers

- Whole-grain cookies

- Whole-grain crackers

- Whole-grain toast with jam or jelly

The most practical way to ensure that your child has enough protein is to be sure they're getting adequate calories from a reasonable variety of foods, including vegetables, grains, legumes, nuts, and seeds (fruits contain little or no protein). Particularly good sources of protein that are also likely to be hits with children include

>> Bean burritos and tacos

>> Hummus or other bean dips with vegetable sticks or tortilla chips

>> Nonfat cheese on crackers

>> Nonfat or soy yogurt

>> Peanut butter on apple chunks or celery sticks

>> Peanut butter sandwiches made with whole-grain bread or crackers

>> Fruit smoothies made with soymilk or skim milk

>> Tempeh sloppy Joes

>> Tofu or nonfat ricotta cheese and vegetable lasagna

>> Tofu salad sandwiches

>> Vegetarian pizza

>> Veggie burgers

>> Veggie hot dogs

TIP

Some scientific evidence suggests that young vegan children's bodies may use protein better if they space meals close together. Eating snacks between main meals, for example, may be helpful.

Keeping up with calcium

Because children and teens grow rapidly, they need plenty of calcium to accommodate the development of teeth and bones. The Food and Nutrition Board of the Academy of Medicine recommends that children and teens ages 9 through 13 get 1,300 milligrams of calcium each day. Several factors, though — including the presence of vitamin D and the absorption and retention of calcium — are as important to maintaining a healthy body as having adequate amounts of calcium in the diet.

Still, it's a good idea to encourage children and teens to eat 6 to 8 servings of calcium-rich foods each day. (Counting servings of calcium-rich foods, rather than counting milligrams of calcium, is a practical way to ensure your children get what they need.)

Calcium-rich foods include dark green, leafy vegetables (such as kale, collard greens, turnip greens, and bok choy), broccoli, legumes, almonds, sesame seeds, calcium-fortified orange juice and plant milk, and nonfat dairy products such as milk and yogurt. I list more foods in Chapter 3.

Aim for big servings — at least a cup at a time — and include one or two servings of a fortified food such as calcium-fortified plant milk or juice. If your kids won't eat their vegetables, keep reading — I cover that later in this chapter.

Iron, too

Many high-calcium foods also happen to be high in iron, so serving these foods to your family gives you a double benefit. Good plant sources of iron include dark green, leafy vegetables, soybeans and other legumes, bran flakes, and blackstrap molasses.

The Food and Nutrition Board of the Academy of Medicine recommends that boys and girls ages 9 to 13 get 8 milligrams of iron in their diets each day. Boys 14 to 18 need a little more — about 11 milligrams of iron each day — and girls in that age range need about 15 milligrams of iron each day. Vegetarians should aim for intakes that are at least this much or somewhat higher to compensate for factors in plant foods that may lessen iron absorption.

Don't forget that it's important for vegetarians to have good food sources of vitamin C present at meals to increase the body's absorption of the iron in those meals. So give your kids plenty of fruits and vegetables to help ensure they get enough calcium, iron, and vitamin C.

Vitamin B12

Everyone, including children and teens, needs a reliable source of vitamin B12. The Food and Nutrition Board of the National Academy of Medicine recommends that boys and girls ages 9 to 13 get 1.8 micrograms of vitamin B12 in their diets each day. Boys and girls 14 to 18 need a little more — 2.4 micrograms each day.

If your kids are eating a vegan or near-vegan diet, they should be eating vitamin B12-fortified foods regularly, such as fortified plant milks or breakfast cereals, or taking a vitamin B12 supplement. If you have any doubt about whether fortified foods are providing enough vitamin B12, the safest bet is to have your kids take a supplement.

Children who regularly include animal products in their diets — milk, eggs, cheese, and yogurt, for example — should have no problem getting necessary amounts of vitamin B12. If you aren't sure if your child is getting enough, ask a registered dietitian nutritionist for individualized guidance.

Vitamin D

The important thing to remember about vitamin D and children is that vitamin D, in concert with calcium, is critical for the normal growth and development of bones and teeth. Our primary source of vitamin D isn't food at all — our bodies produce vitamin D after our skin is exposed to sunlight. Vitamin D-fortified cow's milk and fortified soymilk, oat milk, and almond milk are also good sources.

The Food and Nutrition Board of the National Academy of Medicine s recommends that boys and girls ages 1 to 18 get 15 micrograms (600 IUs) of vitamin D, in their diets each day. I discuss vitamin D in more detail in Chapter 3.

TIP

If you have any doubts about whether your child is at risk of not getting enough vitamin D, ask a registered dietitian nutritionist or your health-care provider for an assessment and recommendations.

Planning healthy meals

In Table 21-1, I provide a vegetarian meal-planning guide for school-aged children up to 13 years of age.

TABLE 21-1 **Meal-Planning Guide for Vegetarian Children from 4 to 13 Years of Age**

Food Category	Number of Servings for Ages 4–8	Number of Servings for Ages 9–13	Example of One Serving
Grains	8 or more	10 or more	1 slice of bread; ½ cup cooked cereal, grain, or pasta; ¾ cup ready-to-eat cereal
Protein Foods	5 or more	6 or more	½ cup cooked beans, tofu*, tempeh, or textured vegetable protein; 1 cup fortified soy-milk*; 1 ounce of *meat analog* (soy-based substitutes such as veggie hot dogs, burger patties, and cold cuts); ¼ cup nuts or seeds*; 2 tablespoons nut or seed butter*
Vegetables	4 or more	4 or more	½ cup cooked or 1 cup raw vegetables*
Fruits	2 or more	2 or more	½ cup canned fruit; ½ cup juice; or 1 medium fruit
Fats	2 or more	3 or more	1 teaspoon butter, margarine (plant-based spread) or oil
Omega-3 Fats	2 per day	2 per day	¼ teaspoon flaxseed oil; 1 teaspoon canola oil; 1 teaspoon ground flaxseed; 3 halves of English walnut

(continued)

TABLE 21-1 *(continued)*

Food Category	Number of Servings for Ages 4–8	Number of Servings for Ages 9–13	Example of One Serving

Starred food items: 6 or more for 4- to 8-year-olds; 8 or more for 9- to 13-year-olds (1 serving = ½ cup calcium-set tofu; 1 cup calcium-fortified soymilk, orange juice, or soy yogurt; ¼ cup almonds; 2 tablespoons tahini or almond butter; 1 cup cooked or 2 cups raw broccoli, bok choy, collards, kale, or mustard greens).

Notes: You can increase the calorie content of the diet by adding greater amounts of nut butters, dried fruits, soy products, and other high-calorie foods. Also, use a regular source of vitamin B12 like Vegetarian Support Formula nutritional yeast, vitamin B12-fortified soymilk, vitamin B12-fortified breakfast cereal, vitamin B12-fortified meat analogs, or vitamin B12 supplements. I also recommend adequate exposure to sunlight —20 to 30 minutes of summer sun on the hands and face two to three times a week — to promote vitamin D synthesis. If sunlight exposure is limited, use supplemental vitamin D.

Adapted from Simply Vegan, Fifth Edition, by Debra Wasserman and Reed Mangels, PhD, RD, 2013. Reprinted with permission from The Vegetarian Resource Group, P.O. Box 1463, Baltimore, MD 21203; phone 410-366-8343; website www.vrg.org.

Teaching Your Children to Love Good Foods

As a kid, what did you do with the vegetables you didn't want to eat? I lined my peas up along the edge of my plate, hidden along the underside of my knife. As you probably know by now, trying to force people to do things they don't want to do is usually a losing battle, and kids are no exception.

You can employ some strategies, however, that may increase the likelihood that your child will eat their vegetables. More important, you can do some things — which I outline in this section — to increase the likelihood that your child will grow up enjoying healthful foods and will make them a part of their adult lifestyle.

Modeling healthy choices

Model the behavior you want your children to adopt. If you'd like your children to eat broccoli and sweet potatoes, for example, let them see you enjoying these foods yourself. But don't pretend to like something you don't, because children can spot a fake. If you don't care for a food, prepare it for the others in your household, and don't make a big show out of the fact that you don't have any on your plate.

Present foods with a positive attitude — an air that says you expect others to like this food. If your child expresses dislike for a food that you want to see them eat, play it low key. They may come around in time. If not, you have no need to fret — you can choose from among hundreds of different vegetables, fruits, and grains. If your child doesn't like one, plenty of other options are out there to take its place.

Giving kids the freedom to choose

Children, like everyone, prefer a measure of freedom. If your child turns up their nose at a particular food, offer one or two other healthful choices. For instance, if your child says no to cooked carrots, offer a few raw carrots with dip instead. If they refuse these, let it go. The next meal will bring new choices, and not eating any vegetables at one meal won't make a difference in your child's health.

Of course, your child may also have special requests. It's okay to entertain them, within reason. In the next section, I talk about the advantages of empowering your children to make good food choices by getting them involved in meal planning.

Getting kids involved in meal planning

Children are more likely to eat what they've had a hand in planning and preparing. Give your child frequent opportunities to get involved in meals.

You can start by taking them shopping. If you buy apples or pears, let them pick out two or three. Let older children have even more responsibility. Send your teen to the opposite side of the produce department to pick out a head of cauliflower. Who cares if it's the best one? It's more important that your kids become involved.

When it comes to cooking, supervise young children and let them help with simple tasks like retrieving canned goods from the pantry or dumping prepared ingredients into a pot. Older kids can help wash and peel fruits and vegetables for salads and can assemble other ingredients for casseroles and stir-fries.

TIP

By planting a garden and tending it together, you can teach children how their foods grow to help them gain an interest in and appreciation for fresh foods. Short on space or time? Try a window-sill herb garden, or grow a pot of tomatoes on your back porch or apartment balcony.

Troubleshooting Common Challenges

Older vegetarian children and teens share diet problems similar to those faced by their nonvegetarian peers. In this section, I offer guidance on the meat-free approach to addressing these issues.

Making the most of school meals

It's gotten much easier in recent years to find a healthy school lunch, including healthy vegetarian options. School systems have poured lots of time, energy, and money into improving their meal programs to bring them into compliance with contemporary dietary recommendations.

Changes in federal regulations have made more health–supporting vegetarian options feasible. For instance, schools can serve plant milk instead of cow's milk, and tofu, tempeh, and soy yogurt count as meat alternatives.

Kids who want vegan options may have fewer choices. What to do? Here are some ideas:

TIP

>> Take a bag lunch. Figure 21-1 shows some ideas to get you started. I also include a list of ten good-tasting and practical ideas for bag lunches in Chapter 25.

>> Get a copy of the cafeteria menu. You and your child can peruse the menu for the best choices each day.

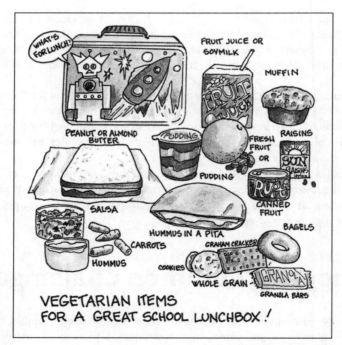

FIGURE 21-1:
Popular vegetarian choices for school lunchboxes.

Illustration by Elizabeth Kurtzman

THE NATIONAL FARM TO SCHOOL PROGRAM

One example of efforts to bring fresher, locally grown produce to schools is the National Farm to School Program, which strives to improve the nutritional quality of school meals and increase options for vegetarians.

The program began with pilot projects in California and Florida in the late 1990s as a movement to connect community farmers and local schools with the goals of supporting local agriculture, improving meals in school cafeterias, and educating students about nutrition.

By 2004, Congress recognized the program in the 2004 Child Nutrition Reauthorization — legislation renewed every five years authorizing federal support for child nutrition programs, such as the National School Lunch Program.

Today, more than 42 percent of schools nationwide include some form of Farm to School programming. Since 2007, the National Farm to School Network (NFSN) has provided vision and leadership for the program, as well as support at the state, regional, and national levels. For more information about Farm to School, go to www.farmtoschool.org.

>> Talk to school food service personnel. The circumstances are different for each student and each school, so try sitting down with food service personnel and discussing practical solutions that both your child and the school can live with.

Supporting a healthy weight

Obesity is a major public health problem for children in North America and around the world. In fact, health professionals worry that today's young people may face more health problems earlier than their parents and grandparents did because of excess weight. The problem is that diets are too high in calories and kids get too little physical activity.

The good news is that vegetarian children are more likely than other children to be at an ideal body weight. Their diets also contain substantially more fiber and less total fat, saturated fat, and cholesterol than diets that include meat.

If your vegetarian child happens to be overweight, give them a junk check (more about that in the next section, "Dejunking your child's diet"). If the diet is already up to snuff, the problem is likely due, at least in part, to lack of exercise.

Pull your child away from the computer or video games and encourage them to get moving. For teens, school sports, hiking and biking outdoors, guided use of a gym, and other team and individual sports such as track, rowing, kayaking, swimming, and tennis are excellent ways of burning calories and increasing cardiovascular fitness and overall strength. Switch activities depending on the season: Snow ski in the winter and swim in the summer. Mix it up to avoid getting into a rut.

Older children and teens are also very body-conscious. Teen boys are more likely than teen girls to feel they're too skinny. Nature will probably take its course, and today's string bean will be tomorrow's 40 regular. It just happens sooner for some than for others.

So if your teen wants to gain weight, the way to do it is simply to eat more of the good stuff. Increase serving sizes at meals and add healthful snacks between meals. Smoothies and juice blends add easy, quick calories. Increasing weight-bearing exercise — within limits, of course — also stimulates the growth of more muscle tissue.

WARNING

Your teen should steer clear of special — and often expensive — protein powders, shakes, bars, or other supplements. Flooding the body with extra protein from supplements won't build muscle. In fact, it could be harmful. Byproducts of protein breakdown have to be filtered from the bloodstream, increasing the workload for the kidneys. Muscle is made from hard work and food — nothing fancier than the nutrients found in an ordinary diet that contains a mix of health-supporting foods.

REMEMBER

Eating disorders are more common in teens — especially girls — than in adults. No cause-and-effect relationship exists between vegetarian diets and eating disorders, such as *anorexia nervosa* (self-starvation) and *bulimia* (bingeing and purging), but research suggests that some people adopt vegetarian diets to mask eating disorders. Eating disorders are medical problems that require help from qualified health and medical professionals. The causes are complex, and treatment requires a team approach.

Dejunking your child's diet

Older children and teens have more freedom than younger children to make their own food choices. Too often, they reach for chips, soft drinks, fast foods, and other junky foods that provide little nutrition in exchange for the calories.

Encourage your child to clean up their diet. Keep fresh fruits on hand at home, and serve bigger helpings of vegetables, whole grains, and legumes. Give your child a big apple to take to school in their backpack. Most important, model a junk-free diet yourself.

TIP

Having some appealing and acceptable — though not nutritionally perfect — alternatives on hand may also be helpful. Diet drinks and noncaloric, flavored seltzer water, for example, are preferable to caloric soft drinks and other sweetened beverages. (All caloric drinks, including fruit juices, contribute to excessive calorie intakes for many children, teens, and adults and may contribute to obesity.) Popping plain corn kernels or steaming a bowl of *edamame* (fresh or frozen soybeans in the pod) and adding a dash of salt may satisfy the craving for a salty snack with only a fraction of the sodium and calories contained in store-bought, processed snacks.

DEALING WITH FOOD ALLERGIES

Food allergies are an extreme response by the body's immune system to proteins in certain foods. Symptoms include hives, rashes, nausea, congestion, diarrhea, and swelling in the mouth and throat. Severe reactions can cause shock and death.

So for some vegetarians, a stray peanut can be life threatening. Other vegetarian foods that are among the most common food allergens include eggs, milk, soy, tree nuts, and wheat.

About 1 in 10 adults and 1 in 13 children have food allergies. Food allergies are different from food intolerances, which seldom cause symptoms so severe. One example is lactose intolerance — the inability to digest the milk sugar lactose. (I discuss lactose intolerance in Chapter 3.)

Food companies are now required by law to use easily recognizable terms on food labels to describe common food allergens. Prior to this law, food companies listed terms such as *albumin* and *casein* on food packages without explaining that they were byproducts of eggs and milk. The law also requires companies to disclose potential allergens if they're present in natural flavorings, natural colorings, and spices added to packaged foods.

Food allergies have no cure. Children may outgrow some food allergies, but allergies to peanuts and tree nuts usually last for life. For more help with food allergies, I recommend:

- Food Allergy Research & Education (FARE), online at www.foodallergy.org

- American Academy of Allergy, Asthma, and Immunology, online at www.aaaai.org

- *Food Allergies For Dummies,* by Robert A. Wood, MD, with Joe Kraynak (Wiley).

- *Food Allergy Survival Guide,* by Vesanto Melina, Jo Stepaniak, and Dina Aronson (Healthy Living Publications).

Chapter **22**

Aging Healthfully: Vegetarian Lifestyles for Adults of All Ages

Many people are healthy and active well into old age these days, though age-related health problems do increase over the years. Within the field of *gerontology*, the study of normal aging, scientists are gaining insights into aspects of aging that most of us take for granted as part of growing old.

Everyone experiences age-related changes, but these changes occur at different rates for different individuals. Some people never develop certain diseases and conditions. Why? Genetic differences among people may be one reason, but lifestyle factors probably play a role, too.

Diet is one lifestyle factor that makes an undeniable difference in the way people age. Physical activity makes a substantial difference, too. Eating a nutritious diet and maintaining a lifelong habit of regular — preferably daily — physical activity may not stop the clock, but it can delay evidence of aging that some people experience later than others.

For example, you may consider constipation, hemorrhoids, and weight gain to be normal parts of the aging process, or you may figure that diabetes and high blood pressure are inevitable at some point.

But vegetarians, as a group, have a different experience.

Vegetarians have lower rates of many chronic diseases and conditions. They generally live longer than nonvegetarians, too. Health and longevity differences may be due, in part, to lifestyle factors typical of some vegetarians, including a higher level of physical activity, not smoking, and eating a health-supporting diet.

In this chapter, I explain how you can leverage an active vegetarian lifestyle to help delay or prevent some age-related changes in your health. I discuss nutritional issues that affect adults as they age, and I cover the basics of eating for optimal athletic performance — whether you're a neighborhood walker or a contender for the Tour de France.

Monitoring Changing Nutrient Needs

Older adults — roughly defined as people age 50 and above — have been at the back of the line when it comes to research on the body's nutritional needs throughout the life cycle. Very little is known about how the aging process affects the body's ability to digest, absorb, and retain nutrients.

For now, recommended intakes for most nutrients for older adults are simply extrapolated from the recommendations for younger people. Scientists do know a bit about how metabolism and the body's need for certain nutrients changes with age, though. Read on to discover the smartest way to get the nutrients you need as you age.

Getting more for less

Yes, what you've always heard is true: Your metabolism declines as you age. Unfair! Unfair! But the sad fact is that you need fewer calories the older you get, assuming that your physical activity level stays the same. In fact, if your activity level decreases, then your calorie needs decline even further. Oh, woe!

It gets worse. If you consume fewer calories, your intakes of protein, vitamins, minerals, and other nutrients also decrease. Unfortunately, as far as anyone knows right now, your nutritional needs don't diminish. Your needs for certain nutrients may actually rise.

WARNING

That means that you have to be extra careful to eat well. You have to get the same amount of nutrition that you got when you were younger (and eating more calories), but you have to get it in less food. That means that you have to eat fewer *empty-calorie foods* — less junk. Fewer sweets, snack chips, cakes, cookies, candy, soft drinks, and alcohol. Empty-calorie foods are nutritional freeloaders — they displace nutrient-dense foods and provide little nutrition in exchange for the calories.

Paying special attention to specific nutrients

More research is needed on how nutritional needs change for people age 50 and beyond, but scientists are sure that needs do change. That may be partly because the body's ability to absorb certain nutrients declines gradually over time.

TECHNICAL STUFF

In fact, a constellation of factors may conspire to compromise vitamin B12 status as people age. Among them is a condition known as *atrophic gastritis,* a chronic inflammation of the stomach that causes changes in the lining of the stomach. This results in both less stomach acid and less *intrinsic factor*, a protein produced by cells in the stomach lining that help you absorb vitamin B12. Scientists estimate that this condition may affect as many as 30 percent of adults over age 50 and as many as 37 percent of people over the age of 80, diminishing their abilities to absorb vitamin B12 and potentially leading to deficiencies of the vitamin.

That's why older adults should eat foods that are fortified with vitamin B12 or take a B12 supplement. This is especially noteworthy for older vegans, who need to be careful to have a reliable source of vitamin B12 in their diets.

REMEMBER

For older vegetarians and nonvegetarians alike, recommendations for calcium, vitamin D, and vitamin B6 are higher than for younger people. If you're an older vegetarian who doesn't drink milk, which is fortified with vitamin D, and your exposure to sunlight is limited, use vitamin D-fortified foods such as some brands of plant milk, or get your vitamin D from a supplement. (Even if you drink vitamin D-fortified milks, your health-care provider may still recommend a vitamin D supplement. Follow their advice.)

The bottom line is that it's important for older folks to be frugal with their calories and save them for nutritious foods, rather than filling up on sweets and junk.

Celebrating the Vegetarian Advantage

You knew you were getting old when your eyebrows started turning gray.

Besides the obvious outward signs of aging — wrinkles, lines, and gray hair — older people have other common complaints. Most have to do in some way with the digestive tract. People start getting constipated, or they have more trouble with heartburn and indigestion. Some of these problems are a result of a decrease in the production of the stomach secretions that aid digestion, or they're in some other way a result of the body not functioning as efficiently as it once did.

But many problems are the result of a lifelong poor diet, or a lack of regular exercise, or any of a host of other destructive habits, such as smoking or abusing alcohol. For instance, if you've been exercising, eating plenty of fiber, and drinking enough water for the past 20 years, you're much less likely than other people to have hemorrhoids or varicose veins.

REMEMBER

The general dietary recommendations for older adults are similar to those for younger people: Get enough calories to meet your energy needs and maintain an ideal weight, and eat a variety of wholesome foods, including fruits, vegetables, whole grains, legumes, and seeds and nuts. Drink plenty of fluids, preferably water, and limit the sweets and junk.

Eating a vegetarian diet can help prevent or delay many of the common problems associated with getting older, and a vegetarian diet can also help alleviate some of the problems after they've developed.

That's something to celebrate — and take advantage of. In this section, I explain how.

Being fiber-full and constipation-free

Constipation is nearly always caused by diet. Regardless of your age, you need plenty of fiber in your diet from fruits, whole grains, vegetables, and legumes. Enough fluids and regular exercise are important factors, too.

Older adults develop problems with constipation when their calorie intakes dip too low. When you eat less, you take in less fiber. If you eat too many desserts and junk foods, you may be getting even less fiber. Older people are also notorious for being physically inactive. Both of these factors — low fiber intake and low activity level — can cause you to become constipated.

Constipation can be made worse if you're taking certain medications, including antacids made with aluminum hydroxide or calcium carbonate, or if you're a habitual laxative user.

If you have problems with constipation, here are some tips to get your system moving again:

>> Add fiber to your diet. Eat plenty of fresh fruit, vegetables, whole-grain breads and cereal products, and legumes.

>> Drink fluids frequently. Water is best. You don't have to count eight glasses per day, but keep a refillable water bottle with you to keep on your desk and in your car.

>> Eat prunes and drink prune juice. Prunes have a laxative effect for many people.

>> Keep fatty foods and junk foods to a minimum. These foods are usually low in fiber and will displace other foods that may contribute fiber to your diet.

>> Hold your fat intake down. If you do, you won't need as many antacids. Fat takes longer to digest than other nutrients, so it stays in the stomach longer and can promote indigestion and heartburn.

>> Get regular physical activity. It keeps your muscles (including those in your abdomen) toned and helps prevent constipation.

Vegetarian diets tend to be lower in fat and higher in fiber than nonvegetarian diets, so it's not surprising that older vegetarians are less likely than older non-vegetarians to have problems with constipation.

Heading off heartburn

Because vegetarian diets tend to be lower in fat than meat-based diets, they can be useful in helping to minimize problems with heartburn. If you're a vegetarian and have trouble with heartburn, examine your diet. You may be eating too many high-fat dairy products or greasy junk foods such as chips, donuts, and French fries.

TIP

In addition to cutting the fat in your diet, you can help prevent heartburn by avoiding reclining immediately after a meal. If you do lie down for a nap after lunch, put a couple of pillows under your back so that you're elevated at least 30 degrees and aren't lying flat. Avoid overeating, and try eating smaller, more frequent meals.

Getting a grip on gas

You may prefer to call it "flatulence." By any name, it's intestinal gas, which can be caused by a number of things, including the higher fiber content of a vegetarian diet.

More than just a social problem, gas can cause discomfort in your abdomen, and it can cause you to belch or feel bloated. Before you incriminate the beans and cabbage, though, a few other causes of gas may be exacerbating your problem, including drinking carbonated beverages, swallowing too much air when you're eating, and taking certain medications.

TIP

If you do think your diet is the problem, you have a few options. Consider these gas-busters:

» Single out the culprits. Beans? Cabbage? Onions? Eliminate one at a time until you reduce your gas production to a level you can live with. The foods that cause gas in one individual don't necessarily cause gas in everyone else, and unfortunately, the foods that do cause gas are among the most nutritious.

» Try using a product such as Bean-zyme or VegLife Peaceful Digestion. They use enzymes to break down some of the carbohydrate that causes gas. The effectiveness varies from person to person.

» Get active. People who exercise regularly have fewer problems with gas.

» Give it time. If you're new to a vegetarian diet, your body will adjust to the increased fiber load over several weeks, and your problem with gas should subside.

» Avoid carbonated beverages.

» Eat slowly and chew your food thoroughly to minimize the amount of air that you take in with each bite.

Living vegetarian is good for what ails you

You're diabetic and you follow a special diet? Maybe you're on a special diet for high blood pressure or heart disease? It doesn't matter. A vegetarian diet is compatible with restrictions for most diets, and in many cases, a vegetarian diet is ideal for people with medical conditions.

For instance, if you have diabetes, you may be able to reduce the amount of medication or insulin you take if you switch to a vegetarian diet. (Be sure to talk to your health-care provider, though, before making any changes in your medications!) The fiber content of vegetarian diets helps to control blood sugar levels.

Anyone taking medications for high blood cholesterol levels should know that the fiber in vegetarian diets helps to lower blood cholesterol levels, too.

REMEMBER

Vegetarians have weights that are closer to ideal than nonvegetarians. Weight control is an important component of the dietary management of diabetes, heart disease, high blood pressure, arthritis, and many other conditions.

TIP

Generally speaking, there's no reason that you can't eat a vegetarian diet, whatever your ailment. If you need help adapting a vegetarian diet to your special needs, contact a registered dietitian nutritionist with expertise in vegetarian nutrition. The Academy of Nutrition and Dietetics online referral service can help you find a dietitian in your area. Go to www.eatright.org.

Staying Active the Vegetarian Way

Regular exercise is an important component of a healthy lifestyle, and it's just as important for older adults as it is for younger people. When you're regularly and vigorously physically active, you burn more calories and are more likely to keep your weight at an ideal level.

You can also eat more! The more food you consume, the more likely it is that you'll get the nutrients you need. You're likely to preserve more bone and muscle tissues, too, when you exercise regularly, especially when the activity is weight-bearing exercise, such as walking or using weight sets.

INSPIRED BY MURRAY ROSE

I was 16 years old and a competitive swimmer when a book by Murray Rose caught my eye and helped to inspire me to change my lifestyle forever. Murray Rose was an Australian swimmer who attributed his athletic endurance to his vegetarian diet.

Rose was a three-time Olympic gold medalist and world record holder in swimming in Melbourne in 1956. He won a gold medal, a silver medal, and another world record at the 1960 Olympic Games in Rome. I'm not sure the switch to a vegetarian diet improved my own athletic performance, but it didn't hurt, and the diet stuck.

Rose was an athlete. I was, too — then. I practiced hard for two hours every day, after which I would swim two lengths of the high school pool underwater. If I tried that today, I'd need the Emergency Medical Service.

In this section, I explain how adults of all ages can eat for optimal athletic performance, whether you're a recreational athlete or a pro.

Nourishing the weekend warrior

In this chapter, I use the term *athlete* to describe a person who is vigorously physically active most days of the week for extended periods of time. Swimmers or runners, or triathletes who are training hard, are considered athletes.

They are in the minority of people who are active.

REMEMBER

If you go to the gym three times a week to work out on the stair climber and lift weights, it's great, but you're not an athlete. It's also not enough activity to make any appreciable difference in your nutritional needs. Ditto for golfers and weekend warriors.

Unless your activity level rises to the level of an elite athlete, it's unlikely that you need to take any special dietary measures on account of your activity.

Giving elite athletes the edge

Like everyone, an athlete's diet should consist primarily of carbohydrates, with adequate amounts of protein and fat. Can athletes do well on a vegetarian diet? You bet. Just ask vegan tennis player Venus Williams, Formula 1 race car driver Lewis Hamilton, long-distance runner Scott Jurek, soccer player Jermain Defoe, boxer David Haye, bodybuilder Barny du Plessis, snowboarder Hannah Teter, weightlifter Kendrick Yahcob Farris, surfer Tia Blanco, mixed martial artist Nate Diaz, or figure skater Meagan Duhamel, among others.

Experts have different opinions about how much protein athletes need. Some question whether physical activity level affects the body's need for protein at all. Others feel that increased physical activity level does necessitate higher levels of protein, depending on the kind of activity. The extra protein isn't needed primarily for muscle development, though, as you may think. Instead, it's needed to compensate for the protein that athletes burn up as fuel.

Some athletes need a tremendous number of calories to meet their energy needs, and if they don't have enough fuel from carbohydrates and fats, their bodies turn to protein for energy. When that happens, they need extra protein in their diets so that enough will be available for building and repairing tissues.

Because athletes need more calories than people who are less active, they tend to consume more protein in the extra food they eat. If you're an athlete, just getting enough calories to meet your energy needs and eating a reasonable variety of foods is probably enough in itself to ensure that you get the protein you need.

This is especially true for endurance athletes, such as swimmers, cyclists, runners, and triathletes. If you're into strength training (weight lifting, wrestling, or football, for example), you need to be more aware of getting enough protein-rich foods in your diet, especially if your calorie intake is low.

Any athlete restricting calories to lose weight while training should also be more careful to get enough protein. The lower your calorie intake, the harder it is to get what you need and the less room there is for junk.

WARNING

A little protein is a good thing, but too much isn't. In times past, it was a tradition for coaches to serve their football players big steaks at the training table before games. A baked potato with butter and sour cream and a tossed salad with gobs of high-fat dressing rounded out the meal. High-protein, high-fat meals like that actually make players sluggish and are generally bad for your health. Instead of a steak, athletes are better off with a big plate of spaghetti with tomato sauce, a heaping helping of stir-fry with vegetables and tofu, or bean burritos with rice and vegetables.

Crunching the carbs

A diet that consists primarily of carbohydrates — vegetables, pasta, rice and other grains and grain products, fruits, and legumes — promotes an athlete's stamina and results in better performance. Athletes who restrict their carbohydrate intake show poorer performance levels. It isn't surprising, then, that vegetarian diets have advantages for athletes, because vegetarian diets tend to consist primarily of carbohydrate-rich foods.

Athletes used to "carb load" before an event. They would restrict their carbohydrate intake and load up on fat and protein for a few days, and then they would gorge on carbohydrate-rich foods for a couple days just before the event. The idea was that this method would maximize their muscles' storage of fuel and result in better performance. Now we know that it's more effective just to eat a high-carbohydrate diet all the time. Most vegetarians are, in effect, in a constant state of carbohydrate loading.

TECHNICAL STUFF

When you eat a diet that's high in carbohydrates, your body stores some of it in your muscles and liver in a form of sugar called *glycogen*. Your body taps into its stockpile of glycogen for energy during athletic events. Whether you engage in endurance events such as swimming and cycling or in shorter, high-intensity activities such as running a sprint or the high hurdles, your muscle and liver glycogen stores are a vital energy supply and a critical determinant of your ability to perform your best.

Getting enough calories and carbohydrate in your diet helps to ensure that the protein in your diet is available for the growth and repair of tissues and that it doesn't have to be sacrificed and burned for fuel. But not just any carbohydrates will do.

Soft drinks, candy, snack cakes, and other junk foods consist mainly of carbohydrates, but these are empty-calorie foods. Anyone who depends on their diet to help them feel and perform their best needs to take pains not to let the junk displace nutrient-dense foods from their diet. Junk-food forms of carbohydrates do provide calories, so they can help keep your body from needing to burn protein for fuel. But you need the nutrients in the more wholesome foods, too. You've got to look at the big picture, not just a little piece of it.

Good choices for carbohydrates include

>> All fruits

>> All vegetables

>> Beans

>> Breads

>> Cold and hot cereals

>> Lentils

>> Pasta

>> Potatoes

>> Rice

>> Plant milks

Some athletes have tremendously high calorie needs, and many carbohydrate-rich foods are bulky. They can be so filling that some athletes can get full at meals before taking in enough calories. If this is your experience, go ahead and include some low-fiber, refined foods in your diet, despite the fact that most other people need more fiber. For instance, you may choose to eat refined breakfast cereals or white bread instead of whole-grain products.

Meeting vitamin and mineral needs

Generally speaking, a well-planned vegetarian diet that emphasizes adequate calories and variety and limits the junk should provide athletes with all the nutrients they need. Under certain circumstances, though, a few nutrients may deserve some special attention.

>> **Calcium:** Athletes have the same needs for calcium as nonathletes, but some female athletes who train intensely may be at risk if their level of training causes *amenorrhea,* the cessation of regular menstrual cycles.

Amenorrhea isn't caused by vegetarian diets; any female athlete may stop having periods when training too intensely. Like postmenopausal women, amenorrheal women have reduced levels of estrogen, and that can lead to accelerated loss of calcium from the bones.

Several factors affect bone health, and the amount of calcium you absorb and retain from your diet is more significant than how much calcium your diet contains in the first place. Nevertheless, if you're a female athlete who has stopped having periods or who skips periods, the recommendations for calcium intake are higher for you. That means you need to push the calcium-rich foods and make less room in your diet for junk. (See Chapter 3 for more information about calcium.)

>> **Iron:** All athletes — vegetarian or not — are at an increased risk of iron deficiency due to iron losses in the body that occur with prolonged, vigorous activity. Female endurance athletes are at the greatest risk, as are athletes who have low iron stores. (See Chapter 3 for a refresher on iron.) You don't need to take a supplement unless blood tests show that you need one. Men, in particular, should avoid taking unnecessary iron supplements because of the connection between high intakes of iron and coronary artery disease.

>> **Other vitamins and minerals:** Vegans, in particular, need to have a reliable source of vitamin B12 in their diets. Some studies also show that exercise raises all athletes' needs for riboflavin and zinc. The most practical advice for any athlete is simply to do your best to eat well to help ensure you get what you need.

Meal planning for peak performance

Whether you're in training or getting ready for an athletic event, what you eat and when you eat it can make a difference in your level of performance.

Here are a few pointers for vegetarian athletes, or any athlete wanting to maximize athletic performance:

>> If your calorie needs are high, add snacks between meals. Dried fruit mixtures, bagels, fresh fruit, soup and crackers, hot or cold cereal with plant milk, a half sandwich, soy yogurt or a smoothie, a bean burrito, or baked beans with toast are all excellent choices.

>> If you have trouble getting enough calories with meals and snacks, reduce your intake of the bulkiest foods, such as salad greens and low-calorie vegetables, and eat more starchy vegetables such as potatoes, sweet

potatoes, peas, beans, and lentils. Liquids can be an especially efficient way to add extra calories — try fruit or soy yogurt shakes and smoothies. Make your own blends, using wheat germ, soy yogurt and plant milk, and frozen or fresh fruit. Remember, too, that some added vegetable fats can be fine for athletes who need a compact source of extra calories.

>> Take a portable snack in your gym bag, backpack, or bike pack for immediately after your workout to replace carbohydrates and protein and provide calories. Fresh fruit, a sports bar, a bagel, or a package of crackers and bottle of fruit juice are good choices.

>> Keep fluids with you when you work out — fruit juice or bottled water are best.

>> Don't work out when you're hungry. Your session will suffer. Take a break and have a light snack first.

>> If you get the pre-event jitters, eat only foods that are easy to digest and low in fiber. Some athletes who get too nervous to eat any solid food before an event may find that it's possible to drink a smoothie or eat some nonfat or soy yogurt.

The following sections give you specific diet information to follow before, during, and after your athletic events.

BEFORE AN ATHLETIC EVENT

If you generally eat a high-carbohydrate vegetarian diet, you're ahead of the game already. When it gets closer to the time of the event in which you'll be competing, it's time to pull a few more tricks out of your sleeve.

In the hours before the event, you want to eat foods that are easy to digest and will keep your energy level up. High-carbohydrate foods are good choices, but now's the time to minimize your fat and protein intakes. Fat, in particular, takes longer to digest than other nutrients. You want your stomach to empty quickly to give your food time to get to the intestines, where it can be absorbed before you burst into action. That's the reason to keep your fat intake low at this point. Avoiding foods that are concentrated in protein is also a good idea immediately before an event because protein also takes a bit longer to digest than carbohydrate. That leaves fruits, vegetables, and grains as the best choices in the hours before an event.

It's also a good idea to avoid foods that are excessively high in sodium or salt because these foods can make you retain fluids, which may impair your performance or make you feel less than your best. Foods that are especially high in fiber are probably best saved for after the event, too, because you'll probably want your large intestine to be as empty as possible during the event. High-fiber foods can cause some people to have diarrhea and others to become constipated before athletic events, especially when they're anxious.

TIP

The best rule is to give yourself one hour before the event for every 200 calories of food you eat, up to about 800 calories. In other words, if you eat a meal that contains 400 calories, it's best to eat it two hours before the event.

Here are some good pre-event light meal and snack ideas:

>> A bagel with jam

>> A banana and several graham crackers

>> A bowl of cereal with plant milk

>> Cooked vegetables over steamed rice

>> Pancakes or waffles with syrup

>> Pasta tossed with cooked vegetables or topped with marinara sauce

>> A plant milk and fruit smoothie

>> Toast or English muffins and soy yogurt

>> A tomato sandwich and a glass of fruit juice

DURING AN ATHLETIC EVENT

Have you ever played a set of tennis in the blazing sun on a hot summer day, or paddled a canoe or kayak for several hours on a river in the middle of August? If so, you may have needed as much as 2 cups of water every 15 minutes to replace the fluids your body lost during heavy exercise in the extreme heat. Many athletes don't pay enough attention to fluid replacement, yet it's critical to your health and optimal performance.

REMEMBER

It's important to drink ½ to 1 cup of water every 10 to 20 minutes while you're exercising and, when possible, when you're competing. If you're working out in a gym, make it a point to take frequent breaks to drink some water. One good gulp or several sips can equal ½ to 1 cup of water. In other settings, keep a water bottle with you on a nearby bench, in your backpack, or strapped to your bike.

Water is the best choice for exercise sessions or athletic events that last up to 90 minutes. After that, there's a benefit to getting some carbohydrates in addition to the water to help boost your blood sugar and prolong the period of time before your muscles tire out. Eating or drinking carbohydrates sooner may also be of some benefit when the activity is of very high intensity, such as racquetball or weight training.

In these situations, it's a good idea to aim for about 30 to 60 grams of carbohydrates per hour. Sports drinks are fine for this purpose and may be more convenient than eating solid food. An added advantage is that they provide fluid as well as carbohydrates. For most brands of commercial sports drinks, that means aiming for ½ to 1 cup every 15 minutes, or twice as much every ½ hour. In lieu of commercial sports drinks, you may prefer to drink fruit juice diluted 1:1 with water. For example, mix 2 cups of apple juice or cranberry juice with 2 cups of water, and drink it over a 1-hour period.

Fruit is also a good choice for a carbohydrate boost. A large banana contains at least 30 grams of carbohydrates, and so do two small oranges.

AFTER AN ATHLETIC EVENT

After the event or exercise session, protein can come back to your table. You need protein for the repair of any damaged muscles. Your body also needs to replenish its stores of muscle and liver glycogen, amino acids, and fluids. So calories, protein, carbohydrate, and fluids are all very important soon after an athletic event. The sooner you begin to replace these nutrients, the better. In fact, studies have shown that your body is more efficient at socking away glycogen in the minutes and hours immediately following the event than it is if you wait several hours before eating.

6

The Part of Tens

IN THIS PART . . .

Review why it makes sense to go vegetarian, including practical advice about how to make it happen.

Apply simple ingredient substitutions.

Identify easy lunchbox ideas.

Create delicious dinner menus.

Chapter **23**

Ten Sound Reasons for Going Vegetarian

I f you need any more persuading to become a vegetarian, this chapter lists ten sound reasons for making the switch.

Talk to veteran vegetarians and you'll probably discover that they were first compelled to kick the meat habit by one of these reasons. After they started on the vegetarian path, other reasons gradually became apparent, adding conviction to the original decision.

Which of these reasons speaks to you?

Vegetarian Diets Are Low in Saturated Fat and Cholesterol

Generally speaking, vegetarian diets tend to be lower in total fat, saturated fat, and cholesterol than nonvegetarian diets. The fewer animal products in the diet, the less saturated fat and cholesterol the diet usually contains. This lower intake of saturated fat and cholesterol probably contributes to the decreased rates of coronary artery disease in vegetarians compared to nonvegetarians. Vegan diets are generally lower in saturated fat than lacto or lacto ovo vegetarian diets, and vegan diets contain zero cholesterol. (Chapter 1 tells you more about the differences between these varying types of vegetarian diets.)

Vegetarian Diets Are Rich in Fiber, Phytochemicals, and Health- Supporting Nutrients

Unless you're a junk food vegetarian, you're likely to get far more dietary fiber on a vegetarian diet than a diet that includes meat.

Fiber-rich vegetarian foods provide the bulk that helps prevent constipation, hemorrhoids, varicose veins, and diverticulosis. Bean burritos, lentil soup, pasta primavera, vegetable stir-fry, and four-bean salad are a few examples. Find easy recipes for all these and more in Part 3.

TECHNICAL STUFF

Fruit-, grain-, and vegetable-rich vegetarian diets are also high in beneficial vitamins, minerals, and phytochemicals such as vitamins E and C, selenium, beta-carotene, lycopene, and isoflavones, which promote and protect your health when you get them naturally from whole foods. These substances are associated with many of the health advantages of vegetarian diets, including a decreased risk for coronary artery disease and cancer.

Vegetarians Are Skinnier

Because vegetarian diets tend to contain lots of bulky fiber foods, the diet helps you fill up before you fill out. In other words, you stop eating before you take in too many calories, because you feel full sooner. Therefore, vegetarians are usually leaner than nonvegetarians. Who needs fancy weight-loss diets when you can be a vegetarian and stay slim the easiest, and healthiest, way of all?

Vegetarians Are Healthier

Not surprisingly, vegetarian diets are associated with a long list of health advantages. Not only are vegetarians slimmer and less prone to coronary artery disease, but they also have lower low-density lipoprotein cholesterol levels, lower blood pressure, lower overall cancer rates, and lower rates of type 2 diabetes.

Science suggests that several characteristics of vegetarian diets are responsible for these health advantages, including lower intakes of saturated fat and cholesterol and higher intakes of fruits, vegetables, whole grains, nuts, soy foods, and beneficial substances such as the aforementioned dietary fiber and phytochemicals.

Vegetarian Diets Are Good for the Environment

Livestock grazing causes *desertification* of the land by causing erosion of the topsoil and drying out of the land. Topsoil is being destroyed faster than it can be created because of people's appetite for meat. All over the world, irreplaceable trees and forests are being lost to make way for cattle grazing. By eating a vegetarian diet, you can help to minimize this devastation.

But that's not all. Emissions from livestock from animal agriculture account for almost one-third of human-caused methane gas emissions, contributing greatly to greenhouse gases responsible for global warming.

Animal agriculture is also one of the greatest threats to the world's supply of fresh water. Factory farms suck up tremendous quantities of water from aquifers deep beneath the earth's surface to irrigate grazing lands for livestock. Animal agriculture also pollutes rivers and streams by contaminating water supplies with pesticides, herbicides, and fertilizers used to grow food for the animals. Nitrogenous fecal waste from the animals themselves compounds the problem. By choosing a vegetarian lifestyle, you can do your part *not* to support this contamination.

The production of meat, eggs, and dairy products also makes intensive and extensive use of fossil fuels (like oil) to transport animal feed and animals and also to run the machinery on the factory farms where animals are raised. By eating fewer animal products, you can do your part to conserve fossil fuels by not supporting the production and distribution of animal-derived goods or food.

Vegetarian Diets Are Less Expensive

Sure, if you opt to buy all your groceries at gourmet stores or the ready-made food section of your local deli, your vegetarian diet can soon become more expensive than a diet that includes meat.

But assuming you eat most of your meals at home and take reasonable care to shop for value, eating vegetarian is an inherently economical way to go. Wholesome, simple vegetarian meals made from fresh, frozen, or canned vegetables and fruits, whole-grain breads and cereals, dried or canned beans and peas, and a smattering of seeds and nuts are all you need. It costs less to build a meal from these ingredients than it does to make meat the focal point of the plate.

Vegetarian Diets Are More Efficient

Vegetarian diets can sustain more people than diets that center on meat and other animal products. That's because it takes far more food energy for an animal to produce a pound of meat or a cup of milk than humans get in return when they eat those foods.

REMEMBER

Eating plants directly — rather than eating them after they've passed through animals first — is a more sustainable and efficient way to nourish the world.

Vegetarian Diets Are the Compassionate Choice

The philosopher and Nobel Peace Prize-winner Albert Schweitzer said, "Until he extends his circle of compassion to include all living things, man will not himself find peace."

And the great artist Leonardo da Vinci said, "I have from an early age abjured the use of meat, and the time will come when men such as I will look on the murder of animals as they now look on the murder of men."

Enough said?

Vegetarian Foods Are Diverse and Delicious

Vegetarians often hear, "If you don't eat meat, what *do* you eat?" If meat eaters only knew. . . .

The variety in food is in the colorful, flavorful, healthful plant kingdom. Cultures around the world serve satisfying and nutritious dishes such as curried vegetables, garlicky pasta, savory spinach pies, thick soups, and spicy couscous mixtures made with a mouth-watering assortment of fresh, meatless ingredients.

TIP

Endless combinations of these foods prepared in creative ways make vegetarian meals exciting. See the recipes in Part 3 for some suggestions to get you started cooking the vegetarian way.

Vegetarian Diets Set a Good Example for Children

Your children notice what you eat. They learn through the models they experience at home and at school. The dietary practices they adopt when they're young carry forward into their adult lives. Who doesn't want the best for their children?

Children everywhere are at high risk for obesity and obesity-related diseases such as type 2 diabetes, high blood pressure, and coronary artery disease. Consider, too, that they'll inherit this earth someday. Encouraging your children to move toward a vegetarian diet is one way to support their health and the health of their world.

Chapter **24**

Ten Simple Substitutes for Vegetarian Dishes

Sometimes, all that stands between a traditional meat-eater's meal and a vegetarian version is one small ingredient. With the creative use of alternatives, you can modernize an old family favorite to accommodate everyone's food preferences, with delicious results!

You'll be surprised at the ways you can accomplish these substitutions. In most cases, even the most discerning foodie won't mind the difference. In fact, kitchen wizards may be stunned to discover the tricks I describe in this chapter. For example, how many people know that you can swap mashed banana for an egg in quick breads and cookies? Or that you can fool your friends by using tofu instead of egg whites in your favorite recipe for an egg salad sandwich?

You may take for granted that you need eggs, milk, and butter to make baked goods, or that spaghetti sauce and sloppy Joes require ground beef, or that vegetarian foods look, smell, or taste "different" from the foods to which you're accustomed.

It doesn't have to be that way. Use the easy techniques I show you in this chapter to assist you in your menu makeovers. I list them roughly in the order in which I think you'll use them — from those you'll use most often to those you may use less often.

In some examples, I show you easy ways to work the meat out. In others, I show how simple it is to work out other animal ingredients such as dairy products and eggs, depending on the extent to which you want to avoid animal ingredients.

Replace Eggs with Mashed Bananas

Replacing eggs with mashed bananas is a no-brainer, as well as a great way to use up those bananas that have gone from just right to too brown.

TIP

In recipes that call for an egg, you can use half of a ripe, mashed banana in place of one whole egg. This trick works best in recipes for foods such as pancakes and muffins in which you wouldn't mind a mild banana flavor. Add 1 to 2 tablespoons of a liquid — plant milk, fruit juice, or water, for example — for each egg omitted to restore the recipe to its original moisture content. Because banana tastes best in foods that are slightly sweet — pancakes, cookies, and muffins — adding sweet liquids such as vanilla plant milk or fruit juice generally works fine. If in doubt, though, use an unsweetened liquid such as any unflavored plant milk or water.

WARNING

I don't recommend this substitution for recipes that rely on eggs to provide lift, as many cakes or a soufflé require. Flat foods such as pancakes, waffles, and cookies, and even dense baked goods such as quick breads and muffins, are perfect candidates for the banana trick, though.

Substitute Plant Milk for Cow's Milk in Any Recipe

You can use plant milk cup for cup instead of cow's milk in most recipes. Nobody will know the difference.

Use unflavored or vanilla flavor in sweet dishes such as rice pudding and smoothies. Use unflavored plant milk in savory recipes like mashed potatoes and cream soups.

REMEMBER

Replacing cow's milk in recipes is an easy way to cut the saturated fat content and make foods such as puddings and soups appropriate for vegans and people who are lactose intolerant.

Use Vegetable Broth in Place of Chicken Stock and Beef Broth

A savory broth is the foundation for many soup recipes. But even vegetable soups — such as minestrone, barley, potato and leek, navy bean, and others — are often made with chicken or beef stock, rendering the recipe out of the question for vegetarians. But it doesn't have to be that way. Replacing chicken or beef broth with vegetable broth is one of the easiest ways to convert a nonvegetarian soup to a version that works for everyone.

Vegetable broths are widely available in a variety of flavors and forms. My favorites, because of their convenience and flavor, are those packaged in aseptic, shelf-stable boxes sold in many supermarkets and natural foods stores. Bouillon cubes, powders, and canned vegetable broths are also available.

TIP

Of course, you can also save money by making your own from scratch at home. You don't need a recipe, because there's no need for precision. First, save vegetable scraps — carrots, onions, celery, bell peppers, and others — in an airtight container in the freezer. When you're ready, simmer them in a large pot of water for at least an hour. Salt and pepper to taste, and add any additional herbs or other seasonings that you like, then drain. After the broth cools down to room temperature, you can freeze it in ice cube trays and save the little blocks of broth to use later as needed.

Vegetable broth works well in most soup recipes, adding just the right amount of richness and flavor. For a change of pace, try using other mixtures available in stores, including tomato and red pepper, ginger carrot, and other tasty variations.

Stir in Plant-based, Veggie Crumbles Instead of Ground Meat

In some recipes, your guests won't know the difference between ground beef and plant-based, veggie crumbles. Not that your bean burritos or meatless spaghetti sauce need the extra ingredient, but if you're aiming for the flavor, look, and feel of fillings and sauces made with ground beef, plant-based, veggie crumbles and similar products are an excellent choice. Use them in the same way you used ground beef or ground turkey in the past. You can brown the crumbles in a skillet or just toss them into a pot of sauce while it's heating.

Find plant-based, veggie crumbles in the freezer section of most supermarkets and natural foods stores. Boca, Gardein, and Morningstar Farms are a few popular brands.

TIP

Make a Nondairy Version of Ricotta or Cottage Cheese

Italian classics like lasagna, manicotti, and stuffed shell pasta are familiar crowd-pleasers. If you make a good-tasting and versatile substitute for ricotta or cottage cheese, your traditional recipes can be suitable for anyone who prefers a nondairy alternative.

Making the substitution for ricotta or cottage cheese is simple. Just mash a block of tofu — any firmness will do — and add a few teaspoons of lemon juice. Mix well. You can mix with your clean hands if you find it helps distribute the lemon juice more evenly throughout the tofu.

TIP

Then, simply proceed with your recipe as usual, incorporating your substitution.

Add fresh, spicy marinara sauce, a crisp green salad, and crusty bread to round out your revamped recipe and make a complete meal.

Take Advantage of Soy "Bacon" and "Sausage"

Soy "bacon" and soy "sausage" have come a long way since food companies first tried to replicate the texture and flavor of the real things. Now they're better than their meat counterparts, because they not only taste great but also are free of nasty nitrates and contain less sodium than the original, with little or no saturated fat and cholesterol. Many of these products are seasoned to taste just like their meat counterparts. Others may taste slightly different or have a different texture. Experiment to see which brands you like best.

Use soy-based products such as Lightlife Smoky Tempeh Strips and Smart Bacon, or Morningstar Farms Veggie Bacon Strips, to make a new-fashioned BLT sandwich. Crumble them over a spinach salad and stir them into German-style potato salad. The same companies make veggie sausage patties and links that you can

TIP

serve with pancakes and waffles. Use sausage crumbles on pizza, or make a healthier sausage biscuit by serving a patty on a toasted English muffin.

There's no going back. Trust me.

Top a Tofu Hot Dog with Vegetarian Chili

Veggie dogs are here to stay — they're that good. You can grill them, boil them, or heat them in the microwave oven. Serve them in a whole-wheat bun or sliced into a pot of baked beans. Top one with some meatless bean chili (you can find the recipe for my Cashew Chili in Chapter 11) and a scoop of freshly minced onions or slaw.

Try Lightlife Smart Dogs, Morningstar Farms Veggie Dogs, and Yves veggie dogs and veggie brats.

Why not enjoy your first health-supporting chili dog? Have two.

Create a Nondairy Substitute for Buttermilk

Buttermilk adds a tangy flavor to pancakes, biscuits, and creamy salad dressings. You can get the same effect without the saturated fat by making your own using unflavored plant milk.

TIP

Just add 2 teaspoons of lemon juice or white vinegar to 1 cup of unflavored plant milk. Stir, and use this mixture cup for cup in place of regular buttermilk made from cow's milk. The acid in the lemon juice or vinegar lends the tangy flavor of buttermilk. No need to wait for the milk to clabber or curdle the way traditional buttermilk is made, though the milk may thicken slightly if left for a few days before using.

Add Flaxseeds Instead of Eggs

TIP

If you want to replace eggs with flaxseeds, here's what to do: Using a small whisk, whip 1 tablespoon of finely ground flaxseeds with ¼ cup of water. This mixture replaces one whole egg. Double it if the recipe calls for two eggs.

That's all there is to it! The flaxseeds gel and bind with the other ingredients in the recipe, sticking everything together, just like an egg would do. It's also a nice way to add some heart-healthy omega-3s to your diet.

REMEMBER

This substitution works well in a variety of recipes whether sweet or savory, including quick breads, muffins, casseroles, and loaves. Don't use it in recipes for foods that rely on eggs for lift, though, including many cakes and soufflés.

Swap Tofu for Hard-Boiled Eggs

Love an old-fashioned egg salad sandwich but want to avoid eggs? No problem.

In traditional recipes, hard-boiled eggs are mashed and mixed with mayo and a little mustard. Some recipes call for minced celery or a teaspoon of pickle relish.

TIP

Follow your favorite recipe, but replace the egg with an equal amount of firm or extra-firm silken tofu. You can even use eggless mayonnaise in place of regular mayonnaise to make this filling suitable for vegans. I include a sample Tofu Salad recipe in Chapter 11.

Chapter **25**

Ten Vegetarian Lunchbox Ideas

Packing your own lunch can save you money and is likely to be healthier than a meal you buy in a restaurant or from a vending machine. But coming up with fresh ideas for tasty foods to take to work or school can be a challenge, whether you're a vegetarian or not.

Free your mind to be creative; creativity is key to packing an appealing bag lunch. Who says you must have a main course, or that lunch has to include a sandwich, an apple, and a bag of chips?

Try some of these delicious ideas and look forward to lunch again.

Almond Butter Sandwich with Granny Smith Apple Slices on Whole-Wheat Bread

Get creative — you can find alternatives to peanut butter. Almond butter is one example.

To make an almond butter sandwich with Granny Smith apple slices, start with two slices of whole-wheat bread. Top one slice with a sticky smear of almond butter. Add thinly sliced apple, finish with the second slice of bread, and cut diagonally into quarters for four little tea sandwiches. These sandwiches are perfect with a serving of leftover pasta salad and a cup of hot tea.

For a change of pace, soy butter, cashew butter, and pumpkin butter make good alternatives to peanut butter. Other ingredients you can substitute or add to the mix include pear, banana, fruit compote, or preserves.

Bean Burrito

To make a tasty bean burrito, start with a flour tortilla and add a scoop of black beans or refried pinto beans. Add chopped lettuce and tomato or a handful of tossed salad from last night's dinner. What's nice is that you can vary the burrito at the same time that you use up leftovers.

You don't have to stop there. Add leftover cooked vegetables or cooked rice. If you like salsa or black olives, include those, too.

Fold up one end of the tortilla, and then roll the whole thing into a neat package. Wrap tightly in aluminum foil or waxed paper. When you're ready to eat, heat and serve. If the idea of warm lettuce bothers you, leave it out or add it later.

My favorite burrito recipe includes mashed sweet potatoes as an option. Find the recipe in Chapter 12.

Easy Wraps

Like burritos and pita pocket sandwiches, wraps are a handy sandwich style because they envelope loose ingredients and help to keep them from falling out.

Use a large flour tortilla or a Middle Eastern, lavash flatbread to make a hummus wrap. (See Chapter 10 for a recipe to make your own hummus.) I like to use hummus as the base because you don't need to warm it before eating, and its stickiness helps bind it with other ingredients, such as leftover salad, chopped tomatoes, grated carrots, black olives, sprouts, and cooked rice.

Sliced low-fat cheese or tempeh strips also make good bases for a wrap sandwich. Add your favorite ingredients, leaving a few inches free of filling on the far end of the bread. Begin rolling from the end closest to you. Extra filling will be squeezed onto the bare end that you strategically left for that purpose. A tightly wrapped sandwich holds together well, but rolling it in waxed paper or aluminum foil helps it survive intact in a backpack or lunchbox until mealtime.

Fresh Fruit Salad with Vanilla Yogurt

In contrast to the granola parfait (see the next section for details), this light, one-dish meal is mostly fresh fruit.

Use whatever's in season — melon balls, blueberries, peach slices, strawberries, or cut-up apples with raisins and cinnamon. Toss fruit with a simple dressing made by mixing nonfat, unflavored, vanilla, or lemon yogurt with a few tablespoons of orange juice and 1 to 2 teaspoons of honey. This is a no-measure recipe. Use enough yogurt (whether plant-based or made from cow's milk) to make a creamy dressing to coat the fruit, and add just enough juice and honey to thin and sweeten the dressing to your liking.

REMEMBER

A big bowl of fresh fruit may be all you need during a day spent sitting at your computer. Fruit is a nutritious, filling, and hydrating choice.

Granola Parfait

Make a granola parfait by using plain or flavored nonfat yogurt and your favorite granola. Simply alternate layers of yogurt and cereal in a narrow glass or plastic cup with a snug lid. This works especially well with unflavored, vanilla, or lemon yogurt, and you can substitute plant-based yogurt for yogurt made with cow's milk, too.

TIP

For extra pizzazz, add a scoop of lemon curd, raspberry preserves, or sliced strawberries, bananas, peaches, melon, or blueberries. Add a shot of nutrients by sprinkling a tablespoon of wheat germ on top.

This works well for a portable breakfast on the run, too.

Leftovers from Last Night's Dinner

Yesterday's vegetable curry or pasta primavera makes a great lunch tomorrow. Round out the meal with a chunky slice of good bread and a piece of fresh fruit. Other tasty vegetarian dinners that reheat and transport well for tomorrow's lunch include

>> Beans and rice

>> Macaroni and cheese casserole

>> Spinach pie (Greek spanakopita)

>> Vegetable lasagna

>> Vegetable pizza

>> Vegetable stir-fry

>> Vegetarian chili

Pita Pocket Sandwich

The nice thing about pita pockets is the way they keep crumbly or messy ingredients all together and off your lap. Buy whole-wheat pita bread instead of white: It tastes better and is more nutritious.

Fill a pita pocket with tofu salad and baby spinach leaves, hummus, and shredded carrots; baked beans and coleslaw; or tossed salad with a drizzling of vinaigrette dressing. You can find the recipe for hummus in Chapter 10 and one for tofu salad in Chapter 11.

TIP

Use waxed paper to wrap your pockets tightly and keep the ingredients intact until you're ready to eat.

Soup Cup

Single-serving soup cups are light and easy to carry. All they require when you're ready to eat is a source of hot water and a spoon. Peel back the top, add piping hot water, stir, and enjoy.

Complement a steamy soup cup with a few whole-grain crackers and a cooling side of fresh fruit salad.

Another variation on the theme: Try a hot cereal cup when you don't have time to eat before you leave home in the morning. Tote it to the office and enjoy it as you ease into your day. Hot oatmeal and multigrain hot cereals are appropriate and healthful alternatives for any meal.

Vegetarian Chili

Like hot soup or cooked cereal, vegetarian chili is hearty and portable. Carry it in a squatty Thermos or in a glass container that you can place in a microwave oven for reheating.

Whole-grain crackers make good scoops for hot chili in lieu of a spoon. Cucumber slices with ranch dressing dip round out this easy meal.

TIP

I include my favorite vegetarian chili recipe — Cashew Chili — in Chapter 11.

Veggie Burger on a Bun

Assemble your burger before you leave home. Heat the patty and place it in a whole-grain bun. Pack lettuce and a tomato slice separately and add them when you're ready to eat. Packing the burger fully assembled risks a soggy sandwich.

Add mustard and ketchup, or vary it by topping your burger with salsa or a scoop of corn relish or mango chutney. Pack a side of crispy carrots and bell pepper slices.

Veggie burgers on a bun even taste good cold. Many brands and varieties are available to choose from to suit most anyone's taste. Experiment with several to find those you like the best.

Chapter **26**

Ten Vegetarian Dinner Menus

For many people, coming up with convenient, good–tasting ideas for dinner is a daily chore and source of anxiety. When "What should we have for dinner tonight?" becomes a burden, it's time to rethink your strategy.

Vow to keep it simple. You'll be surprised at how easy it can be to make "simple" synonymous with elegant and delicious.

The menus that follow are examples that take into consideration basic menu planning principles that stress variety in color, flavor, texture, and temperature, creating combinations of ingredients or foods that complement each other and increase the appeal of the meal.

I draw from recipes included in this book, as well as other simple menu additions that may not even require you to follow a recipe. In some cases, food suggestions are so simple that they may seem more like "assembling a meal" rather than cooking from scratch.

Use the ideas that follow to get you started. As you gain experience, add to this list yourself, and keep it handy for days when you need a dose of inspiration.

Bruschetta with Fresh Basil and Tomatoes, Vegetarian Lasagna, Tossed Green Salad, and a Scoop of Lemon Sorbet

This one is a crowd-pleaser. It works well when you have a family or large group to feed.

The lasagna (recipe in Chapter 12) can be prepared several hours or the day before and kept in the refrigerator until you're ready to bake it. Serve the bruschetta (Chapter 10) as an appetizer while you're tossing the salad.

TIP

Don't forget to set the mood. Soft music, a good bottle of wine, and a fresh table-cloth and napkins make guests — even your own family — feel special.

Cashew Chili, Sliced Bell Peppers and Carrot Sticks with Cucumber and Dill Yogurt Dip, Easy Cornbread and a Cherry Oatmeal Cookie

This chili (Chapter 11) is especially good on a rainy day or as a cold weather meal. The sliced veggies with dip (find the dip recipe in Chapter 10) add cooling crunch and a pop of color. The chili thickens overnight and is even better the next day, making leftovers good news!

Of course, if you have room left after this filling meal, one cookie may not hurt (Chapter 14).

Cuban Black Beans and Rice, Pan-fried Plantains with Brown Sugar, Green Salad with Sliced Cucumbers and Tomatoes

Plantains look like sturdy bananas and are a traditional accompaniment to black beans and rice (recipe in Chapter 12) in the Caribbean. Ripe plantains are soft and sweet and can be sliced lengthwise or into rounds for cooking.

REMEMBER

Attention to the environment can make the meal more enjoyable. Place a few palm fronds in a vase on the table and start your Buena Vista Social Club playlist in the background.

Grilled Vegetable Quesadilla, Mango Salsa and Guacamole with Yellow Corn Tortilla Chips

In this case, we've elevated a starter from Chapter 10 to the role of dinner entrée, rounding out the meal with colorful, flavorful condiments (also from Chapter 10). Of course, our bean burrito from Chapter 12 could easily stand in for the quesadilla here, but I wanted to raise the possibility of some of these foods "trading places," where you use your imagination to configure creative combinations to fit any occasion.

TIP

Consider using blue corn tortilla chips in place of yellow chips if you need color contrast in a meal. In this menu, for example, the dark chips with pale red salsa could be a nice complement to the pale flour tortilla.

Loaded Baked Potato, Spinach and Strawberry Salad, and Mixed Berry Cobbler

Fix the salad while the potatoes are baking in the oven. Consider setting up a "toppings bar" and let dinner guests customize their own potatoes with their favorite toppings. With cobbler for dessert (Chapter 14), this meal is full of comfort and color and is densely packed with good nutrition. Find the baked potato and salad recipes in Chapters 12 and 11, respectively.

This meal works just as well if you substitute sweet potatoes for the usual Russet baking potatoes. If you do serve baked sweet potatoes, consider including crushed pineapple as a topping choice.

Pesto Pasta Primavera, Italian Chopped Salad, Rice Pudding

Add crusty bread for a heartier meal, or omit the salad for a simpler, one-dish meal. Find the recipe for the pasta in Chapter 12; the salad in Chapter 11. The pudding adds a light, cooling finish. Find the recipe in Chapter 14.

You might also consider experimenting with serving this menu as a different kind of one-dish meal. Arrange a bed of salad on a plate and place a scoop of the pasta in the center.

Pasta does not have to be served piping hot. It can be okay for the pasta to cool a bit to reduce the temperature gradient, if serving it atop a base of chopped salad. Think of it as a pasta salad meal.

Roasted Vegetable Pizza, Tossed Green Salad, Chocolate Chip Cookie

You can save leftover pizza (Chapter 12) for lunch the next day . . . in the unlikely event that there is any leftover! The cookie recipe can be found in Chapter 14.

Ready-made pizza crusts are now readily available in many supermarkets. They're a good time-saver, and they are easy to use. You can use a variety of leftovers that may be in your refrigerator — pasta sauce, basil pesto, grated mozzarella cheese, cooked vegetables, and small bits of fresh vegetables such as baby spinach leaves, bell peppers, mushrooms — to top the pizza, adding variety each time you serve this.

Rotini with Chopped Tomatoes and Fresh Basil, Grilled Italian Bread with Roasted Garlic Spread, Easy Vegan Chocolate Cake

This meal is especially good during the summer when backyard tomatoes and basil are in season. I like to serve it with a small dish of mixed olives and plenty of shaved Parmesan cheese.

Find the pasta recipe in Chapter 12, and the garlic spread in Chapter 10. The chocolate cake recipe is in Chapter 14.

TIP

Since you are heating the oven to bake the garlic, you can make good use of the hot oven for toasting thick slices of Italian bread directly on the oven baking rack.

Scrambled Tofu, Seasoned Home Fries, Arugula Salad with Pickled Beets and Candied Pecans

This menu is a take on the much-loved breakfast for dinner. In this case, the scrambled tofu recipe that is found with the breakfast recipes in Chapter 9 is paired with potatoes (Chapter 11) and a colorful salad (also Chapter 11) to round out the meal.

Soy-Ginger Kale with Tempeh, Roasted Roots, Sourdough Roll, Maple Pecan Pumpkin Pie

This is a menu for occasions when you have more time to cook, though none of the foods on this menu are particularly time-consuming to prepare. Your reward will include the delicious aromas in your house. For an even heartier meal, add steamed rice as an accompaniment to the kale and tempeh (recipe in Chapter 12).

The recipes for Roasted Roots as well as Maple Pecan Pumpkin Pie are in Chapter 15.

REMEMBER

A menu this flavorful, making use of so many seasonal, cold-weather foods could work well for wintertime holidays such as Thanksgiving, Winter Solstice, Christmas, or New Year's Day. By adding holiday decorations, table settings and music, you can help establish new food traditions.

Index

About the Author

Suzanne Babich, DrPH, MS, RDN, is a registered dietitian/nutritionist and internationally recognized expert on food, nutrition, and dietary guidance policy. After two decades in practice, she moved into academia and today is the Associate Dean of Global Health, a full, tenured Professor and Acting Chair of the Department of Global Health at the Indiana University Richard M. Fairbanks School of Public Health in Indianapolis, Indiana. She joined IU in 2015 after 14 years on the faculty of the Department of Health Policy and Management and Department of Nutrition at the Gillings School of Global Public Health, University of North Carolina at Chapel Hill.

Social justice and global health equity are her lifelong commitments. She has worked in global health and international higher education for more than 20 years. She has a special interest in international, interdisciplinary education and applications of technology for progressive approaches to public health workforce education and leadership development. She directs the Doctoral Program in Global Health Leadership (DrPH), a unique professional distance doctoral degree program for mid- to senior-level health practitioners working full-time in field positions around the world. An award-winning educator, Dr. Babich has extensive experience in distance education and experiential teaching and learning. She collaborates closely with colleagues around the world and holds faculty positions in the School for Public Health and Primary Care, Maastricht University, The Netherlands and l'Ecole des Hautes Etudes en Santé Publique (EHESP), the French national school of public health, Paris and Rennes. She is Chair of the Board of Accreditation, European Agency for Public Health Education Accreditation (APHEA) and served for 10 years on the U.S.-based Council on Accreditation of Health Management Education (CAHME).

She holds a doctorate in public health from the Department of Health Policy and Management at the Gillings School of Global Public Health, University of North Carolina at Chapel Hill, the top-ranked public school of public health in the U.S. She holds BS and MS degrees in dietetics and human nutrition. A professional science writer and former newspaper columnist, she is (as Suzanne Havala Hobbs) the author of 14 consumer diet and health books and more than 600 newspaper columns and magazine articles translating research into practical recommendations for the public. A vegan-leaning, lacto ovo vegetarian for nearly 50 years, she was the primary author of the Academy of Food and Nutrition (then the American Dietetic Association) 1988 and 1993 position papers on vegetarian diets and the founding chair of the Academy's Vegetarian Nutrition Dietetic Practice Group. She served for many years on the editorial board of *Vegetarian Times* magazine and advisory boards of the nonprofit Vegetarian Resource Group and the Physicians Committee for Responsible Medicine. Her popular newspaper column, *On the Table*, for 12 years explored topics related to food, nutrition, and health policy. The column reached more than 400,000 readers weekly in *The News & Observer* of Raleigh, North Carolina, and in *The Charlotte Observer*.

Dedication

This book is dedicated to my mother, Kay Babich, who started it all as the first vegetarian in the family all those years ago.

And it's dedicated to people everywhere who strive to eat well to support their health and to protect the well-being of our environment and all living things with whom we share our beautiful planet.

Author's Acknowledgments

Heartfelt thanks to the kind, competent, and hardworking team at Wiley Publishing who made this book possible: to Acquisitions Editors Zoe Slaughter and Elizabeth Stilwell, Managing Editor Michelle Hacker, Project Editor Donna Wright, and food photographers Wendy Jo Peterson and Grace Geri Goodale, who expertly guided this book from concept to completion, and to their very talented colleagues, who worked their magic in the design and production departments. I'm grateful to Rachel Nix for her assistance with the recipe testing and nutritional analyses of the recipes. I'm especially indebted to my longtime friend and colleague, Reed Mangels, PhD, for her help with the technical review. Many of my colleagues in the U.S., in Canada, and around the world have dedicated their lives and careers to advancing knowledge in nutrition science, the links between diet and health, and the practice of diet and health policymaking. My work builds on theirs, and I salute the collective efforts of this community of scholars and practitioners.

Publisher's Acknowledgments

Acquisitions Editor: Elizabeth Stilwell

Project Editor: Donna Wright

Technical Editor: Reed Mangels, PhD

Recipe Tester: Rachel Nix, RD

Nutritional Analysis: Rachel Nix, RD

Proofreader: TK

Photographers: Wendy Jo Peterson and
  Grace Geri Goodale

Illustrator: Elizabeth Kurtzman

Production Editor: Mohammed Zafar Ali

Cover Image: Courtesy of Wendy Jo Peterson

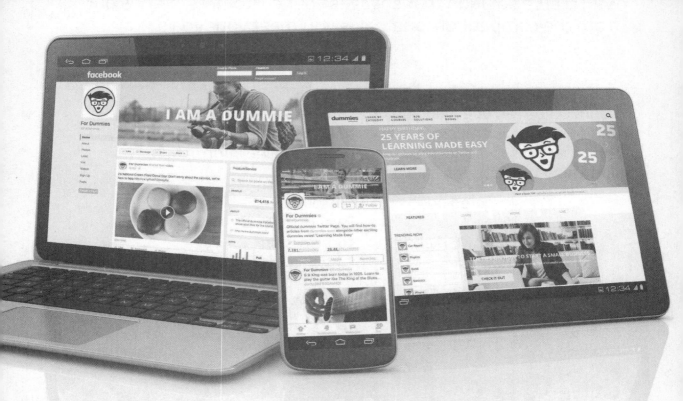
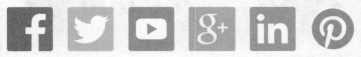
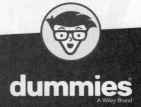

Leverage the power

Dummies is the global leader in the reference category and one of the most trusted and highly regarded brands in the world. No longer just focused on books, customers now have access to the dummies content they need in the format they want. Together we'll craft a solution that engages your customers, stands out from the competition, and helps you meet your goals.

Advertising & Sponsorships

Connect with an engaged audience on a powerful multimedia site, and position your message alongside expert how-to content. Dummies.com is a one-stop shop for free, online information and know-how curated by a team of experts.

- Targeted ads
- Video
- Email Marketing
- Microsites
- Sweepstakes sponsorship

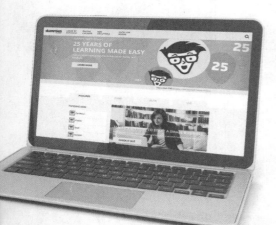

20 **MILLION** PAGE VIEWS
EVERY SINGLE MONTH

15 **MILLION** **UNIQUE**
VISITORS PER MONTH

43%
OF ALL VISITORS
ACCESS THE SITE
VIA THEIR MOBILE DEVICES

700,000 NEWSLETTER SUBSCRIPTIONS
TO THE INBOXES OF
300,000 UNIQUE INDIVIDUALS EVERY WEEK